Oral Healthcare and the Frail Elder
A Clinical Perspective

Oral Healthcare and the Frail Elder

A Clinical Perspective

Editor

Michael I. MacEntee, LDS(I), FRCD(C), Dipl Prosth, PhD

Professor of Prosthodontics and Dental Geriatrics
ELDERS Research Group
Faculty of Dentistry
University of British Columbia
Vancouver, Canada

Associate Editors

Frauke Müller, Dr Med Dent Habil

Professor and Chair
Division of Gerodontology and Removable Prosthodontics
University of Geneva Dental School
Geneva, Switzerland

Chris Wyatt, BSc, DMD, MSc, Dipl Prosth, FRCD(C)

Faculty of Dentistry
University of British Columbia
Vancouver, Canada

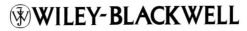
A John Wiley & Sons, Inc., Publication

Edition first published 2011
© 2011 Blackwell Publishing Ltd.

Blackwell Publishing was acquired by John Wiley & Sons in February 2007.
Blackwell's publishing program has been merged with Wiley's global Scientific,
Technical, and Medical business to form Wiley-Blackwell.

Editorial Office
2121 State Avenue, Ames, Iowa 50014-8300, USA

For details of our global editorial offices, for customer services, and for information
about how to apply for permission to reuse the copyright material in this book, please
see our Website at www.wiley.com/wiley-blackwell.

Library of Congress Cataloging-in-Publication Data

Oral healthcare and the frail elder : a clinical perspective / [edited by] Michael I
MacEntee, Frauke Müller, Chris Wyatt.
       p. ; cm.
   Includes bibliographical references and index.
   ISBN 978-0-8138-1264-9 (pbk. : alk. paper)
   1. Older people–Dental care.   I. MacEntee, Michael I.   II. Müller,
Frauke.   III. Wyatt, Chris, 1959–
   [DNLM: 1. Dental Care for Aged.   2. Mouth Diseases.   3. Frail Elderly.
4. Oral Health. WU 490 O6345 2011]
   RK55.A3O733 2011
   617.60084′6–dc22
                                        2010020450

A catalog record for this book is available from the U.S. Library of Congress.

Set in 9.5/12 pt Palatino by Toppan Best-set Premedia Limited

Printed and bound in Singapore by Fabulous Printers Pte Ltd

Disclaimer

1   2011

Contents

Contributor List

B. Lynn Beattie, MD, FRCP(C)
Professor Emeritus
Division of Geriatric Medicine
Department of Medicine
University of British Columbia
Vancouver, BC, Canada

Pierre J. Blanchet, MD, FRCP(C), PhD
Associate Professor
Department of Stomatology
Faculty of Dental Medicine
Universite de Montreal;
Neurologist
Universite de Montreal Hospital Centre (CHUM)
Louis-H. Lafontaine Hospital
Montreal, QC, Canada

Jane Bradbury, BSc, PhD, RPHNutr
Senior Lecturer in Nutrition
School of Life Sciences
Faculty of Science
Kingston University
Kingston upon Thames, United Kingdom

Mario A. Brondani
Assistant Professor
Division of Prosthodontics and Dental Geriatrics, Division of
Community Dentistry
ELDERS Research Group
Faculty of Dentistry
University of British Columbia
Vancouver, BC, Canada

S. Ross Bryant, DDS, MSc, PhD, FRCD(C)
Assistant Professor
Division of Prosthodontics and Dental Geriatrics
ELDERS Research Group
Prosthodontics and Dental Implants Elders Link with Dental Education
Research and Service (ELDERS) Group
Department of Oral Health Sciences Faculty of Dentistry
University of British Columbia
Vancouver, BC, Canada

A. John Campbell, MD, ChB, FRACP, FRCP
Professor of Geriatric Medicine
Dunedin School of Medicine
University of Otago
Dunedin, New Zealand

Marcia Carr, RN, BN, MS, GNC(C), NCA
Clinical Nurse Specialist, Older Adult Program, Fraser Health Authority;
Adjunct Professor, University of British Columbia School of Nursing and
University of Victoria School of Nursing;
Gerontology Research Department, Simon Fraser University;
Assistant Clinical Professor, McMaster University

Laura Hurd Clarke, MSW, PhD
Associate Professor
School of Human Kinetics
University of British Columbia
Vancouver, BC, Canada

Nico H.J. Creugers, DDS, PhD
Professor
Chair, Department of Oral Function and Prosthetic Dentistry
College of Dental Sciences
Radboud University Nijmegen Medical Centre
Nijmegen, The Netherlands

Shafik Dharamsi, BA, BEd, BSDH, MSc, PhD
Assistant Professor
Department of Family Practice
Faculty of Medicine
University of British Columbia
Vancouver, BC, Canada

Leeann Donnelly, DipDH, BDSc(DH), MSc, PhD (Candidate)
Faculty of Dentistry
University of British Columbia
Vancouver, BC, Canada

Ronald L. Ettinger, BDS, MDS, DDSc, DABSCD
Professor
Department of Prosthodontics and Dows Institute of Dental Research
College of Dentistry
University of Iowa
Iowa City, IA

Heather Frenkel, BDS, PhD
Adviser in Special Care Dentistry
Dental Postgraduate Department
University of Bristol Dental School
and
Hospital Lower Maudlin Street
Bristol, United Kingdom

Michael B. Goldberg, MSc, DDS, Dipl Perio
Assistant Professor, Discipline of Periodontology
Faculty of Dentistry
University of Toronto;
Head, Division of Periodontology
Department of Dentistry
Mount Sinai Hospital
Toronto, ON, Canada

Kazunori Ikebe, DDS, PhD
Associate Professor
Department of Prosthodontics and Oral Rehabilitation
Graduate School of Dentistry
Osaka University
Suita Osaka, Japan

Arminée Kazanjian, Dr Soc
Professor
School of Population and Public Health
Faculty of Medicine
University of British Columbia
Vancouver, BC, Canada

Matana Kettratad-Pruksapong, DDS, PhD
Faculty of Dentistry
Thammasat University
Rungsit Campus
Patumthani, Thailand

Shiva Khatami, DDS, Cert. Ortho., PhD
Assistant Professor
Nova Southeastern University
College of Dental Medicine
Fort Lauderdale, FL

H. Asuman Kiyak, MA, PhD
Professor, Oral and Maxillofacial Surgery
Director, Institute on Aging
Adjunct Professor, Psychology
University of Washington
Seattle, WA

Stella Kwan, OBE, PhD, MPH, MDentSci, PGCLTHE, ILTM, BSc(Hons)
Senior Lecturer in Dental Public Health
Director, WHO Collaborating Centre for Research and Development for Oral Health, Migration and Inequalities
Leeds Dental Institute
Clarendon Way
Leeds, United Kingdom

Jim Yuan Lai, BSc, DMD, MSc(Perio), MEd, FRCD(C)
Assistant Professor, Discipline Head and Graduate Director
Discipline of Periodontology
Faculty of Dentistry
University of Toronto
Toronto, ON, Canada

Gilles Lavigne, DMD, FRCD(Oral Med), PhD
Canada Research Chair and Dean
Faculté de médecine dentaire
Université de Montréal;
Sleep and Trauma Unit, Surgery Department
Hopital Sacre Cœur de Montreal
Montreal, QC, Canada

Michael I. MacEntee, LDS(I), FRCD(C), Dipl Prosth, PhD
Professor of Prosthodontics and Dental Geriatrics
ELDERS Research Group
Faculty of Dentistry
University of British Columbia
Vancouver, BC, Canada

Rodrigo Mariño, CD, MPH, PhD
Associate Professor
Oral Health Cooperative Research Centre
Melbourne Dental School
University of Melbourne
Melbourne, Vic., Australia

Debora C. Matthews, DDS, Dipl Perio, MSc
Professor and Chair
Department of Dental Clinical Sciences
Faculty of Dentistry
Dalhousie University
Halifax, NS, Canada

Lynda McKeown, RDH, HBA, MA
Lecturer, Clinical Education
Northern Ontario School of Medicine
Lakehead University
Thunder Bay, ON, Canada

Mary E. McNally, MSc, DDS, MA
Associate Professor
Faculty of Dentistry
Dalhousie University
Halifax, NS, Canada

Victor Minichiello, PhD
School of Health
Faculty of the Professions
University of New England
Armidale, NSW, Australia

Paula Moynihan, BSc, SRD, PhD, PHNutr
Professor of Nutrition and Oral Health
Institute for Ageing and Health
School of Dental Sciences
Newcastle University
Newcastle upon Tyne, United Kingdom

Frauke Müller, Dr Med Dent Habil
Professor and Chair
Division of Gerodontology and Removable Prosthodontics
University of Geneva Dental School
Geneva, Switzerland

Ina Nitschke, Dr Med Dent Habil, MPH
Clinic for Geriatric and Special Care Dentistry
University of Zürich
Zürich, Switzerland

Athena S. Papas, DMD, PhD
Johansen Professor of Dental Research
Head of Division of Public Health Research and Oral Medicine
Tufts University School of Dental Medicine
Boston, MA

G. Rutger Persson, DDS, PhD
Professor
University of Bern
Bern, Switzerland;
Research Professor
University of Washington
Seattle, WA;
Professor
University of Kristianstad
Kristianstad, Sweden

Alison Phinney, PhD, RN
Associate Professor
School of Nursing
University of British Columbia
Vancouver, BC, Canada

Martin Schimmel, Dr Med Dent
Chef de Clinique
Division of Gerodontology and Removable Prosthodontics
University of Geneva Dental School
Geneva, Switzerland

Barry Sessle, MDS, PhD, DSc(hc), FRSC
Professor and Canada Research Chair
Faculty of Dentistry
University of Toronto
Toronto, ON, Canada

Joanie Sims-Gould, PhD, RSW
Postdoctoral Research Fellow
Faculty of Medicine
University of British Columbia
Vancouver, BC, Canada

Stephen T. Sonis, DMD, DMSc
Professor of Oral Medicine
Harvard School of Dental Medicine;
Chief of Oral Medicine and Senior Surgeon
Brigham and Women's Hospital and the Dana-Farber Cancer Institute
Boston, MA

H.C. Tenenbaum, DDS, Dipl Perio, PhD, FRCD(C)
Professor of Periodontology
Faculty of Dentistry;
Professor of Laboratory Medicine and Pathobiology
Faculty of Medicine
University of Toronto
Toronto, ON, Canada

W. Murray Thomson, BSc, BDS, MA, MComDent, PhD
Professor
Department of Oral Sciences and Sir John Walsh Research Institute
School of Dentistry
University of Otago
Dunedin, New Zealand

June M. Tordoff, MPharm, PhD, MRPharmS, RegPharmNZ
Senior Lecturer
School of Pharmacy
University of Otago
Dunedin, New Zealand

Shane N. White, BDentSc, MS, MA, PhD
Professor
UCLA School of Dentistry
Los Angeles, CA

Michael A. Wiseman, DDS, DABSCD
Assistant Professor
Faculty of Dentistry
McGill University
Montreal, QC, Canada

Chris Wyatt, BSc, DMD, MSc, Dipl Prosth, FRCD(C)
Associate Professor, Chair
Division of Prosthodontics and Dental Geriatrics
ELDERS Research Group
Faculty of Dentistry
University of British Columbia
Vancouver, BC, Canada

George Zarb, BChD, MS, DDS, MS, FRCD(C), DSc(HD), MD(HC), PhD(HC)
Emeritus Professor
University of Toronto
Toronto, ON, Canada;
Editor-in-Chief
International Journal of Prosthodontics

Preface: The challenge of frailty

Do not cast me off in the time of old age, forsake me not when my strength is spent.

—Psalms 71:9

A SCENARIO

Mrs. Olivera's reflections on life's course.

Mrs. Olivera (or "Dona" Olivera as she prefers) was born in Nicaragua on July 31, 1923—87 years and 5 months ago, but to her not so long ago. She remembers clearly the pleasures and difficulties of growing up in a suburb of Managua. It was a middle-class suburb insofar as the capital city in Nicaragua had a middle class. The houses were modest, with security bars on all of the windows. Mrs. Olivera was the third of five children—two girls and three boys.

She recalls a joyful upbringing. Her father was a schoolteacher and proudly respected. Her mother was a "pillar of the church" who taught her children to read early and to respect authority. Mrs. Olivera attended her father's primary school until she moved further into the city for a secondary education where her early thoughts of the civilized *el norte* formed.

The celebrations at age 15 of her "coming out" are as vivid today as ever. She described again with glee to Mrs. Catalano, her new neighbor in the nursing home in which she now lives, how she noticed for the first time the furtive glances of "the boy next door" as she danced about in her bright blue dress and new white socks. She was pleased, even if a little mystified, by his attentions, so she smiled back with the big white teeth that were the focus of gentle teasing by her sister and brothers. She was by any measure a handsome and healthy teenager. However, her teeth were also a source of annoyance, and already she had made several long painful trips to have her back teeth pulled at the dental clinic in the city—a very frightening experience. But like all sickness—and there was plenty around—she bounced back, and upon completing school she followed in her father's footsteps to become a teacher.

The furtive glances of her youthful admirer evolved into a mixture of intimate and animated conversations about Nicaragua, the future, and finally marriage. She accepted his offer of marriage—he was now a young lawyer with good prospects she tells Mrs. Catalano again—and her three children arrived joyfully in quick succession with all the hopes and dreams of youth. She remembers it all *como si ayer* as she tells Mrs. Catalano, for she prefers only Spanish now. There were setbacks, the usual childhood illness and fears of young parents, but worst of all was the loss of her front teeth and her confident smile. With each child she lost several teeth that a dentist at the hospital replaced with a partial denture. She did not like the denture—it was ugly and it made her gums bleed, but worse still it caused her husband to send furtive glances elsewhere.

Nonetheless, they grew wealthy, and her parents joined them in their big house closer to the business section of the city. She occupied herself with the usual needs of her children. And then the earthquake struck for 5 min at midnight on the day before Christmas Eve, 1972. At age 49, her routine stopped abruptly, everything fell apart. The house collapsed, and her social security lay in rubble about her. The family survived, but only just. Fortunately, her two sons were in Canada for education, while the youngest, now aged 24, was preparing to follow them. Their fortune—it was real estate she tells Mrs. Catalano regularly—literally took a tumble. However, they were well connected, her husband's law practice remained fruitful with government support, and slowly they resurrected. Her daughter joined the boys in Canada as planned. She visited the children in Vancouver and Toronto and was amazed, if somewhat disturbed, by the affluence and remoteness of *el norte*. It did not live up to her earlier dreams so she worried even more for her children. It was cold and unfriendly, she told Mrs. Catalano, but fortunately, if sadly for her, the children seemed settled.

She did wonder with growing concern about her old age. It was approaching faster than expected—as she was sure Mrs. Catalano would appreciate. She felt secure at home despite her domestic uncertainty and loneliness as life emerged from the rubble of the great shake. But then, she repeats with rising anxiety, the next catastrophe struck from the political instability of the country. The government collapsed and the rebels took power in 1979, 2 weeks before her 56th birthday—it was as if it was yesterday.

Her husband was not much liked by the new revolutionary government, and his growing estate was confiscated. Almost overnight, they had nothing. Her husband's health failed rapidly as he struggled to survive, and he succumbed to a heart attack the following year. Dona Olivera had no income, no home, no children nearby, and now no husband. All seemed in ruins, so she had little option but to join her children in *el norte*.

She bounced unhappily back and forth between Toronto and Calgary on the "charity of her children," as she explained to Mrs. Catalano, until they put her into this home for "old people." It was not where she saw herself as a respectable "Dona" at age 86. In fact, she complains again to Mrs. Catalano, if not for the stroke that put her in a wheelchair she would go back to Managua and start all over again.

To make matters worse, her teeth were "going"—once the center of her good looks and confidence, Mrs. Catalano was reminded. The partial denture did not stay in place when she cracked a smile—not that she has much to smile about—and it is even more difficult to speak English or eat in the company of strangers without front teeth. "Was there no pride left?" she whispered quietly to her friend. Her right hand did not move anymore since the stroke. She could not clean her teeth easily with her left hand, and her breath, she knew, was *repugnante*. She told Mrs. Catalano that she was very concerned about the possibility of losing another tooth each time "that young girl (a middle-aged care-aide who spoke English with a strong accent that Mrs. Olivera could not decipher) tried to push a toothbrush into my mouth."

The doctor gave her "happy" pills for sleeping, but they made her mouth dry and the denture painful and even less secure. Indeed, she was not sure where she had put the denture, or rather where "that young girl" had put it. However, apart from Mrs. Catalano, there is nobody she much wants to see, and she never smiles now. Her daughter visits occasionally, but only, or so it seems, to comment on her mother's dishevelled appearance and missing teeth.

Her daughter offers to take her to a dentist, but Mrs. Olivera believes that the dentist will want to pull the remainder of her teeth—and this frightens her more than anything. It was bad without a respectable smile, and it will be worse, she fears, without teeth to chew.

Now, she laments regularly to her friend Mrs. Catalano, "my family is gone, my teeth are going, so there is not much more life can do to me. Who cares for a small old Dona?" Mrs. Catalano smiles affectionately and knowingly, as she squeezes the Dona's hand, "No, Dona Olivera, I'm sure your daughter and the boys care; now when I was a girl. ..." And so they whisper and wait!

This sad story of reminiscence and distress emerged from my encounters with many elderly people. It relates the depression that can afflict elders who have had a challenging course through life. It draws attention to the prominent role teeth can play in easing or inhibiting social activities. Dona Olivera could benefit from a sympathetic dentist, and her distress might be significantly eased if she could smile and eat with confidence, and if her teeth were clean and her breath fresh. She presents a challenge for anyone attending to her care. Clearly, her poor dental status and mouthcare are part of a complicated array of entwined physical, psychological, and social disabilities. Our book contains many more scenarios to illustrate this point.

I must add here with as much forcefulness as a few words can muster that I have encountered very many patients, friends, and relatives who rejoice in their maturity, achievements, and tranquillity as they age. Indeed, as I wrestle with my own "threescore and a few," I am constantly encouraged by the people I encounter who are frail and optimistic, who laugh and smile—with or without teeth—and who look forward with a balance in life that is both remarkable and enviable. They have been the inspiration for my attempt in this book to invite, cajole, and bully colleagues, young and old, to share their knowledge of how oral healthcare is an integral, and occasionally a very central, part of healthy aging.

My interest in dental geriatrics began early in my academic career as a prosthodontist. I was asked for information about the prevalence and management of oral diseases in elderly denture-wearers, and found surprisingly little published information of practical value to help address the dental needs of an aging population (MacEntee, 1985). Since then, there has been a wide awakening of interest in aging and its potential impact on societies everywhere. We hear far and wide that we, the "boomers," are coming in all our enthusiastic splendor and well-honed sense of entitlement. Yet what we will bring or do in our declining years range from unimagined creativity to widespread poverty.

Already, during my academic career, we have seen the complete loss of teeth and their replacement with complete dentures shift from the norm to the exception among elders of all age groups (Mojon et al., 2004). The impact of this shift in dental status has had and will continue alone to have a very significant effect on the need for mouthcare as we grow frailer and more dependent on others. It is much easier to remove complete dentures than natural teeth for cleaning or when they are troublesome. Already, over the last few decades, the incidence of caries, gingivitis, and gross neglect of oral hygiene among dentulous residents of long-term care facilities borders on epidemic magnitudes (MacEntee, 2006a).

Frailty, according to Gill et al. (2002), includes anyone who needs "more than 10 seconds to walk along a 10-ft [3.0-m] course and back as quickly as possible) or if they could not stand up from a seated position in a hard-back chair with their arms folded." These criteria are presented more parsimoniously for clinical practice in the "Study of Osteoporotic Fractures" (SOF) index, which designates as frail anyone who has lost weight, cannot rise from a chair five times without using the arms, and who has poor energy (Ensrud et al., 2009). In practice, most clinicians can identify someone who is frail and in need of assistance.

Healthcare in old age becomes difficult when frailty and dependency disturbs life's routines, such as oral hygiene and attending a dentist. The difficulties are not directly related to age, although after fourscore years the prevalence of chronic diseases and, with them, frailty increases markedly (Denton and Spencer, 2009).

The premise of this book is that oral health and care of oral health are influenced by frailty. Oral health is itself a complex concept, with practical implications for hygiene, comfort, and of course, general health (MacEntee, 2006a; Brondani et al., 2007). It is challenged when frailty challenges other aspects of healthcare; consequently, it should be managed in the context of general health, although this is not how it is managed in most situations. Instead, we see dentistry and mouthcare as services solely in the professional realm of dentists, dental hygienists, and other oral healthcare specialists. But we have not yet found our appropriate, effective, or comfortable role in the multidisciplinary management of frail elders. Oral healthcare has an integral and occasionally even a critical part in caring for the frail elder. Our book is about this role from a wide array of perspectives. The authors are clinicians, scientists, and researchers, some old and some young; but above all they are all fully aware of their responsibilities in our aging societies.

This book is directed primarily at dentists, dental hygienists, and other professionals who attend to the needs of frail elders, but particularly at those who bring their professional services into long-term care facilities and to homebound elders. It also provides practical information for nurses, care-aides, and physicians to enhance their knowledge of oral healthcare as a routine part of daily healthcare and of the benefits that dental professionals can bring to the multidisciplinary team of professionals who help make aging a dignified and comfortable part of life from the first arthritic twinge to the comforting environment of palliative care.

ACKNOWLEDGMENTS

This book began in my mind as a collaborative effort involving four colleagues who have an active, collaborative, and comprehensive view of dental geriatrics. I contacted Jane Chalmers, Frauke Müller, and Chris Wyatt with my idea, they were enthusiastic, and you have the results before you. I am very grateful for their advice and contributions.

Sadly, as we settled on the general outline and list of authors, Jane was struck with a recurrence of cancer. Nonetheless, she kept her oar in the water and in her usual untiring way she continued creatively to advise us until the cancer spread and we lost her. Jane's contributions did not end there, as is evident from a quick glance at the references to many chapters. She has had a broad influence on the large body of knowledge relating to oral healthcare in old age, and particularly on our management of dementia and cognitive impairment. We trust that this book reflects her spirit.

As the senior editor, I will add that this has been a revealing experience, sometimes joyous and sometime exhausting, but always challenging. As an editorial team, we learned much, and for this we are grateful to all our contributors. I especially thank Mary, my wife, for her tolerance, patience, encouragement, and joyfulness as I excused myself regularly to glare compulsively and indulgently at a computer screen. I am sure she was not alone among the supporters of all the authors who share their experiences and knowledge within these pages. We are grateful!

Michael I. MacEntee

REFERENCES

Brondani MA, Bryant SR, and MacEntee MI. 2007. Elders assessment of an evolving model of oral health. *Gerodontology* 24:189–95.

Denton FT and Spencer BG. 2009. *Chronic Health Conditions: Changing Prevalence in an Aging Population and Some Implications for the Delivery of Health Care Services.* SEDAP Research Paper No. 259. McMaster University QSEP Research Report Series. Table 2. p. 20. Available at http://socserv2.socsci.mcmaster.ca/sedap/p/sedap259.pdf (accessed August 3, 2010).

Ensrud KE, Ewing SK, Cawthon PM, Fink HA, Taylor BC, Cauley JA, Dam TT, Marshall LM, Orwoll ES, Cummings SR, and Osteoporotic Fractures in Men Research Group. 2009. A comparison of frailty indexes for the prediction of falls, disability, fractures, and mortality in older men. *J Am Geriatr Soc.* 57:492–8.

Gill TM, Baker DI, Gottschalk M, Peduzzi PN, Allore H, and Byers A. 2002. A program to prevent functional decline in physically frail elderly persons who live at home. *N Engl J Med* 347:1068–74.

MacEntee MI. 1985. The prevalence of edentulism and diseases related to dentures. A literature review. *J Oral Rehabil* 12:195–207.

MacEntee MI. 2006a. Missing links in oral healthcare for frail elderly people. *J Can Dent Assoc* 72:421–5.

MacEntee MI. 2006b. An existential model of oral health from evolving views on health, function and disability. *Community Dent Health* 23:5–14.

Mojon P, Thomason JM, and Walls AW. 2004. The impact of falling rates of edentulism. *Int J Prosthodont* 17:434–40.

Oral Healthcare and the Frail Elder

A Clinical Perspective

Theories and significance of oral health in frailty

Joanie Sims-Gould, Mario A. Brondani, S. Ross Bryant, and Michael I. MacEntee

WE ARE ALL AGING

Clinicians are becoming increasingly interested in the complexity of the mouth in old age as more people are living longer with natural teeth, and there is an appreciation that the mouth and teeth if neglected, can be a serious source of distress and disease. In this chapter, we address the demographics of our changing populations, we highlight how age impacts the mouth and what we think it means to be frail, and finally, we explain how frailty can contribute to and be aggravated by oral diseases, impairments, and disabilities.

The world population is aging as a consequence of longer life expectancy and a decline in fertility, particularly in developed countries, during the latter half of the past century (Fitzpatrick, 2003; United Nations Department of Economic and Social Affairs, 2010). While people in Europe, North America, and Japan are living longer than ever before, a dramatic increase is expected by 2050 in the proportion and total numbers of older people in Latin America, China, and India (Gutman et al., 2000). The current demographic change is a global phenomenon. In 1950, for example, there were about 131 million people on Earth who were 65 years of age or older, whereas by 1995 the number had tripled to about 371 million. Moreover, if the current growth continues until 2025, the number is likely to double, and by 2050 there will be more than 1.4 billion elders around the globe (Fischer and Heilig, 1997).

The United Nations identified the immense significance of these global demographics in Article 2 of the political declarations made at the Second

Oral Healthcare and the Frail Elder: A Clinical Perspective.
Edited by Michael I. MacEntee © 2011 Blackwell Publishing Ltd.

Table 1.1 Prevalence of self-reported chronic conditions among noninstitutionalized Canadian elders by age group in 2005.

Condition	% of age group	
	65–79 years	80+ years
Arthritis	44.3	51.6
High blood pressure	43.2	47.2
Cataracts	19.6	30.0
Heart disease	17.1	25.3
Urinary incontinence	9.6	16.3
Glaucoma	5.7	9.5
Cancer	4.6	5.7
Stroke	3.6	7.4
Alzheimer's or other dementia	1.1	4.3

Based on the master file of the Canadian Community Health Survey, Cycle 3.1, and adapted from Denton and Spencer (2010).

World Assembly on Ageing in 2002 with the statement "that the world is experiencing an unprecedented demographic transformation and that by 2050 the number of persons aged 60 years and over will increase from 600 million to almost 2 billion and that the proportion of persons aged 60 years and over is expected to double from 10 to 21 per cent. The increase will be greatest and most rapid in developing countries where the older population is expected to quadruple during the next 50 years" (United Nations, 2002a). Even more dramatically, we see the rapid growth of the population older than 80 years, who are growing globally at an annual rate of 3.8%, which is currently twice as high as the 1.9% growth of the population over 60 years of age (United Nations, 2002b). These are dramatic changes that will focus attention even more keenly on aging and associated phenomena.

As numbers change, so too will our social networks, our physical functions, and our cognitive agility. The prevalence of chronic disability is noticeable at age 65 years and increases as age increases (Table 1.1).

Table 1.1 shows data on self-reported health status from elders who are living independently, and undoubtedly, the prevalence of chronic conditions is much higher in the frailer population in nursing homes. The prevalence of dementia, for example, is remarkably low in this noninstitutionalized population. A survey of predominantly Caucasian elders aged 90 years and older in California reported that 45% of women and 28% of men were clinically demented, and the prevalence rates doubled every 5 years for women but not men (Corrada et al., 2008).

THE AGING MOUTH

Normal aging changes the mouth and associated structures in relatively mild ways as physiological capacity is reduced compared with the more extreme reactions precipitated by disease. There is, for instance, age-related loss of mucosal elasticity, submucosal tissue, and tactile sensitivity around the mouth (Landt and Fransson, 1975; Nedelman and Bernick, 1978; Wolff et al., 1991). The sensation of taste also diminishes a little (Easterby-Smith et al., 1994), as does the mass and strength of the jaw muscles (Newton et al., 1993). Within the pulp of vital teeth, there is a decrease in the number of blood vessels and cells and an increase in secondary dentine deposits, all of which compromise a tooth's capacity to recover from physical trauma and caries (Mandojana et al., 2001). Likewise, cells can lose their ability to proliferate and produce protein as they age. Consequently, we can expect a slight relocation of periodontal attachment and loss of bone support around teeth (Papapanou et al., 1989). The occlusal surfaces of teeth show signs of attrition (Bartlett and Dugmore, 2008), and the curved articulating surfaces of the jaw joints flatten a little as they age (Magnusson et al., 2008). However, it has been challenging to distinguish between the contributions of genes and of the environment to age-related changes because, frequently, the difference between normal "wear and tear" and active disease is obscure.

The balance between health and disease, as between impairment and disability, of the mouth is influenced by interactions of human behavior, the environment, and various diseases such as caries, periodontal disease, trauma and, to a lesser extent, cancer (Gutmann and Gutmann, 1995; Reichart, 2000; Levy et al., 2003; Petersen et al., 2005). Consequently, frail elders today present with repaired or missing teeth because of the ravages of caries over many years (Marcus et al., 1996; Thompson and Kreisel, 1998; Wyatt and MacEntee, 1998; Fure, 2003), and many of them have lost all of their natural teeth (Schoenborn and Heyman, 2009). Problems of the mouth can have a very disturbing affect on nutrition, communications, and social interactions at any age (MacEntee et al., 1997; Moynihan et al., 2000), but as frailty increases, oral neglect can contribute to life-threatening conditions in the respiratory, cardiovascular, and endocrine systems (Bonito, 2002; Awano et al., 2008). Although there is controversy around the strength of the contributions, and awareness of the capacity that elderly people have for coping with adversity (Brondani and MacEntee, 2007), there is little doubt that a neglected mouth can be very challenging to general well-being and quality of life (Gift and Redford, 1992; MacEntee, 2007; Sanders et al., 2009).

THE SILENCE OF THE FRAIL ELDERLY

Frailty complicates the care needed to manage oral diseases, and oral diseases complicate the management of frailty (Satcher, 2000a; Chalmers and Ettinger, 2008). Moreover, the neglect of oral health and acceptance of infectious diseases are complicated even further by elders who are too frail to complain (Satcher, 2000b; Helgeson et al., 2002).

Box 1.1 Helena's frailty.

Helena just had her 82nd birthday. She enjoys reading and the time she can spend in her garden on sunny days. She has not walked for 7 years and gets around in an electric wheelchair. She describes her health overall as "the pits," with numerous related concerns, including post-polio syndrome, rheumatoid arthritis, heart problems, breathing problems, and seizures. She has been hospitalized several times in the last year. Fortunately, her family is very supportive.

She lives with Joyce, her 50-year-old daughter, and Ken, her 28-year-old grandson. Joyce works as a registered nurse, while Ken quit his job to help out at home where he does a lot of the physical labor, including helping Helena in and out of her wheelchair. Helena explains that she would not be able to manage at home without Ken. She also receives homecare services four times a day for one hour each visit, including preparations of her meals.

She has six natural lower front teeth but she can eat only pureed food because of difficulties with her upper complete denture, which occasionally she does not wear. However, she has not been to a dentist for the past 5 years because she believes "there is no point." Overall, she has a positive attitude to her life, and she enjoys her family and friends, including the homecare workers.

There is much debate about the establishment of a comprehensive definition that describes the characteristics, causes, and management of frailty (Kaethler et al., 2003; Bergman et al., 2007). Helena's circumstances at age 82 years demonstrate that physical frailty does not necessarily cause social isolation (Box 1.1). Although her upper denture adds a layer of complexity to her health, whether or not she is "frail" and what in fact exacerbates or improves her physical situation is less clear. Is she neglecting her mouth because she is frail? Does her physical disability impede her ability, and therefore her wish, to visit a dentist, or is she so accepting of her mouth and denture problems that she sees no point in visiting a dentist? These are questions that warrant good answers if we are to appreciate fully the role of physical function and oral health in Helena's life.

FRAILTY

Some theories of frailty rest entirely on biological explanations of aging and senescence, whereas others carefully consider social and environmental factors. As a concept in medical care, frailty was seen initially as a biological attribute of health and disability stemming from age-related impairments in multiple biological systems, and it was ascribed pragmatically to people who seemed to cope poorly with the physical challenges of old age (Bergman et al., 2004). This largely biomedical concept was expanded by others to include a wider range of phenomena that increase vulnerability to disease through numerous biological, psychological, cognitive, and social interactions (Rockwood, 2005).

At first glance, Helena fits the biomedical characteristics of frailty because her disability involves her mouth among other physiological systems. But frailty, if we accept the expanded concept, is a multifactorial phenomenon associated with vulnerability to various problems. Consequently, Helena is less likely to be considered frail in a global sense when we consider her social support and her apparent emotional capacity to deal with her physical problems. Almost everyone is physically frail by age 95 years; however, if the physical manifestations of frailty are tempered by an adequate capacity to cope with impairments, even centenarians can be relatively robust while people half their age can present as shockingly frail.

Instrumental definitions and objective measures of frailty, both of which are characteristic of the medicalization of aging, can be restrictive because they dwell mostly on medical needs to the exclusion of environmental and social issues, such as isolation and poverty (Kaufman, 1994; Markle-Reid and Browne, 2003). A more global assessment of Helena's frailty, if such is possible, would highlight her biomedical vulnerability moderated by a complicated and variable social environment. Associating frailty with aging alone has negative implications, such as the unjust stereotyping of Helena as unduly pessimistic about her teeth because she is old. Moreover, quantifying frailty can lead to suggestions of homogeneity and uniformity among elders, which is far from real. Probably, there is more diversity and heterogeneity among older people than among any other age group. Aging and frailty are not simply a shift in the battle of independence versus dependence but rather a change in the capacity for autonomy and personal strengths along a broad continuum of possibilities (Markle-Reid and Browne, 2003).

"Frail" dental patients

The impact of frailty on oral health and mouthcare has been considered mainly as a feature of access to care, with patients classified as functionally independent, frail, or dependent (Ettinger and Beck, 1984). However, the impact can be considered even more simply in the context of independence and dependence. Either way, the classification, or at least the impact, of frailty is based solely on physical capacity to access dental services (Bonito, 2002). It does not explain how frailty influences the mouth and teeth. Helena, for example, is functionally dependent on Ken for help to attend a dentist; therefore, she is frail. Yet she chooses not to go to a dentist because "there is no point," presumably because she has other priorities and feels that a dentist cannot help her. Therefore, her frailty has no direct influence at present on whether or not she goes to a dentist, and so access to dentistry does not influence her sense of frailty. She struggles to swallow food because of difficulties with her denture, and a dentist would probably consider these difficulties as compelling evidence of need for a new or relined upper denture, and possibly, a lower partial denture. Helena, undaunted, copes with the difficulties by eating pureed food, which is an acceptable compromise given the overriding proclamation that her health is "the pits"! For Helena, frailty is a psychosocial phenomenon more than a physical dysfunction.

The frail mouth

People with poor dentition tend to select soft foods (Millwood and Heath, 2000), and because many of them have lost teeth due to caries, they might have a preference also for sweet foods. But is this preference influenced by a long-standing addiction to sugar that has damaged the dentition over many years, and so the addiction continues into old age and is bolstered by the impaired dentition? Disabled elders frequently have mucosal, gingival, and periodontal inflammation because of difficulty with oral hygiene, and they have difficulty managing dentures because their orofacial muscles have weakened. And so, the decline in nutritional state, oral function, and hygiene contributes further to frailty.

Typically, the dentures worn by people who are frail are assessed as clinically inadequate by dental professionals, yet the denture-wearers cope quite effectively with them (Mojon and MacEntee, 1992). Further complications arise from salivary gland hypofunction exacerbated by many of the medications associated with frailty. The result is a salivary deficiency, either in quantity or quality or both, that increases the risk of caries, complicates oral hygiene, precludes denture retention, and significantly reduces the resilience of the oral mucosa (Walls et al., 2000). The onset of dementia detracts even more from the selection of nutritious food and the ability to keep the mouth and dentures clean, which typically leads to caries, gingivitis, candidiasis, and denture stomatitis (Chalmers et al., 2003; Ellefsen et al., 2008). These conditions are rarely a source of obvious complaint or obvious discomfort to people who are demented (Chalmers et al., 2003). However, detection of pain is challenging in the presence of advanced dementia, and the impact on their social interactions and enjoyment of food might be much more distressing than we realize.

COPING WITH FRAILTY AND ORAL DISORDERS

Good oral health implies comfort, hygiene, and the absence of disease, but it also accommodates moderate impairment and disability to which elderly people seem reasonably and surprisingly tolerant (Davis, 1976; Brondani et al., 2007). This implication contrasts with the debate around oral health-related quality of life in which oral disease, impairment, and disability are portrayed as intolerable and disturbing experiences (Slade, 1997; Gilbert et al., 1998; Williams et al., 1998; Locker and Gibson, 2005; Nuttall et al.,

2006). Undoubtedly, this negative perspective on oral disorder and disability fits Helena's physical status, but it is challenged seriously by the social network of her family from which she derives positive support and encouragement to offset her physical disabilities.

CONCLUSIONS

We have explained that oral health can influence frailty, just as frailty can influence oral health. They are inextricably connected, both for good and for bad. The case of Helena portrays the complicated connection between oral health and frailty by raising questions about how and why elderly people adapt and cope with physical impairment and disability. It is common for dentists and other dental personnel to identify multiple mouth problems in this population, but careful consideration to the emotional, social, and environmental contexts in which people live should prompt us to temper our professional care with a sophisticated appreciation for the tolerance that most elders have for their predicament and for the autonomy they wish to retain despite the challenges of frailty.

REFERENCES

Awano S, Ansai T, Takata Y, Soh I, Akifusa S, Hamasaki T, Yoshida A, Sonoki K, Fujisawa K, and Takehara T. 2008. Oral health and mortality risk from pneumonia in the elderly. *J Dent Res* 87:334–9.

Bartlett D and Dugmore C. 2008. Pathological or physiological erosion—Is there a relationship to age? *Clin Oral Investig* 12(Suppl. 1):S27–31.

Bergman H, Béland F, Karunananthan S, Hummel S, Hogan DB, and Wolfson C. 2004. Développement d'un cadre de travail pour comprendre et étudier la fragilité. *Gerontol Soc* 109:15–29.

Bergman H, Ferrucci L, Guralnik J, Hogan DB, Hummel S, Karunananthan S, and Wolfson C. 2007. Frailty: An emerging research and clinical paradigm issues and controversies. *J Gerontol A Biol Sci Med Sci* 62:731–7.

Bonito AJ. 2002. Executive summary: Dental care considerations for vulnerable populations. *Spec Care Dentist* 22:5S–10S.

Brondani MA and MacEntee MI. 2007. The concept of validity in sociodental indicators and oral health-related quality-of-life measures. *Community Dent Oral Epidemiol* 35:472–8.

Brondani MA, Bryant SR, and MacEntee MI. 2007. Elders assessment of an evolving model of oral health. *Gerodontology* 24:189–95.

Chalmers JM and Ettinger RL. 2008. Public health issues in geriatric dentistry in the United States. *Dent Clin North Am* 52:423–46.

Chalmers JM, Carter KD, and Spencer AJ. 2003. Oral diseases in community living older adults with and without dementia. *Spec Care Dentist* 23: 7–17.

Corrada MM, Brookmeyer R, Berlau D, Paganini-Hill A, and Kawas CH. 2008. Prevalence of dementia after age 90: Results from the 90+ study. *Neurology* 71:337–43.

Davis P. 1976. Compliance structure and the delivery of health care: The case of dentistry. *Soc Sci Med* 10:329–37.

Denton FT and Spencer BG. 2010. Chronic health conditions: Changing prevalence in an aging population and some implications for the delivery of health care services. *Can J Aging* 29:11–21.

Easterby-Smith V, Besford J, and Heath RM. 1994. The effect of age on the recognition thresholds of three sweeteners: sucrose, saccharin and aspartame. *Gerodontology* 11:39–45.

Ellefsen B, Holm-Pedersen P, Morse DE, Schroll M, Andersen BB, and Waldemar G. 2008. Caries prevalence in older persons with and without dementia. *J Am Geriatr Soc* 56:59–67.

Ettinger RL and Beck JD. 1984. Geriatric dental curriculum and the needs of the elderly. *Spec Care Dentist* 4:207–13.

Fischer G and Heilig GK. 1997. Population momentum and the demand on land and water resources. *Phil Trans R Soc Lond B* 352:869–89.

Fitzpatrick RM. 2003. Society and changing patterns of disease. In: Scambler G (ed.), *Sociology as Applied to Medicine*, 5th edn. Edinburgh: W.B. Saunders, pp. 3–17.

Fure S. 2003. Ten-year incidence of tooth loss and dental caries in elderly Swedish individuals. *Caries Res* 37:462–9.

Gift HC and Redford M. 1992. Oral health and the quality of life. *Clin Geriatr Med* 8:673–83.

Gilbert GH, Duncan RP, Heft MW, Dolan TA, and Vogel WB. 1998. Multi-dimensionality of oral health in dentate adults. *Med Care* 36:988–1001.

Gutman GM, Wister A, and Carrierre Y. 2000. *Fact Book on Aging in BC*, 3rd edn. Vancouver, BC: Gerontology Research Center, Simon Fraser University, pp. 3–10.

Gutmann JL and Gutmann MS. 1995. Cause, incidence and prevention of trauma to teeth. *Dent Clin North Am* 39:1–13.

Helgeson MJ, Smith BJ, Johnsen M, and Ebert C. 2002. Dental considerations for the frail elderly. *Spec Care Dentist* 22:40S–55S.

Kaethler Y, Molnar FJ, Mitchell SL, Soucie P, and Man-Son-Hing M. 2003. Defining the concept of frailty: A survey of multi-disciplinary health professionals. *Geriatr Today* 6:26–31.

Kaufman SR. 1994. The social construction of frailty: An anthropological perspective. *J Aging Stud* 8:45–58.

Landt H and Fransson B. 1975. Oral ability to recognize forms and oral muscular coordination ability in dentulous young and elderly adults. *J Oral Rehabil* 2:125–38.

Levy SM, Warren JJ, Chowdhury J, DeBus B, Watkins CA, Cowen HJ, Kirchner H, Lester H, and Jed S. 2003. The prevalence of periodontal disease measures in elderly adults, aged 79 and older. *Spec Care Dentist* 23:50–7.

Locker D and Gibson B. 2005. Discrepancies between self-ratings of and satisfaction with oral health in two older adult populations. *Community Dent Oral Epidemiol* 33:280–8.

Markle-Reid M and Browne G. 2003. Conceptualizations of frailty in relation to older adults. *J Adv Nurs* 44:58–68.

MacEntee MI. 2007. Quality of life as an indicator of oral health in old age. *J Am Dent Assoc* 138:47S–52S.

MacEntee MI, Hole R, and Stolar E. 1997. The significance of the mouth in old age. *Soc Sci Med* 45:1449–58.

Magnusson C, Ernberg M, and Magnusson T. 2008. A description of a contemporary human skull material in respect of age, gender, temporomandibular joint changes, and some dental variables. *Swed Dent J* 32:69–81.

Mandojana JM, Martin-de las Heras S, Valenzuela A, Valenzuela M, and Luna JD. 2001. Differences in morphological age-related dental changes depending on post mortem interval. *J Forensic Sci* 46:889–92.

Marcus SE, Drury TF, Brown LJ, and Zion GR. 1996. Tooth retention and tooth loss in the permanent dentition of adults: United States, 1988–1991. *J Dent Res* 75:684–95.

Millwood J and Heath MR. 2000. Food choice by older people: the use of semi-structured interviews with open and closed questions. *Gerodontology* 17:25–32.

Mojon P and MacEntee MI. 1992. Discrepancy between need for prosthodontic treatment and complaints in an elderly edentulous population. *Community Dent Oral Epidemiol* 20:48–52.

Moynihan PJ, Butler TJ, Thomason JM, and Jepson NJ. 2000. Nutrient intake in partially dentate patients: the effect of prosthetic rehabilitation. *J Dent* 28:557–63.

Nedelman C and Bernick S. 1978. Age changes in mucosa and bone. *J Prosthet Dent* 39:494–501.

Newton JP, Yemm R, Abel RW, and Menhinick S. 1993. Changes in human jaw muscles with age and dental state. *Gerodontology* 10:16–22.

Nuttall NM, Slade GD, Sanders AE, Steele JG, Allen PF, and Lahti S. 2006. An empirically derived population-response model of the short form of the Oral Health Impact Profile. *Community Dent Oral Epidemiol* 34:18–24.

Papapanou PN, Wennström JL, and Gröndahl K. 1989. A 10-year retrospective study of periodontal disease progression. *J Clin Periodontol* 16:403–11.

Petersen PE, Bourgeois D, Ogawa H, Estupinan-Day S, and Ndiaye C. 2005. The global burden of oral diseases and risks to oral health. *Bull World Health Organ* 83:661–9.

Reichart PA. 2000. Oral mucosal lesions in a representative cross-sectional study of ageing Germans. *Community Dent Oral Epidemiol* 28:390–8.

Rockwood K. 2005. What would make a definition of frailty successful? *Age Ageing* 34:432–4.

Sanders AE, Slade GD, Lim S, and Reisine ST. 2009. Impact of oral disease on quality of life in the US and Australian populations. *Community Dent Oral Epidemiol* 37:171–81.

Satcher D. 2000a. *Oral Health in America: A Report of the Surgeon General.* Department of Health and Human Services: U.S. Public Health Service. Available at www.nidcr.nih.gov/DataStatistics/SurgeonGeneral/sgr/home.html (accessed October 12, 2009).

Satcher D. 2000b. *Oral Health in America: A Report of the Surgeon General. Chapter 5: Older Adults and Mental Health.* Department of Health and Human Services: U.S. Public Health Service. Available at www.surgeongeneral.gov/library/mentalhealth/chapter5/sec1.html (accessed October 12, 2009).

Schoenborn CA and Heyman KM. 2009. *Health Characteristics of Adults Aged 55 Years and Older: United States, 2004–2007.* U.S. Department of Health and Human Services, National Center for Health Statistics, Centers for Disease Control and Prevention. Available at www.cdc.gov/nchs/data/nhsr/nhsr016.pdf (accessed January 18, 2010).

Slade GD. 1997. *Measuring Oral Health and Quality of Life.* Chapel Hill: University of North Carolina, Dental Ecology, pp. iii–v.

Thompson GW and Kreisel PS. 1998. The impact of the demographics of ageing and the edentulous condition on dental care services. *J Prosthet Dent* 79:56–9.

United Nations. 2002a. *World Population Aging 1950–2050. I. Demographic Determinants of Population Ageing.* Available at www.un.org/esa/population/publications/worldageing19502050/pdf/8chapteri.pdf (accessed October 12, 2009).

United Nations. 2002b. *World Population Aging 1950–2050. IV. Demographic Profile of the Older Population.* Available at www.un.org/esa/population/publications/worldageing19502050/pdf/90chapteriv.pdf (accessed October 12, 2009).

United Nations Department of Economic and Social Affairs. 2010. *The World at Six Billion.* Available at www.un.org/esa/population/publications/sixbillion/sixbilpart1.pdf (accessed January 7, 2010).

Walls AW, Steele JG, Sheiham A, Marcenes W, and Moynihan P. 2000. Oral health and nutrition in older people. *J Public Health Dent* 60:304–7.

Williams KB, Gadbury-Amyot CC, Bray KD, Manne D, and Collins P. 1998. Oral health-related quality of life: a model for dental hygiene. *J Dent Hyg* 72:19–26.

Wolff A, Ship JA, Tylenda CA, Fox PC, and Baum BJ. 1991. Oral mucosal appearance is unchanged in healthy different-aged persons. *Oral Surg Oral Med Oral Pathol* 71:569–72.

Wyatt CCL and MacEntee MI. 1998. Dental caries in chronically disabled elders. *Spec Care Dentist* 17:196–202.

Ethical considerations for the oral healthcare of frail elders

Mary E. McNally, Shafik Dharamsi, S. Ross Bryant, and Michael I. MacEntee

INTRODUCTION

Meeting care needs is a central ethical concern in healthcare. (As there is no commonly accepted pattern of differentiating the terms *ethical* and *moral*, they will be treated as synonyms in this chapter.) Significant lapses in care may even be considered a moral failing for those who value health and healthcare as a social good (Dharamsi and MacEntee, 2002). As the chapters of this book unfold, we will see that meeting the oral healthcare needs of frail elders is complex and the supports required to mitigate potential lapses in care are vast. The purpose of this chapter is to focus on key ethical dimensions within this unique realm of healthcare. While one-on-one decisions about the health needs and clinical care of individual patients will feature prominently, we recognize that collective decisions, such as those that establish priorities for resource allocation and health education, are also integral to meeting health needs. In our view, decisions made about healthcare have ethical dimensions because outcomes ultimately affect the human condition—whether as an individual or as part of a larger social group.

Since the realm of healthcare ethics is so vast, we will not attempt to provide an ethical framework sufficient to examine all dimensions of care. Rather, we will use clinical scenarios to elucidate a number of key themes and challenges that are commonly encountered when dental professionals attend to the needs of frail elders.

The chapter has three sections. First, we provide a clinical context for the chapter by describing three scenarios. Second, we respond to relevant ethical themes arising from the cases where we address: patient autonomy

Oral Healthcare and the Frail Elder: A Clinical Perspective.
Edited by Michael I. MacEntee © 2011 Blackwell Publishing Ltd.

as it relates to informed choice and capacity; unclear treatment outcomes; and neglect and abuse. Finally, we raise the broader issue of social responsibility, considering the role of dental professionals, implications for education, and the larger role of society in responding to the oral healthcare needs of frail elders.

CLINICAL CONTEXT

Issues of chronic care and aging have been debated and discussed by ethicists for some time (Daniels, 1991; Callahan, 1995), although both applied and theoretical bioethics have focused primarily on issues of acute care and medical research. The literature is replete with ethical frameworks and strategies for examining and responding to the complex and dramatic issues of acute care. More recently, attention is being directed toward ethical issues arising in chronic care, particularly among vulnerable underserved groups such as the aged (WHO, 2002; Pedersen et al., 2008). Our focus is on identifying morally relevant and unique features of oral health and oral healthcare among frail elders.

Oral health is an essential part of daily comfort, hygiene, and general health (MacEntee et al., 1997). A defective dentition can dramatically disturb eating, speaking, general appearance, and comfort, whereas poor oral hygiene raises significant social and personal concerns for most people (MacEntee, 2007). Pain and discomfort, no matter what the source, impede enjoyment, comfort and dignity. For people who are frail and dependent, the need for oral care typically ranges from daily personal care to complicated therapeutic and restorative treatments. It follows then that effective care requires a coordinated response to address the challenges of "hands-on care" along with the policy and organizational processes supporting care. The following scenarios introduce a number of the issues, with a short description of relevant ethical themes. Typical of real challenges, the scenarios consider the care of individuals residing in a variety of living arrangements, and who represent a range of personal abilities and support.

Mr. Scholten's clinical scenario

Mr. Scholten, who is 83 years old and financially secure, lives in a residential care facility because of severe rheumatoid arthritis. His only other significant medical issue is hypertension. He and his family noticed his teeth deteriorate over the past 2 years coincident with his increasing difficulties with mobility and managing his own personal care. He had no dental pain or discomfort; however, his family encouraged him to consult Dr. Green, the dentist who attends the facility. He was motivated to accept this advice because his broken teeth were becoming an embarrassment when dining and participating in other social activities. On the day of his appointment, his blood pressure was 180/115 mmHg. He reported that he used to take blood pressure medications on his physician's orders but stopped several years previously. He told Dr. Green that, "I have lived a good long life, and I pray for good health. But, it is really in God's hands. I am not going to take medications anymore." The examination revealed a healthy periodontium, generally, but several teeth had active caries. Dr. Green recommended that certain teeth be extracted, and that he needed fillings in several others, and possibly a removable partial denture in both jaws to replace missing teeth. He also explained that the treatment would not be overly invasive, but that he would be uncomfortable providing it when the blood pressure was so high.

Commentary on Mr. Scholten

The ethically relevant features of Mr. Scholten's situation center on his autonomy and the choices for care in light of the potential risks and benefits of dental treatment. He wants to improve his quality of life by having his dental concerns addressed, but he also wants to avoid medications. This raises a serious ethical conflict for the dentist. In the interest of his patient's autonomy, is it appropriate for the dentist to put Mr. Scholten at risk by rendering treatment in the presence of uncontrolled hypertension? Might this be considered substandard care in the context of appropriate clinical practice? On the other hand, if Mr. Scholten is fully informed about the risks and wants the dental treatment, is there moral justification for the dentist to simply refuse?

Mr. Jackson's clinical scenario

Mr. Jackson is an 82 year-old retired farmer and widower. Since moving to the city 10 years ago to be closer to his children, he has been a semiregular patient at a local dental clinic. Recently, he attended the clinic for a routine examination and hygiene. Normally, he is very talkative, bright, and smartly dressed. On this visit, however, Dr. Smith, his dentist, noticed that he was dishevelled and very distracted. He found also that Mr. Jackson had an abscessed molar tooth with a vestibular swelling and tenderness on palpation. He knew that the tooth would be difficult to extract and would require another appointment. In the meantime, Dr. Smith prescribed an antibiotic to reduce the risk of cellulitis. Although he had concerns about Mr. Jackson's well-being and state of mind, his patient seemed to understand the explanation about the tooth. Therefore, he dismissed Mr Jackson's appearance as simply a consequence of the early morning appointment.

Mr. Jackson did not appear for the follow-up appointment, and when the receptionist phoned him, Mr. Jackson said, "I guess I must have forgotten ... I forget a lot of things these days." They rebooked the appointment for the following week, but again, Mr. Jackson failed to keep it, and he sounded confused and upset when the receptionist phoned again. He complained that Dr. Smith did something to his tooth because it was painful and his face was swollen. Consequently, he did not want Dr. Smith to do any more harm and refused another appointment.

Commentary on Mr. Jackson

Autonomy is also the primary issue associated with Mr. Jackson. However, in this case, there is doubt about Mr. Jackson's capacity to understand and make decisions about his health status and treatment needs. Dr. Smith initiated an appropriate course of treatment to benefit Mr. Jackson, but the lack of follow-up could have serious consequences. Dr. Smith will now have to engage the appropriate substitute decision maker if Mr. Jackson truly lacks the capacity.

Mrs. Alders' clinical scenario

Mrs. Alders is a 93-year-old patient with multiple health problems, including dementia and chronic obstructive pulmonary disease. Although she has been cared for by her family for the past 13 years, her 71-year-old daughter can no longer cope with the increasing demands associated with the dementia. Mrs. Alders was admitted recently to a residential care facility approximately 100 km from her daughter's home. On admission to the facility, a dental screening revealed very poor oral hygiene, rampant caries, and extensive structural break-down and mobility of almost all of her remaining 16 teeth. There were no obvious signs of dental pain or distress during the screening examination. She can eat soft foods without difficulty but needs help to carry the food from the plate to her mouth. Her mouth is very dry most of the time, likely a side affect of multiple medications. Combative behavior due to the dementia makes it very difficult for care-aides to clean her teeth or for Dr. West, the facility's attending dentist, to provide the dental treatment. Dr. West offered to extract all of Mrs. Alders' teeth under general anaesthesia in a hospital 45 km from the facility. However, Mrs. Alders would have to travel to the hospital for an examination by an anesthetist before the surgery could be scheduled, and she or her family would have to pay directly for the transport and costs related to examination and treatment. Her daughter refuses to consent because she does not want her mother to be distressed by the extractions or the multiple visits to hospital.

Commentary on Mrs. Alders

Mrs. Alders is representative of many dependent frail elders whose oral health deteriorates and poses a threat to her general health and well-being. She is unable to attend to her daily mouthcare, and apparently, the nursing staff and her daughter cannot provide this care for her. In addition, access to a hospital for dental surgery is difficult, and the cost and complexity of dental care is burdensome for her family. This raises ethical questions within the larger social context about how oral healthcare is organized, managed, and financed. Where, for example, does the responsibility lie to facilitate her daily mouthcare? What is appropriate care for someone who is cognitively disabled and almost completely dependent on others for basic needs? Is it appropriate to extract her remaining teeth or could the loss of so many teeth increase Mrs. Alders' distress and well-being. Alternatively, is it ethically acceptable to withhold dental treatment until she becomes distressed and impaired by toothache or acute infection?

RESPONDING TO ETHICAL ISSUES

The dual phenomena of an aging population with a seemingly endless array of techniques to improve and prolong life have prompted discussions about ethical decisions bearing on the terminal stages of frailty. Advance directives, withholding and withdrawing life-sustaining treatment, and assisted suicide are among the more serious issues that challenge families, clinicians, ethicists, and lawyers to examine the value of human life in a medically sophisticated environment. The responsibility of dentists for providing care toward the end of life in the midst of severe frailty also requires serious thought about the value placed on the care of people who are debilitated or dying, and on the ethical dimensions of decisions influencing this care.

Typically, ethical problems in healthcare arise when a decision must be made in the context of an unresolved moral tension between alternative choices (Purtilo, 1993). Mr. Scholten, for example, challenges the dentist with the struggle between his wish to avoid medications and the dentist's concern about the risks of treatment impacting dangerously on uncontrolled hypertension. Although intuitive judgments are made everyday by clinicians, ethical problems may require a more systematic approach to support moral decisions (Ozar and Sokol, 2002). In the case scenarios we describe, determining a morally defensible course of action requires that various ethical approaches be examined in the context of patient needs and values as well as clinical best practices. This process can be difficult when there are divergent opinions about the best theoretical approaches to a given question or dilemma (Baylis et al., 1995). Indeed, many ethical problems have multiple conflicting solutions with no obvious resolution (Ozar and Sokol, 2002).

Standards of ethics in contemporary healthcare arise for the most part from perspectives grounded in a variety of theories and strategies. They help to frame appropriate responses to a variety of problems, such as delivery of care, biomedical research, codes of professional conduct, organizational ethics, and resource allocation. This theoretical orientation not only affects the ways in which we analyze and resolve particular problems but it also influences issues that we recognize as morally significant and the solutions that are morally acceptable (Baylis et al., 1995).

The most prominent approaches taken in contemporary bioethics are supported by a variety of ideas, including consequence-based ethics, deontological (rights and duties oriented) ethics, virtue ethics, and feminist ethics (Baylis et al., 1995; Kluge, 1999). *Consequentialist* theories, such as utilitarianism, evaluate the moral appropriateness of an action by determining the moral desirability of its consequences. Although there are many variations, the basic principle of utility requires that we would "act in such a way as to maximize the balance of good over harm for the greatest number of people" (Kluge, 1999). In contrast, *deontological* theories determine the moral rightness or wrongness of an action in terms of whether or not it adheres to fundamental moral rules that can be justified independently of consequences (Baylis et al., 1995). There is great debate about which moral rules or principles are consistently justifiable in healthcare. Current approaches recognize that a number of relevant principles must be considered and balanced against each other depending on the situation (Kluge, 1999).

Central to modern biomedical ethics are the four principles "nonmaleficence," "beneficence," "respect for autonomy," and "justice" (Beauchamp and Childress, 2001). This set of principles provides a useful framework through which to analyze and consider ethical issues in healthcare. Each principle indicates a duty related to a specific choice of behavior or action in the absence of a conflicting duty. In keeping with the Hippocratic tradition, nonmaleficence indicates that we "do no harm," while beneficence requires removal and prevention of harm, and promotion of good. The high value placed in most cultures on respect for human dignity and self-determination leads to respect for a patient's autonomy and wishes. Finally, justice is concerned with the fair distribution of benefits and burdens in society. In healthcare generally, but particularly when considering vulnerable populations, attainment of accessible and adequate care reflects a reconciliation of various tensions and responsibilities in the pursuit of justice. Overall, the four principles are guides that leave room for the development of more context-specific rules and policies. The American Dental Association's Code of Ethics provides a useful example of how these principles can be applied in relevant ways to dentistry and oral healthcare (ADA, 2005).

Virtue ethics provides a way of thinking about ethics where actions are not governed by obligations or rules of conduct. Virtues represent a "habit of acting, perceiving, and valuing in the best way possible for the situation" (Ozar and Sokol, 2002). Moral virtues are character traits with high moral value. Applied to healthcare, virtue ethics is concerned with recognizing and developing character traits and daily habits that lead to right actions without careful reflection (Ozar and Sokol, 2002). Virtues such as benevolence, integrity, and compassion are often identified in codes of ethics to exemplify what is valued by the profession as a whole. They represent what it means to be a "good dentist" and offer evidence of moral competency (Welie and Rule, 2006).

Feminism considers the social experiences of women as distinct from the experiences of men, and feminist ethics offers approaches for responding to the distinctions that challenge the dominant male traditions (Tong, 1995). It has been invaluable in bringing attention to the impact of traditional power arrangements and discriminations that affect women (Young,

1990; Sherwin, 1992). It helps focus the meaning of care, relationships, and dependency (Tronto, 1993; Sherwin 1998), and of social and political justice (Young, 1990; Tronto, 1993). Feminist concepts of social justice, that include a positive obligation to alleviate unjust burdens of illness, poverty, and discrimination, for example, are particularly relevant to frail elders. It is prudent, according to feminist ethics, to realize in healthcare that we have a particular responsibility to disadvantaged or vulnerable groups (Young, 1990; McNally, 2003).

PATIENT-CENTERED ETHICS

Autonomy and capacity

Patient autonomy is a relevant feature of the three clinical scenarios described. Autonomy refers to self-determination, whereas the principle of "respect for autonomy" involves treating people so they can act autonomously (Beauchamp and Childress, 2001). Ideally, respect for autonomy involves attitudes and actions that allow patients to make choices in their own best interest and free from constraints. It provides the ethical basis for informed choice and confidentiality in treatment and research so that patients and subjects are capable with sufficient information of exercising "choice" (Dickens, 2004). (The term "informed consent" is used widely for autonomous authorization of a treatment or research intervention; however, "informed choice" is a more appropriate term [Dickens, 2004].) Engaging in the process of informed choice is both an ethical and a legal duty in healthcare. It consists of three obligatory components: disclosure, voluntariness, and capacity. *Disclosure* provides relevant information for an informed choice. *Voluntariness* allows choice free from constraints or undue influence, while *capacity* attests to an understanding of the consequences of decisions (Etchells et al., 1996a; Dickens, 2004).

Our three clinical scenarios represent very distinct challenges to autonomy and informed choice, largely around the issue of capacity. Mr. Scholten's choice to refuse medical advice for the treatment of his hypertension reflects his personal values, which probably seems irrational to his dentist, and could be misconstrued as Mr. Scholten's incapacity for acting in his own best interest. However, neither agreement nor disagreement between the clinician and the patient, nor refusal of treatment substantiates incapacity (Etchells et al., 1996b; Dickens, 2004).

In contrast, Mrs. Alders clearly lacks capacity to make decisions for herself. She relies on her daughter to make decisions for her. This is a substitution grounded also in the principle of autonomy as a means of extending a patient's self-control with assistance from someone who is likely to know and is willing to act on how the patient would decide if capable (Lazar et al., 1996; Ozar and Sokol, 2002). Mrs. Alders' daughter is probably well aware that her mother would prefer not to be transported to a distant hospital for dental surgery, and she is obliged to estimate the benefits and burdens of choices in her mother's best interest if she is not sure which treatment her mother would select.

In some respects, Mr. Jackson's capacity poses the most challenging of our three cases. This is not so much because respect for his autonomy competes with the benefits and risks of treatment as in the other cases, but rather because it may not be clear that he is capable of making decisions in his own best interests. He has neglected the dentist's advice and may be confused about the treatment recently provided. Ideally, these events should prompt the dentist to recommend an assessment to facilitate continuing care. Standard tests of cognitive function, such as the Mini Mental State Examination (Folstein et al., 1975), provide a general impression of a patient's cognitive capacity (Etchells et al., 1996b). The reality, however, is that there are varying degrees of capacity (Ozar and Sokol, 2002), and capacity can even fluctuate from time to time (Lazar et al., 1996) For instance, people with mild to moderate dementia might be able to make reasonable decisions about dental care if they understand fully and accept what is proposed, although they might be quite incompetent in other matters (Dickens, 2004). Similarly, the cognitive capacity of a patient recovering from a reversible illness, such as delirium, adverse drug reaction, depression, or stroke, can improve with time (Lazar et al., 1996).

It is not clear whether Mr. Jackson has a disability that is transient or whether he is exhibiting early signs of a progressive dementia. His dentist has an ethical obligation to continue care. Ideally, he would consult with Mr. Jackson's family. If the family were unavailable or unable to attend to Mr. Jackson, the dentist must also consider contacting appropriate supports such as a social worker if there are concerns about his ability to live independently. This is a delicate situation because respect for autonomy also requires an obligation to protect his privacy (Kleinman et al., 1997). Consequently, it would be prudent to seek Mr. Jackson's permission before contacting anyone on his behalf.

There is concern that incapacity is assigned too widely in an "all or none" approach to decision making, not only about finances and healthcare but also about all personal decisions, including hygiene and other routine needs (Flegel and MacDonald, 2008). It is easy to accept that a tooth extraction in the presence of frank infection will benefit a patient by preventing further morbidity, even if a substitute makes the decision. Difficulties surface when the clinical situation is more complicated or the outcomes less threatening, as is often the case with mouthcare. If, for example, a frail person with dementia refuses help with oral hygiene, is it appropriate for a care-aide to exert control? Often, there is no simple or correct answer. How to proceed must always be considered by balancing the known benefits of an intrusion against the patient's dignity and desire for control over personal matters. Offering choice about engaging in activities such as oral hygiene, with or without assistance, goes a long way toward respectful and ethical caring even when a patient's capacity is limited. Certainly, capacity for decision making must not be predicated upon age or type of disease. Rather, "it is a function of the person and the decision at hand" (Flegel and MacDonald, 2008).

Understanding how to manage patients who lack capacity will continue to grow in importance as the population ages with increasing levels of dependency. Dentists experienced with institutional care have reported for example, that "sometimes … consent … can change from moment to moment. They want something done, but five minutes later they're asking you if you're one of their grandchildren. They clearly don't remember that you're the dentist and that they've consented to treatment. It's a tough one" (Bryant et al., 1995). Complicating this further, family members may not easily acknowledge the concern; "I've had families say, 'Mum can decide, she's quite capable', and … it's clear to me that, 'No, Mum can't decide.' … It's difficult when the families are sort of in denial about what decisions can and can't be made" (Bryant et al., 1995).

Unclear treatment outcomes

In addition to capacity issues, unpredictable treatment outcomes or the vague wishes of a competent patient can create moral angst for clinicians attempting to address a need for care (Purtilo, 1993). It is difficult to accurately weigh the harms and benefits of treatment for people who are frail because outcomes can have such an unclear prognoses. Frail elders tend to experience dietary, medicinal, and behavioral risk factors that favor a recurrence of oral disease even when dental treatment is available (Chalmers et al., 2003). Moreover, it is rarely clear how extensive dental treatment needs to be to reestablish or preserve personal dignity (Mojon and MacEntee, 1992; Sanders et al., 2009). For example, dentists experienced in treating frail elders often ask: "is it better to leave broken off, decaying teeth, or impose an ordeal of treatment on them?" or "is the patient really going to benefit from having a denture?" (Bryant et al., 1995). Mrs. Alders' situation typifies this challenge. Her poor oral health can diminish her general well-being and be source of discomfort. This is a concern to her family and presents an unstable situation for her dentist to manage. Since it is not clear how the quality of her life would be enhanced by treatment, a palliative approach to dental maintenance and hygiene may be the most ethically sound choice. Conversely, if there is stronger evidence that dental disease poses a more significant threat to her general health, it becomes more reasonable and justifiable to extract the teeth. Either way, the clinician is guided by a duty to provide benefit to Mrs. Alders and to minimize harm whether it is a result of a toothache, a serious infection, or from unnecessary treatment. Clearly, input from Mrs. Alders' daughter to compensate for Mrs Alders' incapacity is essential to balance these difficult tensions.

The continuum of care options between "ideal" treatments at one extreme and "practical" or "palliative" care at the other is the subject of differing ethical views among dentists (Bryant et al., 1995). Some dentists attribute professional distress in this context to an education that led them to believe that there is an ideal treatment irrespective of the level of frailty. (Bryant and coworkers 1995) provided an example of this distress from one dentist who explained "if a healthy young adult were to walk into the office, I would have an ideal treatment plan. The ideal with the senior in the institution would be exactly the same … That's how dental school trains us"; and from another who rationalized that although "we're all taught ideal treatment … that is a mistake … I didn't have an ideal in mind for all my patients … you can call it a compromise. We call it 'rational treatment planning' [coined by Ettinger and Beck (1984)] … Gets rid of some of my guilt."

Formal ethical decision making may not be a conscious or common activity among dentists. However, experienced dentists who provide care for frail elders seem able to balance difficult decisions by weighing judiciously the physical risks associated with choices for care against the ethical requirement and psychosocial benefits of respecting autonomy. Returning to our case scenarios, Mr. Scholten represents someone who has capacity to make choices and for whom "ideal treatment" is feasible. Mrs. Alders' situation suggests that less ambitious treatment goals are warranted. Nevertheless, some dentists might feel that invasive treatment is inappropriate for Mr. Scholten given his general health, while others would be uncomfortable doing nothing for Mrs. Alders. Unsettling questions for both patients include how much intervention is too much and how much is too little? Ettinger and Beck (1984) caution that dentists who manage the dental needs of frail elders should know that "too much or too little treatment … may have more serious consequences than treatment errors in almost any dental specialty." Although not entirely clear about the range of knowledge needed by dentists to treat frail elders, they propose a "rational dental care model" to "approach these complicated diagnostic situations" (see Chapter 11). The model offers sound moral and practical considerations not only for diseases and interventions but also for the values, preferences, capacity, and autonomy of patients. More recently, the practice of "minimal intervention dentistry" has been proposed to minimize harm to frail elders by focusing on risk assessment, prevention, and early detection of disease, along with conservative restoration of teeth (Chalmers, 2006a, b). Some might consider minimalist or ultraconservative dentistry as being paternalistic or discriminatory toward people who are frail and dependent. However, minimal interventions do not preclude a broad scope of treatment options if they suit a patient's medical and personal circumstances. If, for example, Mr. Scholten's hypertension was controlled, there is no moral or ethical reason that he could not have teeth extracted, restored, and replaced safely in any way that dentistry has to offer. The same cannot be presumed for Mrs. Alders.

In caring for frail elders, choices are often made where the patient's health and autonomy and the dentist's sense of ideal treatment seem compromised. Unfortunately, if the complexity of these difficult choices is not fully understood, it can cause feelings of professional discomfort and inadequacy among dentists, and it can limit the contribution of many dentists and dental hygienists to the care of frail elders (MacEntee et al., 1992; Bryant et al., 1995). It is a fact of life that choices must be made even in the face of uncertainty, and it is not morally defensible to withdraw from service simply because the outcomes are uncertain (Pellegrino, 1993).

Elder abuse and neglect

Abuse and neglect are unethical by any moral standard. Recent awareness of the seriousness of this problem in geriatrics serves as a reminder of the insidious and hidden forms of neglect and abuse that abound. Elder abuse refers to "mistreatment" of older people by those in a position of trust, power, or responsibility, while neglect refers to a "failure to meet the needs" of an older person who cannot meet those needs alone (National Clearinghouse on Family Violence, 1999). Although neglect and abuse are harmful and should always prompt an ethical response to "right the wrong," careful considerations of the appropriate processes are equally important. For example, Mrs. Alders' dentist could conclude that her poor oral health is a preventable harm that could reasonably be construed as neglect. More seriously, the prolonged nature of this neglect may be labeled as deliberate "mistreatment" and could reasonably be identified as physical abuse. We know that Mrs. Alders' aging daughter was unable to cope with the demands of her mother's personal care. Perhaps she had inadequate resources, education, or social supports to address her mother's needs. If, on the other hand, she simply "could not be bothered," the suggestion of deliberate mistreatment is not out of the question. How we would engage in righting the wrongs that led to Mrs. Alders' poor oral health requires reflection on a broad range of factors—including the definition of abuse.

Elder abuse takes on many forms and is variously described to include financial, physical, emotional, psychological, sexual, systemic or ageism, and spiritual abuse (Lachs et al., 1997; National Seniors Council, 2007; Wiseman, 2008). Age, race, poverty, functional disability, and cognitive impairment are known factors associated with greatest risk as well as elders who are female, isolated, dependent, cared for by someone with an addiction, or living in a residential care facility. It is a global phenomenon (Penhale, 2006) with between 4% and 10% of older adults in North America subjected to some form of abuse (National Seniors Council, 2007), although there is reason to suspect underreporting, especially from within residential care facilities (National Clearinghouse on Family Violence, 1999).

From a legal perspective, obligatory reporting of adults in need of protection tends to be monitored and enforced inconsistently in different jurisdictions (Gibson, 2004). Certainly, there is an ethical responsibility to report abuse. Dental professionals, like other healthcare providers, should be familiar with their legal obligations and with the local legal, social, and medical support available to victims of abuse or neglect. A legal obligation to report may be accompanied by an exception to the duty of confidentiality in the interests of protecting adults at risk. In other words, no action would lie against a person who provides information unless it is given maliciously or without reasonable and probable cause. Unfortunately, in jurisdictions where legislation is not clear, concerns about possible breaches of privacy can inhibit reports of suspected cases of abuse (National Seniors Council, 2007). Protecting privacy is a duty that is incorporated under the principle of "respect for autonomy." It is an obligation that cannot be taken lightly when faced with the decision of whether or not to report an elder who seems to be in harm's way and in need of protection (Wiseman, 2008).

Returning to our clinical scenarios, it is possible that Mr. Scholten's refusal to take antihypertensive medications could be construed as "self-neglect" since he is not availing himself of necessary medical care. However, earlier, we argued that he has capacity to decide on how he wants to live; therefore, we must accept also that he does not need protection from himself, even if we disagree with his choices. Mr. Jackson's predicament is less clear. We are unsure of his capacity, so we must be vigilant to ensure that we remain respectful of his autonomy when we decide whether or not to contact his family or other social and legal supports on his behalf.

Dental professionals who care for older adults occasionally recognize incidents of abuse and neglect, and have a role to play in reporting it. Familiarity with the population groups at greatest risk, coupled with a comprehensive strategy as described for screening, detecting, intervening, and monitoring to protect patients in our care, is a good starting point from which to address and respond to elder abuse and neglect (Wiseman, 2008).

SOCIALLY RESPONSIBLE ORAL HEALTHCARE

As we have demonstrated, the relationship between a healthcare professional and a patient is a defining feature of ethical healthcare (Kluge, 1999). It provides a standpoint from which to observe health and personal needs, the types of care that are available and offered, whether there are adequate resources to meet needs, and how improvements to health are achieved. Although our case scenarios emphasize the role of the clinician in navigating complex ethical decisions about care, they also draw attention to broader social issues. Mrs. Alders' situation represents the increasingly typical and complicated circumstances facing frail elders that have prompted calls for more socially responsible and sensitive oral healthcare. The conventional private practice model of dental care may well be incapable of meeting her particular needs, but it is not yet clear how best to manage her problems given current resources and professional organization. What is clear, from an ethical standpoint, is that lapses in care that led to Mrs. Alders' circumstances represent an injustice (Dharamsi and MacEntee, 2002; McNally, 2003). While an in-depth analysis of the meaning of justice in this context is beyond the scope of this paper, we highlight a number of relevant responses (see WHO [2002] and President's Council on Bioethics [2005] for a more comprehensive analysis).

Clinical and personal care must be extended to include a multidisciplinary approach, involving a broad range of healthcare providers (Pearson and Chalmers, 2004; MacEntee, 2006). Where overall access to adequate care is limited or even nonexistent, we must also examine how social and political factors influence care needs (Pyle, 2002; McNally, 2005). It is clear that healthcare is valued as a common social good when a community decides to support healthcare and to educate healthcare professionals with public funds. Indeed, healthcare systems are largely about society's values where it is recognized that society has a role to play in establishing public policy that supports the health of its citizens. The moral significance here is the decision making that ultimately affects the welfare of others (Kenny, 2002). A common feature of all healthcare systems, no matter how they are organized, managed, and financed, is that poor health, including oral health, is significantly associated with low-income, disabled, dependent, minority, and other vulnerable groups, including frail elders (Dharamsi and MacEntee, 2002; Treadwell and Northridge, 2007). Moreover, dentistry and other oral healthcare services are excluded from publicly funded health services in most countries. Despite the likelihood that "[s]ubsidization of the poor by inclusion of dental care in social health insurance models appears to offer the most potential for equitable access," the current policies almost everywhere is away from publicly funded dentistry (Leake and Birch, 2008).

PROFESSIONAL RESPONSIBILITIES

Politics also play out within the health professions. Dentistry, like other professions, works within the context of a social contract that allows self-regulation of service, standards, and practices. In exchange, it is reasonable for the society served by the profession to expect that its members are ethical, competent, and altruistic. Here, altruism requires dentists to place the needs and interests of patients ahead of their own (Welie, 2004). It is also reasonable for society to expect that the dental professions, as a collective, have a key role in addressing significant lapses in care. Dentists are aware of this contractual responsibility (Weiss et al., 1993; Bryant et al., 1995; Dharamsi et al., 2007), although when challenged by patients like Mrs. Alders, many of them are unsure about how best to respond (Ettinger and Beck, 1984, Bryant et al., 1995). Moreover, even with a collective acknowledgment of responsibility to the public, it is not clear how that could be translated to individual practitioners. As long as there is a market for the private practice, fee-for-service model, dentists will continue to enjoy a great deal of professional autonomy. Dentists are greatly empowered by this autonomy and as a result, can be selective about whom they care for and what type of care they choose to provide.

Educating professionals for social responsibility enables the development of practice that accounts for the common good while at the same time respecting diversity and individuality (Nemerowicz and Rosi, 1997). Accordingly, an increased emphasis on social responsibility that includes community-oriented service by students is a strategy that holds much promise (MacEntee et al., 2005; Yoder, 2006). Additional possibilities for creating an "education for justice" include raising consciousness about the issues of oral health disparities by providing accurate evidence; sharing inspiring stories of exemplary role models who make positive contributions to social justice; seeking out creative models and programs that successfully respond to disparities; and acknowledging limits to resources to focus goals of care that ensures that all members of society have reasonable access to adequate care (Winslow, 2006).

Understanding the influence of professional and organizational culture within dental schools and reflecting on appropriate systematic responses are both essential steps in developing further the moral competencies needed to address the challenges posed by our three clinical scenarios (Rule and Welie, 2006).

CONCLUSIONS

Systems of social assistance offer protection from unavoidable social, political, and financial challenges. Within such systems, healthcare professionals and the broader political structures are expected to act cooperatively for the public good. Yet arguments and conflicts continue about who should control the system, how providers are paid, what services should be included, and who should have access to financial assistance. There are legitimate concerns about the costs of healthcare overall. In spite of convincing arguments that favor support for the frail and vulnerable segments in society, the practicalities of rationing remain unresolved (Veatch, 1991; Daniels, 2001; Dharamsi and MacEntee, 2002). Ultimately, an inclusive system of oral healthcare for frail elders will be possible only with the willing participation of a broad range of health and social professions along with advocates for policy and administrative change. What seems likely is that the need to manage the large numbers of individuals who will be in the situations represented by Mr. Scholten, Mr. Jackson, and Mrs. Alders over the coming decade will compel change and innovation to manage the challenges of our aging populations.

REFERENCES

ADA. 2005. *Principles of Ethics and Code of Professional Conduct.* American Dental Association. Available at http://www.ada.org/sections/about/pdfs/ada_code.pdf (accessed May 31, 2010).

Baylis F, Downie J, Freedman B, Hoffmaster B, and Sherwin S. 1995. Theory and method in health care ethics. In: Baylis F, Downie J, Freedman B, Hoffmaster B, and Sherwin S (eds.), *Health Care Ethics in Canada*. Toronto, ON: Harcourt Brace & Co., pp. 4–9.

Beauchamp T and Childress J. 2001. *Principles of Biomedical Ethics*, 5th edn. New York: Oxford University Press.

Bryant SR, MacEntee MI, and Browne A. 1995. Ethical issues encountered by dentists in the care of institutionalized elders. *Spec Care Dentist* 15:79–82.

Callahan D. 1995. *Setting Limits: Medical Goals in an Ageing Society with a Response to My Critics*. Washington, DC: Georgetown University Press.

Chalmers JM. 2006a. Minimal intervention dentistry: Part 1. Strategies for addressing the new caries challenge in older patients. *J Can Dent Assoc* 72:427–33.

Chalmers JM. 2006b. Minimal intervention dentistry: Part 2. Strategies for addressing restorative challenges in older patients. *J Can Dent Assoc* 72:435–40.

Chalmers JM, Carter KD, and Spencer AJ. 2003. Oral diseases in community living older adults with and without dementia. *Spec Care Dentist* 23:7–17.

Daniels N. 1991. Equal opportunity and health care rights for the elderly. In: Bolle TJ III and Bondeson WB (eds.), *Rights to Health Care*. Boston: Kluwer Academic Publishers, pp. 201–12.

Daniels N. 2001. Justice, health, and healthcare. *Am J Bioeth* 1:2–16.

Dharamsi S and MacEntee MI. 2002. Dentistry and distributive justice. *Soc Sci Med* 55:323–9.

Dharamsi S, Pratt DD, and MacEntee MI. 2007. How dentists account for social responsibility: Economic imperatives and professional obligations. *J Dent Educ* 71:1583–92.

Dickens B. 2004. Informed choice. In: Downie J, McEwen K, and MacInnis W (eds.), *Dental Law in Canada*. Markham: LexisNexis Canada Inc., pp. 219–36.

Etchells E, Sharpe G, Walsh P, Williams JR, and Singer PA. 1996a. Bioethics for clinicians: 1. Consent. *Can Med Assoc J* 155:177–80.

Etchells E, Sharpe G, Elliott C, and Singer PA. 1996b. Bioethics for clinicians: 3. Capacity. *Can Med Assoc J* 155:657–61.

Ettinger RL and Beck JD. 1984. Geriatric dental curriculum and the needs of the elderly. *Spec Care Dentist* 4:207–13.

Flegel KM and MacDonald N. 2008. Decision-making capacity in an age of control. *Can Med Assoc J* 178:127.

Folstein M, Folstein SE, and McHugh PR. 1975. "Mini-mental state" a practical method for grading the cognitive state of patients for the clinician. *J Psychiatr Res* 12:189–98.

Gibson E. 2004. Privacy and confidentiality issues for dental professionals. In: Downie J, McEwen K, and MacInnis W (eds.), *Dental Law in Canada*. Markham ON: Butterworths LexisNexis Canada Inc., pp. 251–69.

Kenny NP. 2002. *What Good is Health Care? Reflections on the Canadian Experience*. Ottawa, ON: CHA Press.

Kleinman I, Baylis F, Rodgers S, and Singer P. 1997. Bioethics for clinicians: 8. Confidentiality. *Can Med Assoc J* 156:521–4.

Kluge EW. 1999. *Readings in Biomedical Ethics: A Canadian Focus*, 2nd edn. Scarborough, ON: Prentice-Hall Canada Inc.

Lachs MS, Williams C, O'Brien S, Hurst L, and Horwitz R. 1997. Risk factors for reported elder abuse and neglect: A nine-year observational cohort study. *Gerontologist* 37:469–74.

Lazar NM, Greiner GG, Robertson G, and Singer PA. 1996. Bioethics for clinicians: 5. Substitute decision-making. *Can Med Assoc J* 155:1435–7.

Leake JL and Birch S. 2008. Public policy and the market for dental services. *Community Dent Oral Epidemiol* 36:287–95.

MacEntee MI. 2006. Missing links in oral health care for frail elderly people. *J Can Dent Assoc* 72:421–5.

MacEntee MI. 2007. Quality of life as an indicator of oral health in older people. *J Am Dent Assoc* 138(Suppl. 1):47S–52S.

MacEntee MI, Weiss RT, Waxler-Morrison NE, and Morrison BJ. 1992. Opinions of dentists on the treatment of elderly patients in long term care facilities. *J Public Health Dent* 52:239–44.

MacEntee MI, Hole R, and Stolar E. 1997. The significance of the mouth in old age. *Soc Sci Med* 45:1449–58.

MacEntee MI, Pruksapong M, and Wyatt CCL. 2005. Insights from students following an educational rotation through dental geriatrics. *J Dent Educ* 69:1368–76.

McNally M. 2003. Rights access and justice in oral health care: Justice toward underserved patient populations—the elderly. *J Am Coll Dent* 70:56–60.

McNally M. 2005. Oral health matters: What will it take to leave no senior behind? *J Can Dent Assoc* 71:465–7.

Mojon P and MacEntee MI. 1992. Discrepancy between need for prosthodontic treatment and complaints in an elderly edentulous population. *Community Dent Oral Epidemiol* 20:48–52.

National Clearinghouse on Family Violence. 1999. *Abuse and Neglect of Older Adults in Institutions: A Discussion Paper*. Ottawa, ON: Public Health Agency of Canada. Available at www.phac-aspc.gc.ca/ncfv-cnivf/familyviolence/html/agediscussion_e.html (accessed April 28, 2009).

National Seniors Council. 2007. *Report of the National Seniors Council on Elder Abuse*. Ottawa, ON: Government of Canada. Available at www.seniorscouncil.gc.ca/eng/research_publications/elder_abuse/2007/hs4_38/page00.shtml (accessed April 28, 2009).

Nemerowicz G and Rosi E. 1997. *Education for Leadership and Social Responsibility*. London: The Falmer Press.

Ozar DT and Sokol DJ. 2002. *Dental Ethics at Chairside: Professional Principles and Practical Applications*, 2nd edn. Washington, DC: Georgetown University Press.

Pearson A and Chalmers J. 2004. Oral hygiene care for adults with dementia in residential aged care facilities. *JBI Rep* 2:65–113.

Pedersen R, Nortvedt P, Nordhaug M, Slettebo A, Grothe KH, Kirkevold M, Brinchmann BS, and Andersen B. 2008. In quest of justice? Clinical prioritisation in healthcare for the aged. *J Med Ethics* 34:230–5.

Pellegrino ED. 1993. The metamorphosis of medical ethics. A 30-year retrospective. *J Am Med Assoc* 269:1158–62.

Penhale B. 2006. Elder abuse in Europe: An overview of recent developments. *J Elder Abuse Negl* 18:107–16.

President's Council on Bioethics. 2005. *Taking Care: Ethical Caregiving in our Aging Society*. Available at http://bioethics.georgetown.edu/pcbe/reports/taking_care/ (accessed May 31, 2010).

Purtilo RB. 1993. *Ethical Dimensions in the Health Professions*, 2nd edn. Philadelphia: W.B. Saunders Co.

Pyle MA. 2002. Changing perceptions of oral health and its importance to general health: Provider perceptions, public perceptions, policymaker perceptions. *Spec Care Dentist* 22:8–15.

Rule JT and Welie JVM. 2006. Justice, moral competencies and the role of dental schools. In: Welie JVM (ed.), *Justice in Oral Health Care: Ethical and Educational Perspectives*. Milwaukee, WI: Marquette University Press, pp. 233–59.

Sanders AE, Slade GD, Lim S, and Reisine ST. 2009. Impact of oral disease on quality of life in the US and Australian populations. *Community Dent Oral Epidemiol* 37:171–81.

Sherwin S. 1992. *No Longer Patient: Feminist Ethics and Health Care*. Philadelphia: Temple University Press.

Sherwin S. 1998. *The Politics of Women's Health: Exploring Agency and Autonomy*. Philadelphia: Temple University Press.

Tong R. 1995. What's distinctive about feminist bioethics? In: Baylis F, Downie J, Freedman B, Hoffmaster B, and Sherwin S (eds.), *Health Care Ethics in Canada*. Toronto, ON: Harcourt Brace & Co., pp. 22–30.

Treadwell HM and Northridge ME. 2007. Oral health is the measure of a just society. *J Health Care Poor Underserved* 18:12.

Tronto JC. 1993. *Moral Boundaries: A Political Argument for an Ethic of Care*. New York: Routledge.

Veatch RM. 1991. Should basic care get priority? Doubts about rationing the Oregon way. *Kennedy Inst Ethics J* 1:187–206.

Weiss RT, Morrison BJ, MacEntee MI, and Waxler-Morrison NE. 1993. The influence of social, economic, and professional considerations on services offered by dentists to long-term care residents. *J Public Health Dent* 53:70–5.

Welie JVM. 2004. Is dentistry a profession? Part 1. Professionalism defined. *J Can Dent Assoc* 70:529–32.

Welie JVM and Rule JT. 2006. Overcoming isolationism. Moral competencies, virtues and the importance of connectedness. In: Welie JVM (ed.), *Justice in Oral Health Care: Ethical and Educational Perspectives*. Milwaukee, WI: Marquette University Press, pp. 97–125.

WHO. 2002. *Ethical Choices in Long-Term Care: What Does Justice Require?* World Health Organization Collection on Long-Term Care. Available at www.who.int/chp/knowledge/publications/ethical_choices/en/index.html (accessed April 28, 2009).

Winslow GR. 2006. Just dentistry and the margins of society. In: Welie JVM (ed.), *Justice in Oral Health Care: Ethical and Educational Perspectives*. Milwaukee WI: Marquette University Press, pp. 81–96.

Wiseman M. 2008. The role of the dentist in recognizing elder abuse. *J Can Dent Assoc* 74:715–20.

Yoder KM. 2006. A framework for service-learning in dental education. *J Dent Educ* 70:115–23.

Young IM. 1990. *Justice and the Politics of Difference*. Princeton, NJ: Princeton University Press.

Oral pain and movement disorders in aging

3

Pierre J. Blanchet, Barry Sessle, and Gilles Lavigne

> ### Clinical scenario
>
> Mrs. G. is an edentulous 77-year-old woman being treated for chronic hypertension who experienced a major depressive illness recently. She had no prior psychiatric history and has never taken psychotropic drugs. She was referred to a psychiatrist, and during her first psychiatric assessment, she complained of moderately intense oral pain and displayed repetitive spontaneous chewing movements. The psychiatrist diagnosed a major depression and tardive dyskinesia, and prescribed quetiapine (Seroquel®, Astra Zeneca Group of Companies, London, UK), which is a second-generation antipsychotic drug. Shortly after this, Mrs. G's physician referred her for a dental assessment.

INTRODUCTION

Orofacial pain is a common problem that occurs in at least 1 in 10 adults but in more than half of the elderly population (Madland and Feinmann, 2001). It is classified according to source or cause of the pain (Table 3.1). The complex category encompasses three distinct entities: (1) primary headache disorders; (2) neuralgias; and (3) persistent idiopathic orofacial pain, which includes burning mouth syndrome, arthromyalgia, atypical odontalgia, and atypical facial pain (Woda et al., 2005).

Chronic orofacial pain in people over 60 years presents particular diagnostic and management challenges (Riley et al., 1998). It can originate

Table 3.1 Source and distribution of chronic orofacial pain in older people (adapted from Woda et al., 2005).

Source	Distribution
Primary headache disorders	
Migraine	3%–5% lifetime prevalence for
Cluster headache	chronic daily headache
Tension-type headache	
Hemicrania continua	
Others	
Neuralgias	
Essential trigeminal neuralgia (tic	Prevalence: 1.6% >age 84
douloureux)	(women: 6.3%; men: 2.7%)
Symptomatic trigeminal neuralgia	Rare
Postherpetic neuralgia	20% 3 months after rash
Glossopharyngeal neuralgia	Rare
Central neuralgia	11% after stroke
Persistent idiopathic orofacial pain	
Burning mouth syndrome (stomatopyrosis)	1.7% (1%–15%)
Arthromyalgia (temporomandibular disorder)	7.7%
Atypical odontalgia (phantom tooth pain)	3%–6% postendodontic treatment
Atypical facial pain	3%

peripherally from an intraoral, extraoral, musculoskeletal, or neural source, or in the central nervous system (CNS). Either way, the pain is confounded by age-related changes exacerbated by dental disorders, tooth loss, denture use, malnutrition, cancer, and by various drugs. Trigeminal and postherpetic neuralgias, along with other atypical orofacial pains, occur primarily in the older age group. Indeed, age-related changes in the CNS, and neurodegenerative conditions affecting monoamine transmission and cognitive processes, such as Parkinson's and Alzheimer's diseases, have a significant influence on how pain is processed, reported, and assessed (Cole et al., 2008). Moreover, oral dyskinesias in people who wear dentures can be particularly painful. Chronic pain upsets quality of life by disturbing cognitive, psychological, and functional status of elders as they grow frail (Nitschke and Müller, 2004), although we should not underestimate the adaptive and coping skills of people in old age (Vickers and Boocock, 2005; Brondani et al., 2007).

    This chapter presents the relevant disease processes by which chronic orofacial pain and disorders of oral movement occur along with related management approaches suitable for frail elders.

PAIN ASSESSMENT IN ELDERS

We know quite well how elderly people report or complain about pain in general (Hadjistavropoulos et al., 2007), but we know much less about responses to chronic orofacial pain. Self-reporting is the most reliable source of information about an older patient's pain, even in the presence of mild to moderate dementia. However, several factors contribute to underdetection of pain and delayed pain management. Elders commonly have difficulty communicating their pain and distress, probably because of denial, stoicism, or neurological impairment; however, compared with younger adults, they are usually less angered or distressed by chronic pain (Vickers and Boocock, 2005). Single pain assessment scales are unreliable for patients with moderate to severe dementia, particularly when complicated by delirium or depression (Hadjistavropoulos et al., 2008). Consequently, reports from caregivers along with signs of grimacing, guarding, or reluctance to eat are more reliable indicators of pain (Ettinger, 2000; Pautex et al., 2006). Patients who cannot communicate or who are agitated and unresponsive to neuroleptic drugs can use a map or drawing of the face to help locate and record the source of the pain. Similarly, a short trial of acetaminophen or narcotics helps to clarify the extent of the pain. These situations, along with fear of analgesic-induced side effects and dependence, can delay diagnosis and adequate pain relief, which can in turn lead to delirium or cognitive deterioration in frail elders (Morrison et al., 2003). Consequently, all complaints of pain should be taken seriously, and changes in mood, eating, social behavior, or sleep should prompt a search for a source of pain.

CHANGES IN PROCESSING PAIN

Overall, older people have a similar or slightly higher pain threshold but lower pain tolerance compared with younger people (Gagliese, 2007). Loss of natural teeth does not seem to alter thresholds of orofacial pain (Blanchet et al., 2008), although tooth loss and old age decrease the density of myelinated fibers in the trigeminal nerve (Nonaka et al., 2001; Ishikawa et al., 2005). Damage to the neural pathways that detect noxious stimuli can result in orofacial neuropathic pain or "neuralgia."

Neuralgias are caused by various events ranging from peripheral nerve damage to increased excitability of neurons in the CNS (Woda and Salter, 2008). Central transmission of noxious stimuli may be facilitated by advancing age due to reductions in neurotransmitters, such as serotonin and norepinephrine (Iwata et al., 2004; Karp et al., 2008). Dopamine is also implicated in descending inhibition pathways, but how it contributes to pain in the dopamine-deficient Parkinson's nervous system is unclear (Mylius et al., 2009).

OROFACIAL PAIN

Orofacial pain, which occurs in about one in five elders in the United States, arises primarily from diseases affecting the teeth, periodontium, jaw joints, and oral mucosa (Riley et al., 1998). Jaw pain and facial pain seem to occur more frequently in women than in men. Painful mucosal ulcers and stomatitis are particularly common in elderly denture-wearers (Jainkittivong et al., 2002). Chronic periodontitis is not usually painful (Brunsvold et al., 1999), whereas inflammatory vesiculoerosive diseases (e.g., lichen planus; erythema multiforme, mucous membrane pemphigoid), oral mucositis from chemotherapy and head-neck radiation therapy, and some malignant and premalignant lesions are usually very painful (Silverman, 2007).

Neuralgic pain

Central and peripheral neuropathic pain is persistent and caused by a primary lesion or dysfunction of the nervous system. About 1% of the general population suffer from it, but it is more prevalent in elderly people with arteriosclerosis, cerebral vascular disease, diabetes, cancer, chronic inflammatory conditions, shingles, or immune deficiencies. The peripheral type is associated typically with trigeminal neuralgia, postherpetic neuralgia, and painful diabetic neuropathy (Schmader, 2002; Hadjistavropoulos et al., 2007).

Trigeminal neuralgia

This neuralgia, also called *tic douloureux*, is a very distressing pain that strikes suddenly, intensely, recurrently, and uncontrollably (De Simone et al., 2008). It occurs with a lifetime prevalence of up to 1.6% in the general population, but more so among women than men (3:2), and the 1-year prevalence when aged 85–94 years reaches about 6% in women and 3% in men (Schwaiger et al., 2009). People older than 50 years are more susceptible to trigeminal neuralgia probably because cerebellar vascular loops pulsate at this age against the trigeminal nerve, especially as the root of the nerve enters the pons in the brainstem where there can be a loss of central myelin (Rappaport et al., 1997). Consequently, excitation of the small-diameter afferent sensory nerve fibers of the face can cause paroxysmal pain. However, the exact cause and pathogenesis of the neuralgia are unclear. The painful jabs are always acute, intense, and excruciating, often described as electrical discharges. Typically, they are brief, but can occur in clusters lasting 1–2 min. They recur several times a day, followed by a refractory period. Most often the pain is unilateral, limited to the infraorbital portion of the maxillary branch of the trigeminal nerve, and begins in the upper lip, gums, or teeth, on the side of the nose, or occasionally around the mental nerve. Accurate diagnosis is based on very definite painful attacks in response to tactile stimulation of specific trigger zones, while neurological responses are normal between attacks. Facial pain manifesting in other ways is unlikely to be trigeminal neuralgia.

Management of trigeminal neuralgia

Anticonvulsants, such as carbamazepine or oxcarbazepine, are the first approach to managing trigeminal neuralgia. It might be necessary to supplement the anticonvulsant with a muscle relaxant, such as a gamma-aminobutyric acid (GABA)-enhancing drug (e.g., baclofen, clonazepam), or to switch to a different anticonvulsant (e.g., lamotrigine, pregabalin, or levetiracetam). However, when pharmacotherapy is unsuccessful, relief for the neuralgia might be obtained with percutaneous controlled radiofrequencies to produce a lesion in the Gasserian ganglion, surgical microvascular decompression of the nerve rootlets, or radiosurgery to relieve the pain (Sekula et al., 2008). Botulinum toxin has been used intradermally to reduce the pain of trigeminal neuralgia (Zuniga et al., 2008) and other types of focal chronic neuropathic pain including postherpetic neuralgia (Ranoux et al., 2008). It can reduce pain intensity and mechanical allodynia, while sparing thermal sensibility.

However, there is no consensus on how best to manage trigeminal neuralgia in people who are frail. If anticonvulsant medications fail, obviously, the less invasive and risky percutaneous approach is preferable, although this can produce a numb and very painful area on the face (anesthesia dolorosa) in a small proportion (<5%) of patients (Rasmussen, 1965). It remains a difficult challenge.

Other trigeminal lesions

Ischemic, compressive (e.g., tumors, aneurysms), demyelinating (e.g., multiple sclerosis), traumatic, or infiltrative lesions associated with the trigeminal nerve origin can cause symptoms of trigeminal neuralgia, although without the trigger spots or the refractory relief. However, even if these atypical forms respond to anticonvulsants, further investigations are needed to locate the source of the problem because of neoplastic possibilities (e.g., meningioma). Numbness of the chin or other discomforts in the gum and teeth innervated by the inferior alveolar nerve suggests a malignancy within the mandible unless there is a more obvious dental source of the symptoms. Typical neuralgic pain associated within the distribution of other cranial nerves (e.g., glossopharyngeal neuralgia in the tonsillar fossa) can occur, but very infrequently, and it is treated much like trigeminal neuralgia.

Postherpetic neuralgia

More than two-thirds of herpes zoster cases occur in people over 60 years of age. The general incidence of herpes zoster based on data from a health maintenance organization in the United States in the early 1990s was estimated at 215 per 100,000 person-years (100,000 person-years = 10,000 persons followed for 10 years; or 20,000 persons for 5 years), representing a 64% increase compared with the preceding 30 years (Donahue et al., 1995). It is also about sixfold higher in older people, possibly because of an age-related decline in cell-mediated immunity to the varicella zoster virus. Older persons who are immunocompromised are particularly at risk.

Acute pain is often experienced prior to the appearance of the shingles rash (Figure 3.1).

The rash resolves within 4 weeks and the pain decreases, but painful responses to normal stimuli along with an itch are common. The prevalence of pain at 1 month after the onset of the rash rises sharply after age 50 years (Choo et al., 1997; Stankus et al., 2000). Postherpetic neuralgia—pain persisting more than 3 months after the onset of the rash—occurs in about one in five people over 50 years of age, but drops to less than 1 in 10 people after a year. The ophthalmic division of the trigeminal nerve is more usually affected than the other two divisions.

Management of postherpetic neuralgia

Unfortunately, the acute antiviral treatment (famciclovir, valaciclovir) for herpes zoster does not reliably prevent the neuralgia even if taken within 72h following onset of the rash. A vaccine reduced the incidence of neuralgia by about two-thirds in older populations (Oxman et al., 2008). However, the standard management includes anticonvulsants (e.g., gabapentin, pregabalin), tricyclic antidepressants (e.g., amitriptyline), 5% or 10% lidocaine topical cream or patch, and tramadol, an opioid analgesic (Moulin et al., 2007; Tyring, 2007). Botulinum toxin has been used intra-

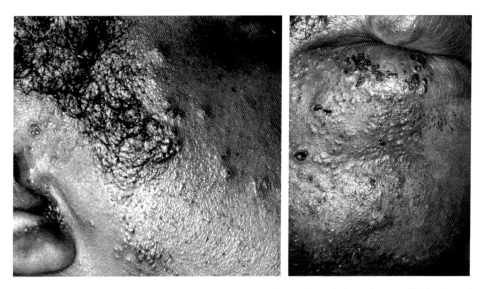

Figure 3.1 Herpes zoster "shingles" rash distributed along the mandibular branch of the trigeminal nerve. (Photograph courtesy of Dr. Michelle Williams, Vancouver, BC, Canada.).

dermally with some success (see management of trigeminal neuralgia above). Anticonvulsants and topical lidocaine are the first-line treatment, while the narcotics are reserved for refractory pain.

Central neuralgia

Acquired lesions along the trigeminothalamic nociceptive pathways can cause severe facial pain resembling trigeminal neuralgia or continuous unpleasant sensations (dysesthesias). In contrast to essential trigeminal neuralgia, a sensory deficit occurs in or adjacent to the painful area, and the pain more commonly involves both sides of the body. Central neuralgia occurs in about 1 in 10 people following a stroke (Bowsher, 2001). Sensitivity to thermal pain decreases following thalamic strokes, and heat-pain thresholds are lower in patients with Parkinson's disease (Djaldetti et al., 2004). There is no doubt that central pain is a dreadful condition and notoriously refractory to treatment even with narcotics or anticonvulsants such as pregabalin (Gray, 2007).

Persistent idiopathic orofacial pain

Acute orofacial pain is usually from a toothache but conditions identified as persistent idiopathic orofacial pain (Table 3.1) are less localized or likely to respond favorably to dental treatment. Consequently, they are often attributed incorrectly to psychological disturbances (Lipton et al., 1993).

Burning mouth syndrome

A burning sensation in the mouth lasting at least 4–6 months without mucosal lesions or other clinical findings occurs occasionally between 50 and 70 years of age. This "burning mouth syndrome" (stomatodynia, stomatopyrosis) disturbs a small (1%–15%) proportion of the population, with women more commonly (sevenfold) affected than men (Ship et al., 1995). Typically, the pain involves the tip and anterior two-thirds of the tongue, but it can involve the lips, hard palate, and edentulous alveolar ridge. Pain levels can be intense with a typical crescendo pattern peaking in the evening, reduced when eating, and absent overnight. The onset is usually spontaneous without an obvious cause, although in one-third of cases it is associated with recent dental treatment, illness, or drug treatment. Xerostomia, dysgeusia, and decreased taste can accompany the pain, but it is unclear whether these are part of the primary condition.

Other conditions have been associated with the syndrome, notably oral mucositis, nutritional (e.g., vitamin B complex, zinc) deficiencies, anemia, diabetes, hormonal changes, Sjögren's syndrome, neuropsychiatric disorders, and antibiotic treatments (Ship et al., 1995). It has also been associated with Parkinson's disease (Clifford et al., 1998) and dopamine deficiency (Jääskeläinen et al., 2001).

There is some evidence that the burning sensation originates in the tongue because of abnormal sensory thresholds for heat (Grushka and Sessle, 1991) and taste (Grushka and Sessle, 1991; Eliav et al., 2007), and small-fiber sensory neuropathy in biopsy specimens from the tongue of people who complain of the burning sensation (Lauria et al., 2005).

Management of burning mouth syndrome
Patients with burning mouth syndrome can be managed successfully with a low dose of a tricyclic antidepressant (e.g., amitriptyline 10–75 mg) at bedtime, or 300–600 mg of an anticonvulsant (e.g., gabapentin) three times daily. Other pharmacological treatments have been suggested but with limited evidence, such as clonazepam 1 mg tid sucked for 3 min (Gremeau-Richard et al., 2004); or alphalipoic acid supplements 200 mg three times daily (Femiano and Scully, 2002).

Atypical odontalgia

Constant and moderately intense toothache localized initially to one or more teeth in the absence of pathoses (phantom tooth pain) is uncommon in elderly people. It tends to occur more in the upper posterior teeth of women between 40 and 50 years, and even in the teeth with endodontic treatment (Melis et al., 2003).

Management of atypical odontalgia
Unfortunately, this atypical pain is unresponsive to narcotics but tricyclic antidepressants can help. Overall, it is best to avoid unnecessary dental procedures.

Facial arthromyalgia

Complaints of sore jaw muscles are unusual in elderly people, although many of them have clinical signs of dysfunction, such as clicking jaw joints (MacEntee et al., 1987). Fortunately, people who are frail are rarely bothered by limitations in jaw movements or clicking joints. Temporomandibular pain in older people comes usually from chronic inflammation due to osteoarthritis, synovitis, rheumatoid arthritis, and giant cell arteritis, and from fibromyalgia, disk displacement, hyperkinetic disorders, and very rarely, from malignant or metastatic diseases. An intractable, persistent, and unilateral experience of pain in the temporal area that extends to the ear and jaw but unrelated to chewing is identified as hemicrania continua if there are autonomic features (e.g., conjunctival infection and tearing, nasal congestion and discharge, droopy swollen eyelid). These patients typically present under age 60. In other patients, this painful experience more insidiously can portend ipsilateral lung cancer.

Management of facial arthromyalgia

Treatment for pain associated with the temporomandibular region is cause-specific, relying primarily on behavioral therapy and physiotherapy supplemented by intraoral occlusal splints or prostheses (Fricton and Schiffman, 2008). Giant cell arteritis should be treated diligently before ischemic complications such as blindness and tongue necrosis occur. Otherwise, short-term medications, such as muscle relaxants, sedatives, nonsteroidal anti-inflammatory drugs (NSAIDs), opioids, and low-dose tricyclic antidepressants, offer limited success. Complete responsiveness to indomethacin is expected in hemicrania continua. Partial response may suggest a coexisting source of pain (e.g., temporomandibular joint disorder).

Atypical facial pain

This relatively rare group of serious and malignant conditions does not fit the description of typical orofacial neuralgias and occurs without obvious organic abnormalities. They produce moderate to severe chronic facial pain. Psychological factors increases the pain sensitivity and expressions associated with them, but they do not necessarily have a psychogenic or benign source. The pain is often dull and continuous, and poorly localized in the deep nonmuscular areas of the face, such as the zygoma. Unlike typical neuralgia, it does not follow a dermatomal distribution. It is a throbbing, boring, or nagging pain located unilaterally or bilaterally, worsened by stress or fatigue, and precipitated possibly by minor facial injuries. Essentially, atypical pain is a challenging diagnosis made largely by excluding other disorders (Madland and Feinmann, 2001).

Management of atypical facial pain

Chronic atypical facial pain does not respond to analgesics and anticonvulsants. Patient education, counseling, and antidepressants offer the best chance of success. Although antipsychotic drugs might be used as add-on therapy in refractory pain (Seidel et al., 2008), they are usually unsuitable for people who are frail.

MOVEMENT DISORDERS AND OROFACIAL PAIN

Oral movement disorders are either hyperkinetic (dystonia, dyskinesia, stereotypy, bruxism) or hypokinetic (parkinsonian) in nature, affecting the tongue, lips, and lower jaw, and are occasionally painful (Ford et al., 1994; Blanchet et al., 2008). A brief description is provided to promote early recognition and referral (Table 3.2). Dental management of oral movement disorders is often difficult in view of the prevailing knowledge gap and array of complications (Table 3.3) that can occur (Lobbezoo and Naeije, 2007).

Table 3.2 Movement disorders and orofacial pain.

Disorder	Definition	Manifestation of pain
Hyperkinetic		
Dystonia	Sustained muscle contractions producing lip retraction; tongue rolling and thrusting; jaw opening with deviation and spasms; jaw closure with trismus; jaw jerks	Myogenous Dental Atypical facial pain Tension-type headache Biting injury Temporomandibular pain
Dyskinesia	Aimless, repetitive, sometimes patterned, brief movements affecting the labial, lingual, and mandibular musculature (e.g., buccolinguomasticatory syndrome)	Aching Gum, lips, tongue, or jaw pain Burning mouth syndrome; biting or friction injuries Temporomandibular pain Central pain
Stereotypies	Repetitive, coordinated, patterned movements producing grimaces, lip movements, licking, biting, and chewing	Unusual gum/mucosal pain Temporomandibular pain
Bruxism	Teeth clenching and grinding	Dental Myogenous Tension-type headache Temporomandibular pain
Hypokinetic		
Parkinson	Akinesia with rigidity, resting (inferior lip, tongue, mandible) tremor, abnormal postural reflexes; voluntary oral movements of reduced amplitude and speed, dysphagia, drooling	Intraoral, face, jaw pain Burning mouth syndrome May be unilateral and fluctuating Muscle cramps Dystonic pain Central neuropathic pain Akathitic discomfort

Oromandibular dystonia

Dystonia is made of excessive prolonged muscle contractions causing twisting or jerky movements and spasms. Oromandibular dystonia is recognizable by sustained lip retraction and grimacing, tongue rolling and thrusting, jaw closure with trismus, jaw opening or lateral deviation, and jaw jerks, sometimes generating teeth clenching with grinding noise (bruxism). Sensory signals provided by holding something in the mouth (seed, gum, straw), or a local light touch, may reduce the spasms. This is called *geste antagoniste*. Pain may occur, but is generally not a prominent feature, and constant pain is atypical. Nonetheless, dystonia has been associated with painful muscle spasms, burning mouth syndrome, atypical

Table 3.3 Potential complications from oral dyskinesias (adapted from Lobbezoo and Naeije, 2007).

Dental
   Tooth wear
   Tooth and denture fractures
   Displacement/impaired retention of prostheses
Bone/joint/muscle
   Accelerated bone loss with edentulism
   Temporomandibular joint degeneration
   Mandibular luxation
   Masseter hypertrophy—square jaw
Pain
Functional impairment
   Speech
   Dysphagia
   Drooling
   Chewing difficulties
   Eating disorder/weight loss
Social embarrassment
   Isolation
   Depression

facial pain, and tension-type headache (Galvez-Jimenez et al., 2004). Oromandibular dystonia causes painful biting injuries and temporomandibular pain. The etiology of most adult-onset focal dystonia is unknown, but focal brain lesions and exposure to drugs that block central dopamine receptors (e.g., antipsychotics, antiemetics) are causative in some cases. Severe lingual dystonia suggests the presence of a secondary cause such as postanoxic encephalopathy and drug-induced dystonia (Schneider et al., 2006). Rare cases can develop after dental treatment.

Management of oromandibular dystonia
Jaw-closing dystonia that is lessened by an object between the teeth might benefit from a soft occlusal overlay that opens the vertical dimension of occlusion by a few millimeters, prevents tooth abrasion, and reduces stress on the temporomandibular joint (Frucht et al., 1999; Osborne et al., 1989). Intramuscular botulinum toxin is an excellent option (Tan and Jankovic, 1999; Møller et al., 2003), but reports of injections into the genioglossus muscle to control tongue movements are rare (Hennings et al., 2008).

Oral dyskinesia

Oral dyskinesia or "buccolinguomasticatory syndrome" is beset by aimless, irregular, repetitive, involuntary, and sometimes patterned movements affecting the labial, lingual, and mandibular musculature. It is precipitated commonly by a wide range of medications, particularly antipsychotics, antiparkinsonian medications (levodopa mainly), antidepressants, psycho-stimulants, anticonvulsants, and antihistaminics. However, it appears also in unmedicated people with cognitive disabilities such as Huntington's and Alzheimer's diseases (Mölsä et al., 1984).

Tardive dyskinesia may be a source of generalized aching and orofacial pain, particularly in elders with tardive akathisia—an unpleasant and occasionally unbearable sensation of restlessness (Ford et al., 1994). It is seen in about one-third of patients on long-term antipsychotic drugs (e.g., haloperidol), and can persist even after withdrawing the drug, particularly in elderly patients. As with burning mouth syndrome, the pain of tardive dyskinesia involves the gum, lips, tongue, and the jaw, and in severe manifestations there can be pain secondary to biting or denture trauma, clenching, or temporomandibular dysfunction but does occur without obvious oral lesions (Osborne et al., 1989).

Management of oral dyskinesia

Management strategies for drug-induced oral dyskinesia should focus on prevention. Early detection of vermicular (wormlike) tongue movements and "tardive pain" should be reported immediately to the treating physician who should gradually withdraw the offending drug whenever possible. Among nonpharmacological treatment strategies, the possible contribution of orodental factors should not be ignored since they worsen orofacial tardive dyskinesia ratings and are amenable to correction (Myers et al., 1993; Sutcher et al., 1998). Mandibular two-implant overdentures have not been evaluated in this context. The potential for adverse effects resulting from antidyskinetic drugs is greater in elders; however, disabling tardive dyskinesia may benefit from the brain monoamine depleter tetrabenazine (Ford et al., 1994; Ondo et al., 1999), the anticonvulsant levetiracetam (Woods et al., 2008), or the GABA-enhancing drug clonazepam (Bobruff et al., 1981). Botulinum toxin (Botox®, Allergan Inc., Irvine, CA; Xeomin®, Merz Pharmaceuticals GmbH, Frankfurt, Germany) is an increasingly popular option but with very limited good evidence on its tolerance by frail elders (Rapaport et al., 2000). Refractory cases might respond to bilateral deep brain stimulation of the internal globus pallidus of the basal ganglia (Damier et al., 2007). Long-standing oral dyskinesias produce premature wear and instability of dentures, and can damage the supporting mucosa and jaw bone.

Stereotypies

Oral stereotypies are characterized by repetitive, coordinated, and patterned movements with grimaces and lip movements, licking, biting, and chewing. They occur in a variety of neuropsychiatric conditions including schizophrenia, mental retardation, and Alzheimer's disease. They resemble the tics displayed in Gilles-de-la-Tourette syndrome, and have been observed as *"edentulous orodyskinesia"* in a small proportion of elderly edentulous people possibly because of defective dentures (Koller, 1983; Blanchet et al., 2008). Edentulous orodyskinesia, unlike tardive dyskinesia, has no extraoral or dystonic movements, nor does the tongue writhe or thrust at rest.

Management of stereotypies

Replacing, relining, and adjusting the dentures can be helpful. Implant-supported overdentures have been proposed with success in edentulous orodyskinesia (Payne and Carr, 1996). Pain treatment is generally not required for repetitive or ritualistic oral movements. Medications for moderate to severe tics in selected cases include tetrabenazine, clonazepam, clonidine, and botulinum toxin.

Bruxism

We do not know the cause of this parafunctional clenching or grinding teeth condition, which is associated frequently with muscle soreness and pain (Rompre et al., 2007; Lavigne et al., 2008). The prevalence of wakeful bruxism is about 20% in adults, while sleep bruxism declines with advancing age from 8% in adults to 3% in elderly populations. Wakeful bruxism is heterogeneous and may result from a habit, anxiety, or movement disorder (stereotypy, tic, oromandibular dystonia, drug-induced dyskinesia). Originally occlusal or orofacial structural discrepancies were blamed for sleep bruxism, but now we believe that they play only minor roles, if any, compared with other autonomic nervous system or behavioral influences such as anxiety and stress (Kato et al., 2003). It appears to be modulated centrally by various neurotransmitters, which probably explains the link to smoking, alcohol, caffeine, and drugs, such as amphetamines, antipsychotics, antidepressants, and antiparkinsonian medications.

Management of bruxism

The approach and treatment response of wakeful bruxism depend on the underlying cause. Botulinum toxin is an increasingly popular option, but with very limited good evidence on its toleration by frail elders. In sleep bruxism, there is scant evidence to support one management strategy over another; however, offending drugs should be removed if at all possible, while lifestyle instructions and education might help to reduce alcohol, tobacco, and caffeine intake, and enhance relaxation techniques (Lavigne et al., 2005). Occlusal overlays might help some patients, but the value of this strategy is unclear in any age group (van der Zaag et al., 2005). Clonazepam has benefited sleep bruxism (Saletu et al., 2005), but the long-term toleration of this drug by elders, especially if they are frail, needs careful assessment.

Parkinson's disease

Parkinson's disease is the second most common neurodegenerative disorder in humans after Alzheimer's disease, affecting 1%–2% of the population over age 50 years. It results from cell loss in the nervous system, affecting noticeably the dopaminergic neurons. Its motor features include akinesia (paucity of movement), bradykinesia (slowness of movement), rigidity, and postural instability, often associated with a resting tremor. These deficits disturb and slow oromandibular movements, which impair speech, chewing, and swallowing. Dysphagia, with silent or symptomatic aspirations, is a particular worry in advanced disease. Other sensory, autonomic, and cognitive manifestations, as well as anxiety and depression, are frequent. Moreover, the levodopa replacement therapy used routinely to restore in part dopamine neurotransmission, induces dyskinesia resembling tardive dyskinesia in at least two-thirds of treated patients. The disease lowers pain thresholds (Djaldetti et al., 2004; Mylius et al., 2009), which are restored with levodopa replacement (Gerdelat-Mas et al., 2007).

Pain is a common feature of Parkinson's disease, which can be of dystonic or central neuropathic origin. A sense of burning or throbbing pain in the gums, teeth, tongue, inner cheek, face, and jaw is experienced occasionally (Ford et al., 1996; Clifford et al., 1998). However, unlike burning mouth syndrome, the sensations are often confined to one side of the mouth. Oral pain fluctuates with periods of low levodopa (Goetz et al., 1986).

Management of Parkinson's disease

An oral examination is needed to rule out other sources of pain, but invasive dental interventions are best avoided if Parkinson's disease is suspected. Antiparkinsonian drug therapy does not necessarily abolish oral pain, but strategies to smooth out fluctuations in performance during the day, and careful use of low-dose dopamine receptor agonists (*dopaminomimetics*), can help.

CONCLUSION

The physiological, pathological, pharmacological, emotional, and social characteristics of aging and frailty increase the risk of chronic orofacial pain. Idiopathic or secondary hyperkinetic and hypokinetic disorders of the mouth are underrecognized sources of peripheral and central pain. Medications that directly or indirectly modulate dopamine neurotransmission and acquired disorders of the nervous system can alter the processing and expression of this pain. Detection and management of orofacial pain in patients with severe dementia rely on clinical examinations and information from other health professionals and family members. Nonverbal behaviors that are abnormal help detect and manage painful conditions.

Chronic nonneuralgic orofacial pain is heterogeneous, multifactorial, often drug resistant, and managed ideally by a multidisciplinary team. In general, invasive, irreversible occlusal and surgical interventions are inappropriate. However, obvious dental and prosthodontic disorders, such as faulty dentures or broken teeth, should be adjusted and repaired to provide stable occlusal contacts to limit the damage from movement disorders of the jaws.

CLINICAL SCENARIO CONTINUED

Continuation of the clinical scenario

Mrs. G., upon her physician's advice, consults you about her mouth pain and the "tardive dyskinesia" diagnosed by her psychiatrist. She seems in good general condition but she mentions that she has been aware of excessive "mouthing movements" for the last 7 years. She explains further that her dyskinesia started shortly after she acquired new dentures, which never felt comfortable, secure, or "balanced." She revisited the clinician who made the dentures but he was unable to improve them and concluded that her mouth was too difficult for dentures because of her age. Consequently, she became resigned to her dental problem and wore the dentures only when mixing socially.

On examination, you notice that her pain and dyskinetic movements are triggered when she wears the dentures, and they cease when she removes them. She does not display the tongue movements when opening her mouth that are typical of drug-induced dyskinesia.

You diagnose denture-related dyskinesia with secondary frictional mucosal irritation. Subsequently, her pain and dyskinesia disappear when you make new dentures for her that are occlusally stable bilaterally and retained securely without discomfort.

REFERENCES

Blanchet PJ, Popovici R, Guitard F, Rompre PH, Lamarche C, and Lavigne GJ. 2008. Pain and denture condition in edentulous orodyskinesia: Comparisons with tardive dyskinesia and control subjects. *Mov Disord* 23:1837–42.

Bobruff A, Gardos G, Tarsy D, Rapkin RM, Cole JO, and Moore P. 1981. Clonazepam and phenobarbital in tardive dyskinesia. *Am J Psychiatry* 138:189–93.

Bowsher D. 2001. Stroke and central poststroke pain in an elderly population. *J Pain* 2:258–61.

Brondani MA, Bryant SR, and MacEntee MI. 2007. Elders assessment of an evolving model of oral health. *Gerodontology* 24:189–95.

Brunsvold MA, Nair P, and Oates TW Jr. 1999. Chief complaints of patients seeking treatment for periodontitis. *J Am Dent Assoc* 130:359–64.

Choo PW, Galil K, Donahue JG, Walker AM, Spiegelman D, and Platt R. 1997. Risk factors for postherpetic neuralgia. *Arch Intern Med* 157:1217–24.

Clifford TJ, Warsi MJ, Burnett CA, and Lamey PJ. 1998. Burning mouth in Parkinson's disease sufferers. *Gerodontology* 15:73–8.

Cole LJ, Far1rell MJ, Gibson SJ, and Egan GF. 2010. Age-related differences in pain sensitivity and regional brain activity evoked by noxious pressure. *Neurobiol Aging* 31(3):494–503.

Damier P, Thobois S, Witjas T, Cuny E, Derost P, Raoul S, Mertens P, Peragut JC, Lemaire JJ, Burbaud P, Nguyen JM, Llorca PM, Rascol O, and French Stimulation for Tardive Dyskinesia (STARDYS) Study Group. 2007. Bilateral deep brain stimulation of the globus pallidus to treat tardive dyskinesia. *Arch Gen Psychiatry* 64:170–6.

De Simone R, Ranieri A, Bilo L, Fiorillo C, and Bonavita V. 2008. Cranial neuralgias: from physiopathology to pharmacological treatment. *Neurol Sci* 29:S69–78.

Djaldetti R, Shifrin A, Rogowski Z, Specher E, Melamed E, and Yarnitsky D. 2004. Quantitative measurement of pain sensation in patients with Parkinson's disease. *Neurology* 62:2171–5.

Donahue JG, Choo PW, Manson JE, and Platt R. 1995. The incidence of herpes zoster. *Arch Intern Med* 155:1605–9.

Eliav E, Kamran B, Schaham R, Czerninski R, Gracely RH, and Benoliel R. 2007. Evidence of chorda tympani dysfunction in patients with burning mouth syndrome. *J Am Dent Assoc* 138:628–33.

Ettinger RL. 2000. Dental management of patients with Alzheimer's disease and other dementias. *Gerodontology* 17:8–16.

Femiano F and Scully C. 2002. Burning mouth syndrome (BMS): Double blind controlled study of alpha-lipoic acid (thioctic acid) therapy. *J Oral Pathol Med* 31:267–9.

Ford B, Greene P, and Fahn S. 1994. Oral and genital tardive pain syndromes. *Neurology* 44:2115–9.

Ford B, Louis ED, Greene P, and Fahn S. 1996. Oral and genital pain syndromes in Parkinson's disease. *Mov Disord* 11:421–6.

Fricton JR and Schiffman EL. 2008. Management of masticatory myalgia and arthralgia. In: Sessle BJ, Lavigne GJ, Lund JP, and Dubner R (eds.), *Orofacial Pain: From Basic Science to Clinical Management*, 2nd edn. Hanover Park, IL: Quintessence Publishing Co., pp. 179–85.

Frucht S, Fahn S, Ford B, and Gelb M. 1999. A geste antagoniste device to treat jaw-closing dystonia. *Mov Disord* 14:883–6.

Gagliese L. 2007. What do experimental pain models tell us about ageing and clinical pain? [Comment]. *Pain Med* 8:475–7.

Galvez-Jimenez N, Lampuri C, Patino-Picirrillo R, Hargreave MJA, and Hanson MR. 2004. Dystonia and headaches: Clinical features and response to botulinum toxin therapy. In: Fahn S, Hallett M, and DeLong MR (eds.), *Dystonia 4: Advances in Neurology*, vol. 94. Philadelphia: Lippincott Williams & Wilkins, pp. 321–8.

Gerdelat-Mas A, Simonetta-Moreau M, Thalamas C, Ory-Magne F, Slaoui T, Rascol O, and Brefel-Courbon C. 2007. Levodopa raises objective pain threshold in Parkinson's disease: A RIII reflex study. *J Neurol Neurosurg Psychiatry* 78:1140–2.

Goetz CG, Tanner CM, Levy M, Wilson RS, and Garron DC. 1986. Pain in Parkinson's disease. *Mov Disord* 1:45–9.

Gray P. 2007. Pregabalin in the management of central neuropathic pain. *Expert Opin Pharmacother* 8:3035–41.

Gremeau-Richard C, Woda A, Navez ML, Attal N, Bouhassira D, Gagnieu MC, Laluque JF, Picard P, Pionchon P, and Tubert S. 2004. Topical clonazepam in stomatodynia: A randomised placebo-controlled study. *Pain* 108:51–7.

Grushka M and Sessle BJ. 1991. Burning mouth syndrome. *Dent Clin North Am* 35:171–84.

Hadjistavropoulos T, Herr K, Turk DC, Fine PG, Dworkin RH, Helme R, Jackson K, Parmelee PA, Rudy TE, Beattie LB, Chibnall JT, Craig KD, Ferrell B, Ferrell B, Fillingim RB, Gagliese L, Gallagher R, Gibson SJ, Harrison EL, Katz B, Keefe FJ, Lieber SJ, Lussier D, Schmader KE, Tait RC, Weiner DK, and Williams J. 2007. An interdisciplinary expert consensus statement on assessment of pain in older persons. *Clin J Pain* 23(Suppl.):S1–43.

Hadjistavropoulos T, Voyer P, Sharpe D, Verreault R, and Aubin M. 2008. Assessing pain in dementia patients with comorbid delirium and/or depression. *Pain Manag Nurs* 9:48–54.

Hennings JM, Krause E, Bötzel K, and Wetter TC. 2008. Successful treatment of tardive lingual dystonia with botulinum toxin: Case report and review of the literature. *Prog Neuropsychopharmacol Biol Psychiatry* 32:1167–71.

Ishikawa H, Ezure H, Goto N, Kamiyama A, and Yanai T. 2005. Morphometric difference in the human maxillary nerve fibers between dentulous and edentulous jaw subjects. *Okajimas Folia Anat Jpn* 81:129–34.

Iwata K, Tsuboi Y, Shima A, Harada T, Ren K, Kanda K, and Kitagawa J. 2004. Central neuronal changes after nerve injury: Neuroplastic influences of injury and aging. *J Orofac Pain* 18:293–8.

Jääskeläinen SK, Rinne JO, Forssell H, Tenovuo O, Kaasinen V, Sonninen P, and Bergman J. 2001. Role of the dopaminergic system in chronic pain—A fluorodopa-PET study. *Pain* 90:257–60.

Jainkittivong A, Aneksuk V, and Langlais RP. 2002. Oral mucosal conditions in elderly dental patients. *Oral Dis* 8:218–23.

Karp JF, Shega JW, Morone NE, and Weiner DK. 2008. Advances in understanding the mechanisms and management of persistent pain in older adults. *Br J Anaesth* 101:111–20.

Kato T, Montplaisir JY, Guitard F, Sessle BJ, Lund JP, and Lavigne GJ. 2003. Evidence that experimentally induced sleep bruxism is a consequence of transient arousal. *J Dent Res* 82:284–8.

Koller WC. 1983. Edentulous orodyskinesia. *Ann Neurol* 13:97–9.

Lauria G, Majorana A, Borgna M, Lombardi R, Penza P, Padovani A, and Sapelli P. 2005. Trigeminal small-fiber sensory neuropathy causes burning mouth syndrome. *Pain* 115:332–7.

Lavigne GJ, Manzini C, and Kato T. 2005. Sleep bruxism. In: Kryger M, Roth T, and Dement WC (eds.), *Principles and Practice of Sleep Medicine.* Philadelphia: Elsevier Saunders, pp. 946–59.

Lavigne GJ, Khoury S, Abe S, Yamaguchi T, and Raphael K. 2008. Bruxism physiology and pathology: An overview for clinicians. *J Oral Rehab* 35:476–94.

Lipton JA, Ship JA, and Larach-Robinson D. 1993. Estimated prevalence and distribution of reported orofacial pain in the United States. *J Am Dent Assoc* 124:115–21.

Lobbezoo F and Naeije M. 2007. Dental implications of some common movement disorders: A concise review. *Arch Oral Biol* 52:395–8.

MacEntee MI, Weiss R, Morrison BJ, and Waxler-Morrison NE. 1987. Mandibular dysfunction in an institutionalized and predominantly elderly population. *J Oral Rehabil* 14:523–9.

Madland G and Feinmann C. 2001. Chronic facial pain: A multidisciplinary problem. *J Neurol Neurosurg Psychiatry* 71:716–9.

Melis M, Lobo S, Ceneviz C, Zawawi K, Al-Badawi E, Maloney G, and Mehta N. 2003. Atypical odontalgia: A review of the literature. *Headache* 43:1060–74.

Møller E, Werdelin LM, Gilbert M, Dalager T, Prytz S, and Regeur L. 2003. Treatment of perioral dystonia with botulinum toxin in 4 cases of Meige's syndrome. *Oral Surg Oral Med Oral Pathol Oral Radiol Endod* 96(5):544–9.

Mölsä PK, Marttila RJ, and Rinne UK. 1984. Extrapyramidal signs in Alzheimer's disease. *Neurology (Cleveland)* 34:1114–16.

Morrison RS, Magaziner J, Gilbert M, Koval KJ, McLaughlin MA, Orosz G, Strauss E, and Siu AL. 2003. Relationship between pain and opioid analgesics on the development of delirium following hip fracture. *J Gerontol* 58:76–81.

Moulin DE, Clark AJ, Gilron I, Ware MA, Watson CP, Sessle BJ, Coderre T, Morley-Forster PK, Stinson J, Boulanger A, Peng P, Finley GA, Taenzer P, Squire P, Dion D, Cholkan A, Gilani A, Gordon A, Henry J, Jovey R, Lynch M, Mailis-Gagnon A, Panju A, Rollman GB, Velly A, and Canadian Pain Society. 2007. Pharmacological management of chronic neuropathic pain-consensus statement and guidelines from the Canadian Pain Society. *Pain Res Manag* 12:13–21.

Myers DE, Schooler NR, Zullo TG, and Levin H. 1993. A retrospective study of the effects of edentulism on the severity rating of tardive dyskinesia. *J Prosthet Dent* 69:578–81.

Mylius V, Engau I, Teepker M, Stiasny-Kolster K, Schepelmann K, Oertel WH, Lautenbacher S, and Moller JC. 2009. Pain sensitivity and descending inhibition of pain in Parkinson's disease. *J Neurol Neurosurg Psychiatry* 80:24–8.

Nitschke I and Müller F. 2004. The impact of oral health on the quality of life in the elderly. *Oral Health Prev Dent* 2(Suppl. 1):271–5.

Nonaka N, Goto N, Ezure H, Goto J, and Yamamoto T. 2001. The mandibular nerve in edentulous jaw humans: Analysis of myelinated nerve fibers. *Okajimas Folia Anat Jpn* 78:141–3.

Ondo WG, Hanna PA, and Jankovic J. 1999. Tetrabenazine treatment for tardive dyskinesia: Assessment by randomized videotape protocol. *Am J Psychiatry* 156:1279–81.

Osborne TE, Grace EG, and Schwartz MK. 1989. Severe degenerative changes of the temporomandibular joint secondary to the effects of tardive dyskinesia: A literature review and case report. *J Craniomandibular Pract* 7:58–62.

Oxman MN, Levin MJ, and the Shingles Prevention Study Group. 2008. Vaccination against herpes zoster and postherpetic neuralgia. *J Infect Dis* 197(Suppl. 2):S228–36.

Pautex S, Michon A, Guedira M, Emond H, Le Lous P, Samaras D, Michel JP, Herrmann F, Giannakopoulos P, and Gold G. 2006. Pain in severe dementia: Self-assessment or observational scales? *J Am Geriatr Soc* 54:1040–5.

Payne AGT and Carr L. 1996. Can edentulous patients with orofacial dyskinesia be treated successfully with implants? A case report. *J Dent Assoc S Afr* 51:67–70.

Ranoux D, Attal N, Morain F, and Bouhassira D. 2008. Botulinum toxin type A induces direct analgesic effects in chronic neuropathic pain. *Ann Neurol* 64:274–84.

Rapaport A, Sadeh M, Stein D, Levine J, Sirota P, Mosheva T, Stir S. Elitzur A, Reznik I, Geva D, and Rabey JM. 2000. Botulinum toxin for the treatment of oro-facial-lingual-masticatory tardive dyskinesia. *Mov Disord* 15:352–5.

Rappaport ZH, Govrin-Lippmann R, and Devor M. 1997. An electron-microscopic analysis of biopsy samples of the trigeminal root taken during microvascular decompressive surgery. *Stereotact Funct Neurosurg* 68:182–6.

Rasmussen PR. 1965. *Facial Pain*. Copenhagen: Munksgard.

Riley JL, Gilbert GH, and Heft MW. 1998. Orofacial pain symptom prevalence: Selective sex differences in the elderly? *Pain* 76:97–104.

Rompre PH, Daigle-Landry D, Guitard F, Montplaisir JY, and Lavigne GJ. 2007. Identification of a sleep bruxism subgroup with a higher risk of pain. *J Dent Res* 86:837–42.

Saletu A, Parapatics S, Saletu B, Anderer P, Prause W, Putz H, Adelbauer J, and Saletu-Zyhlarz GM. 2005. On the pharmacotherapy of sleep bruxism: Placebo-controlled polysomnographic and psychometric studies with clonazepam. *Neuropsychobiology* 51:214–25.

Schmader KE. 2002. Epidemiology and impact on quality of life of postherpetic neuralgia and painful diabetic neuropathy. *Clin J Pain* 18:350–6.

Schneider SA, Aggarwal A, Bhatt M, Dupont E, Tisch S, Limousin P, Lee P. Quinn N, and Bhatia KP. 2006. Severe tongue protrusion dystonia: Clinical syndromes and possible treatment. *Neurology* 67:940–3.

Schwaiger J, Kiechl S, Seppi K, Sawires M, Stockner H, Erlacher T, Mairhofer ML, Niederkofler H, Rungger G, Gasperi A, Poewe W, and Willeit J. 2009. Prevalence of primary headaches and cranial neuralgias in men and women aged 55–94 years (Bruneck Study). *Cephalalgia* 29:179–87.

Seidel S, Aigner M, Ossege M, Pernicka E, Wildner B, and Sycha T. 2008. Antipsychotics for acute and chronic pain in adults. *Cochrane Database Syst Rev* 4:CD004844.

Sekula RF Jr, Marchan RM, Fletcher LH, Casey KF, and Jannetta PJ. 2008. Microvascular decompression for trigeminal neuralgia in elderly patients. *J Neurosurg* 108:689–91.

Ship JA, Grushka M, Lipton JA, Mott AE, Sessle BJ, and Dionne RA. 1995. Burning mouth syndrome: an update. *J Am Dent Assoc* 126:842–53.

Silverman S Jr. 2007. Mucosal lesions in older adults. *J Am Dent Assoc* 138(Suppl. 9):41S–46S.

Stankus SJ, Dlugopolski M, and Packer D. 2000. Management of herpes zoster (shingles) and postherpetic neuralgia. *Am Fam Physician* 61:2437–8.

Sutcher H, Soderstrom J, Perry R, and Das A. 1998. Tardive dyskinesia: Dental prosthetic therapy. *Panminerva Med* 40:154–6.

Tan EK and Jankovic J. 1999. Botulinum toxin A in patients with oromandibular dystonia: Long-term follow-up. *Neurology* 53:2102–7.

Tyring SK. 2007. Management of herpes zoster and postherpetic neuralgia. *J Am Acad Dermatol* 57(Suppl. 6):S136–42.

van der Zaag J, Lobbezoo F, Wicks DJ, Visscher CM, Hamburger HL, and Naeije M. 2005. Controlled assessment of the efficacy of occlusal stabilization splints on sleep bruxism. *J Orofac Pain* 19:151–8.

Vickers ER and Boocock H. 2005. Chronic orofacial pain is associated with psychological morbidity and negative personality changes: a comparison to the general population. *Aust Dent J* 50:21–30.

Woda A and Salter MW. 2008. Mechanisms of neuropathic pain. In: Sessle BJ, Lavigne GJ, Lund JP, and Dubner R (eds.), *Orofacial Pain: From Basic Science to Clinical Management*, 2nd edn. Hanover Park, IL: Quintessence Publishing Co., pp. 53–9.

Woda A, Tubert-Jeannin S, Bouhassira D, Attal N, Fleiter B, Goulet J-P, Gremeau-Richard C, Navez ML, Picard P, Pionchon P, and Albuisson E. 2005. Towards a new taxonomy of idiopathic orofacial pain. *Pain* 116:396–406.

Woods SW, Saksa JR, Baker CB, Cohen SJ, and Tek C. 2008. Effects of levetiracetam on tardive dyskinesia: a randomized, double-blind, placebo-controlled study. *J Clin Psychiatry* 69:546–54.

Zuniga C, Diaz S, Piedimonte F, and Micheli F. 2008. Beneficial effects of botulinum toxin type A in trigeminal neuralgia. *Arq Neuropsiquiatr* 66:500–3.

Dry mouth and medications

W. Murray Thomson, Kazunori Ikebe, June M. Tordoff, and A. John Campbell

INTRODUCTION

On first consideration, saliva is a distinctly "uncool" fluid. As Mandel (1990) so eloquently pointed out, "saliva is not one of the popular bodily fluids. It lacks the drama of blood, the sincerity of sweat and the emotional appeal of tears." However, as with so many other essentials, it is only when we do not have enough of it that we appreciate what it is that we have lost. In this chapter, we take the reader through an overview of the salivary system and the role of saliva before describing the measurement, occurrence, and consequences of dry mouth. Finally, we examine the practical aspects of dry mouth and its management in residential care facilities.

SALIVARY GLANDS

The salivary system is composed of a number of tubuloalveolar exocrine glands that secrete their products into ducts. There are two main types: three bilateral *major* salivary glands and numerous *minor* salivary glands. The three *major* salivary glands are the parotid, submandibular, and sublingual glands.

The parotid gland, which is the largest, is situated in front of the ear and behind the mandibular ramus. The parotid or Stenson's duct produces serous secretions opposite the upper second molar tooth. The submandibular gland produces a mixture of mucous and serous secretions under the body of the mandible with its duct (Wharton's duct) running across

Oral Healthcare and the Frail Elder: A Clinical Perspective.
Edited by Michael I. MacEntee © 2011 Blackwell Publishing Ltd.

the floor of the mouth to open beneath the anterior part of the tongue. The sublingual gland, which is the smallest of the three major glands, produces mostly mucous secretions from small ducts (Bartholin's ducts) on the floor of the mouth beneath the tongue (Whelton, 2004).

The minor salivary glands are located in the buccal and labial mucosa, the posterior palate, and the lateral border of the tongue to lubricate the mouth primarily with mucous secretions.

Unstimulated saliva is hypotonic; it becomes isotonic when secreted initially, but it becomes hypotonic as it flows through the ducts (Figure 4.1) (Aps and Martens, 2005).

At rest, about 60% of salivary flow comes from the submandibular gland, 25% from the parotid gland, 7%–8% from the sublingual gland, and another 7%–8% from the minor glands. When salivary flow is stimulated, the contribution of the parotid can rise to about 50%.

A key to understanding dry mouth is to understand the innervation of the salivary glands and the physiology of salivary flow. The autonomic nervous system plays an important role, and the glands have both sympathetic and parasympathetic nerve supplies. Salivation is mainly under parasympathetic control from the salivary nuclei situated in the pons and the medulla of the brainstem. However, sympathetic stimulation also causes salivation via adrenergic stimulation, but with characteristics different from saliva obtained from parasympathetic (cholinergic) stimulation. β-Adrenergic stimulation produces low volumes of highly viscous saliva with very high concentration of mucin, whereas α-adrenergic stimulation also produces low volumes of highly viscous saliva but with low concentration of mucin. Cholinergic stimulation results in a high volume of saliva with low concentrations of protein and mucin, so that it is not viscous (Aps and Martens, 2005). In theory, sustained β-adrenergic stimulation by β-adrenergic agonists such as bronchodilators used in asthma could lead to relatively small amounts of viscous saliva, which would dry

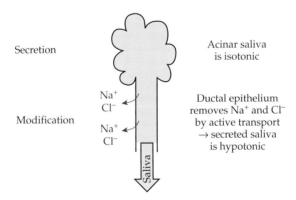

Figure 4.1   Modification of glandular secretions in transit through the glandular ducts.

the mouth even if the quantity or volume of saliva is undisturbed. Drugs with an anticholinergic effect can reduce the flow of saliva, especially after chronic exposure. The concept of "overall anticholinergic burden" (Chew et al., 2008), although unproven empirically, is useful, whereby the greater the dose of anticholinergic drug, the greater the likelihood and severity of a dry mouth in patients medicated for disorders of the gastrointestinal, genitourinary, or respiration, or for Parkinson's disease or bradycardia.

Basic mechanical (touch) and chemical (taste) stimuli in the mouth also excite the salivary nuclei, as do higher-level stimulation and inhibition (Edgar et al., 2004), which is why anxiety can cause the mouth to feel dry, and thinking about good food can increase salivation.

THE ROLE OF SALIVA IN HEALTH AND DISEASE

Dentists are becoming more aware of the importance of saliva as they treat older patients who have medical problems and various medications that can dry the mouth as a side effect.

The complexity of saliva is best appreciated through its many functions in the oral and gastrointestinal environment (Table 4.1). It is essential for the preservation of a healthy oropharynx (Whelton, 2004). It helps swallowing, oral cleansing, speech, digestion, and taste (Turner and Ship, 2007). We can eat without saliva, but mealtimes may be difficult, uncomfortable, and embarrassing (Mandel, 1987). Saliva is stimulated reflexively by smell,

Table 4.1   Functions of saliva (adapted from Whelton, 2004).

Function	Description
Lubrication	A protective coating on intraoral surfaces enables them to move together smoothly.
Cleansing	Moistening helps to move food around the mouth and ease swallowing.
Ionic reserve	Saturation with calcium and phosphate ions helps to remineralize teeth.
Buffering	Ionic concentration helps to neutralize the pH of the dental biofilm after eating.
Microbial control	Antimicrobial activity with IgA and lysozyme, for example, help control infections.
Agglutination	Agglutinins such as mucins and glycoproteins aggregate and help clear oral bacteria.
Pellicle formation	Proteins form a protective barrier on teeth.
Digestion	Enzymes such as α-amylase digest starches.
Gustation	Solvent action helps taste buds to function.
Hydration	Oral dehydration triggers the urge to drink and promotes a reduction in urine output from the kidneys.

taste, and mastication as it prepares and coalesces food into a bolus for digestion and swallowing (Turner and Ship, 2007). The high water content of the parotid secretions moistens the food, while mucins from the submandibular, sublingual, and minor glands facilitate ingestion (Table 4.1).

Saliva solubilizes many components of food and serves as a medium for the components to interact with receptors on taste cells (Mandel, 1987). It stimulates gustatory receptors on taste buds and delivers substances ("tastants") that stimulate the sense of taste at the receptors (Turner and Ship, 2007). Therefore, reduced flow of saliva can distort the sensation of taste (dysgeusia). No specific constituent of saliva has been connected directly to dysgeusia, although specific electrolytes and minerals are necessary for a normal sensation of taste (Ship, 2004; Mese and Matsuo, 2007; Yoshinaka et al., 2007).

The mix of salivary constituents protects the soft and hard tissues of the mouth against mechanical, thermal, and chemical irritants (Mandel, 1987; Whelton, 2004), whereas the stimulated flow of saliva plays an important lubricating role when chewing with complete dentures (Ikebe et al., 2007). Swallowing occurs in oral, pharyngeal, and esophageal stages, and each stage requires lubrication of the mucosal tissues to ensure a safe and efficient swallow. Low salivary flow, in contrast, is associated with dysphagia, which can lead to aspiration pneumonia from gram-negative anaerobes that originated in the mouth (Loesche et al., 1995).

Salivary lubrication is attributed to strong layers of mucin glycoproteins that, together with proteases, protect the mucosa from drying and from penetration or ulceration by particles of sharp food, or even by infiltration by carcinogens. Epidermal growth factors in submandibular saliva help damaged mucosa to repair by reducing clotting time and accelerating contraction of the wound. Saliva contributes to lavage and debridement of wounds by reducing the aggregation and adherence of pathogens, and by direct antibacterial, antifungal, and antiviral activity (Mandel, 1987). The physical flow of saliva stimulated by muscular activity around the mouth, along with the secretory IgA system, interferes with the adherence of bacteria to teeth, mucosa, and dentures, while mucins and proteins (lysozyme, lactoferrin, and lactoperoxidase) can kill or disable bacteria (Tabak et al., 1982).

Salivary bicarbonate maintains a neutral pH in the mouth, neutralizes acidity from esophageal reflux, and regulates the pH of the biofilm on teeth. Other constituents, such as fluoride ions, increase the enamel's resistance to caries.

Cariogenic microorganisms colonize teeth rapidly without saliva to regulate pH and control bacteria (Turner and Ship, 2007). A persistently low flow of salivary after eating and drinking refined carbohydrates promotes the carious demineralization of dental enamel and dentin.

Chronically reduced salivary output can lead to painful mucositis and candidiasis from *Candida albicans* and other fungi (Ship, 2004). The fungi present usually as pseudomembranous erythema that frequently extends extraorally at the corners of the mouth as "angular cheilitis" and occasionally produce a burning sensation of the tongue or other parts of the mouth. Oral candidiasis is opportunistic and can worsen with a weakened immune system.

WHAT IS DRY MOUTH?

The term "dry mouth" is a catchall phrase encompassing either or both the sensation of a dry mouth and the situation where the output of saliva is low (Cassolato and Turnbull, 2003). In this chapter, we are concerned with *chronic* dry mouth typically lasting 3 months or more (Last, 2001) rather than the more acute, transient condition associated with dehydration or fear.

DRY MOUTH AND QUALITY OF LIFE

A dry mouth can seriously affect quality of life in any age group through any or all of its consequences (Table 4.2). It is particularly difficult, for example, for people with salivary gland hypofunction (SGH) to eat dry food, such as biscuits or crackers, without liquids to help swallow the food. Taste disturbances are common when saliva is abnormal; consequently, patients with chronic SGH secondary to Sjögren's syndrome or head and neck radiotherapy, for example, experience abnormal sensations of taste or gustation (Turner and Ship, 2007).

Dry mouth has two possible manifestations, which makes it particularly difficult to define and diagnose (Table 4.2). Xerostomia is the subjective feeling of a dry mouth, assessed only by directly questioning the patient (Fox et al., 1987), whereas SGH refers directly to abnormally low salivary flow when measured by sialometry (Navazesh, 1993). Moreover, the subjectivity of one rarely coincides with the measurement of the other, which complicates clinical assessments considerably (Thomson et al., 1999a). Different medications are associated with the two aspects; however, there is much that we do not understand about the effect of saliva on the sensation of a dry mouth, and this lack of concordance could be due partly to differences in the quality of saliva.

A dry mouth also contributes to halitosis, a burning sensation around the mouth and tongue, and an intolerance to acidic and spicy foods (Atkinson and Wu, 1994); such effects compromise nutritional status and quality of life. People with xerostomia, for example, tend to avoid crunchy or dry foods (such as vegetables or bread) and sticky foods (such as peanut butter) (Loesche et al., 1995), while denture-wearers without saliva are likely to have loose dentures due to inadequate peripheral seal, and sores from abrasive movements of the dentures on the mucosa.

Similarly, speech and eating difficulties from a dry mouth can impair social interactions and engagements (Ship et al., 2002). However, this

Table 4.2 Consequences of xerostomia and salivary gland hypofunction.

Consequences	Xerostomia[a]	Salivary gland hypofunction[b]
Dry mouth	x	x
Dysphagia	x	x
Denture problems	x	x
Caries	x	x
Dysgeusia	x	x
Speech difficulties	x	
Nocturnal oral discomfort	x	
Oropharyngeal infections	x	x
Oropharyngeal burning	x	
Mucus accumulation	x	x
Food retention in the mouth	x	
Plaque accumulation	x	
Altered oral microflora	x	x
Mucosal changes	x	
Thirst	x	
Oral dysfunction	x	
Sleeping difficulties		x
Traumatic oral lesions		x
Oropharyngeal candidosis		x
Mucositis		x
Problems chewing		x
Gingivitis		x
Halitosis		x
Dry lips		x

[a] Adapted from Turner and Ship (2007).
[b] Adapted from Gupta et al. (2006).

severe response is more common in patients who have undergone radio-therapy for head and neck cancer (Hamlet et al., 1997; Logemann et al., 2003; Dirix et al., 2006). Nearly all patients, several months after radiation therapy, will complain of a dry mouth, and many will have oral pain, a disturbed sense of taste, and difficulty chewing, swallowing, and speaking, while those with natural teeth will be at high risk of caries, and denture-wearers will feel that their dentures are loose and very uncomfortable (Epstein et al., 1999). Overall, they will feel that the mouth dryness inter-feres badly with their daily activities and quality of life (Ikebe et al., 2007).

MEASURING DRY MOUTH

SGH pertains to salivary flow rate relative to a threshold value, whereas xerostomia relates to how people feel.

Measuring salivary flow rate

Valid and reliable measurements of salivary flow rate are challenging. The two parameters of measurement are unstimulated and stimulated salivary flow (Figure 4.2).

If both are measured in a single session, the unstimulated flow is recorded first because, when you stimulate flow, you cannot readily return to the unstimulated state for a long while. The highest unstimulated salivary flow rates occur in the late afternoon, and the lowest rate during the night (Dawes, 1972). Thus, measures of the stability of a patient's salivary flow over time should be repeated at approximately the same time of day.

Flow from individual glands (or pairs of glands) is measured by "cannulating" each gland, whereas total salivary flow is measured more easily by collecting "whole saliva" as it pools in the floor of the mouth. However, whole saliva is more relevant clinically because SGH is usually a multi-glandular condition (Sreebny and Broich, 1987) and it offers practical relevance to dental demineralization and caries (Navazesh and Christensen, 1982). There appears to be little or no clinical justification for collecting anything other than whole saliva.

Unstimulated flow can be measured only with whole saliva because it is impossible to cannulate a salivary duct without stimulating flow. The four methods for measuring unstimulated salivary flow are termed (somewhat prosaically) the "drain," the "spit," the "suction," or the "swab" (Navazesh and Christensen, 1982). The "drain" allows saliva to drain passively out of the mouth into a receptacle for a specified time (usually 3 min). The "spit" requires the patient to collect saliva in the mouth for a specified period and then spit it into a receptacle. The "suction" uses a tube to suck saliva from the floor of the patient's mouth, whereas the "swab" uses preweighed swabs, such as dental cotton rolls, on the floor of the mouth to collect saliva for a specified time, after which the rolls are weighed again to measure the quantity of saliva collected. Neither the "suction" nor the

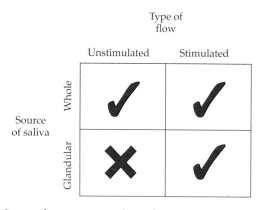

Figure 4.2 Options for measuring salivary flow.

"swab" method is suitable for collecting unstimulated saliva, as the collection process is itself likely to stimulate salivary flow. The "spit" method is preferable for most patients; however, irrespective of the method, the mouth must be cleansed with water and the patient allowed to sit quietly in order to eliminate further stimulation of the glands prior to collection. The volume of saliva collected can be measured directly from the container or more reliably by weighing it (Thomson, 2005).

Normal flow rates

Typical or average whole-saliva flow rates are about 0.3 mL/min for unstimulated whole saliva, and 1.7 mL/min for stimulated saliva (Dawes, 2004). The relative glandular contributions differ according to the type of flow (Aps and Martens, 2005), with the submandibular glands providing more than two-thirds (~70%) of unstimulated flow, while the parotid glands dominate the stimulated flow.

Measuring xerostomia

A number of different questions are useful when asking patients about their symptoms. For example, we have found it particularly useful to know, "*How often does your mouth feel dry?*", with four response options "*Never*," "*Occasionally*," "*Frequently*," or "*Always*." A response of "*Frequently*" or "*Always*" usually categorizes a patient as xerostomic. Fox et al. (1987) used four separate questions to identify people with *both* xerostomia and SGH, whereas Pai et al. (2001) used a visual analogue scale to measure subjective assessments of dry mouth.

The Xerostomia Inventory

We developed the 11-item "XI" or "Xerostomia Inventory" to reflect the experiential and behavioral aspects of dry mouth, which represents the severity of chronic xerostomia when combined into a single (continuous scale) score ranging from 11 to 55, with 55 representing the most severe symptoms (Table 4.3).

The inventory scale was validated by comparing over a 6-month period older people against patients undergoing radiotherapy for head/neck cancer (Thomson and Williams, 2000), and it has been used as an outcome measure in several clinical trials (Johnstone et al., 2001; Bots et al., 2005). Recent applications of the XI demonstrate that an increase of six or more points in a summary score represents a clinically meaningful deterioration in xerostomia (Thomson, 2007).

MEDICATIONS AND DRY MOUTH

Older people, particularly as they grow frail, take more medications (a situation known as "polypharmacy") than any other age group for symptom-

Table 4.3 The xerostomia inventory (adapted from Thomson et al., 1999b).

Item[a]

- I sip liquids to aid in swallowing food.
- My mouth feels dry when eating a meal.
- I get up at night to drink.
- My mouth feels dry.
- I have difficulty in eating dry foods.
- I suck sweets or cough lollies to relieve dry mouth.
- I have difficulties swallowing certain foods.
- The skin of my face feels dry.
- My eyes feel dry.
- My lips feel dry.
- The inside of my nose feels dry.

[a]Response options: "Never" = 1; "Hardly ever" = 2; "Occasionally" = 3; "Fairly often" = 4; "Very often" = 5.

atic relief of the symptoms associated with various chronic diseases. Many of those medications either produce the symptoms of xerostomia or reduce salivary flow (Sreebny and Valdini, 1988). Exactly what medications are involved, and whether they produce SGH, xerostomia, or both, can be very confusing. Because of this, we apply the term "xerogenic" to medications that are associated with dry mouth, as it is a more inclusive term than either "xerostomic" or "hyposalivatory." *Xerostomic* drugs produce the symptoms of dry mouth, whereas *hyposalivatory* drugs reduce salivary flow. By contrast, *xerogenic* drugs can exert their action either by reducing the volume of saliva secreted or by altering the threshold for perceiving a dry mouth so that xerostomia is experienced (or, of course, by doing both).

Interpreting and synthesizing the literature on medications and dry mouth can be difficult because of differences in population samples, study design, and analysis, particularly relating to how the dry mouth is diagnosed and the medications measured. In practical terms, it is difficult to distinguish between the effects of the medication and the side effects of a disease. For example, a dry mouth associated with bronchodilators might be caused by the sustained β-adrenergic stimulation of the drug that produces a low volume of viscous saliva, or it might be related more directly to mouth breathing in a physical effort to compensate for bronchospasms. There is, therefore, both a physical and a pharmacological explanation for the dry mouth.

Three general approaches have been taken to study the xerogenicity of medications:

- First, we can look very generally for associations between symptoms of dry mouth and the overall *number* of medications consumed. This approach has confirmed that medications do indeed increase the risk of xerostomia, but they do not tell us which medications are responsible (Locker, 1993; Nederfors et al., 1997).

- Second, we can look for associations with specific *classes* of medications that we believe cause xerostomia or SGH. Three classifications for this approach are available, but they vary greatly in both the number and types of medications listed, and the evidence is weak for including many of the categories (Grad et al., 1985; Handelman et al., 1986; Sreebny and Schwartz, 1997). Nevertheless, a list of xerogenic medications is clinically useful for physicians, dentists, pharmacists, and others who manage the needs of frail people, but we need further evidence on the validity of this approach.
- Third, and leaving aside any preconceptions about xerogenicity, we can look for evidence of xerostomia among takers of the medications available in various therapeutic categories (Table 4.4). This approach allows us to identify pharmacological alternatives in an effort to prevent or reverse the consequence of a dry mouth. However, the information available should be interpreted with caution because the evidence on the xerogenicity of the medications listed in Table 4.4 needs further investigation.

Polypharmacy is a major problem in older populations, and it is probably a major contributor to xerostomia and SGH. In general, the more medications taken, the greater the likelihood of a dry mouth (Ship, 2004), probably because of the overall anticholinergic burden (Chew et al., 2008).

Clinical scenario 1

Mr. Tom Swift is a 75-year-old retired teacher living with his wife in their own home. Recently diagnosed with glaucoma, he had been using timolol eye drops for three months. He visited Dr. Dredge, his dentist, to complain of a sore mouth and poorly fitting dentures.

Dr. Dredge asked him about dry mouth, how often this might occur, and whether it had occurred recently. Tom said he had had a dry mouth occasionally over the years, but that it was worse recently, and that he sucked boiled sweets to prevent it. Dr. Dredge asked Tom about the medication he consumed, and together they compiled a list (Table 4.5).

The dentist recommended a spray of water from a small atomizer bottle (Figure 4.3), and asked Tom to return in 2 weeks.

Meanwhile, the dentist checked Tom's medication against a list of medicines associated with dry mouth (Table 4.4) and discussed these with a clinical pharmacist. They noted that timolol eye drops, omeprazole, metoprolol, and enalapril were each associated with dry mouth and considered alternatives.

Two weeks later, Tom was still troubled by a dry sore mouth and ill-fitting dentures. Dr. Dredge wrote to Tom's physician, who suggested referral to an ophthalmologist, who in turn changed the eye drops to a prostaglandin analogue (latanoprost) which is not associated with dry mouth. Tom's sore mouth improved quickly, and with occasional use of the water spray, he was able to keep his now mild symptoms of dry mouth under control. Changing to latanoprost improved the symptoms somewhat, but did not eliminate them.

Table 4.4 Reported associations between dry mouth and drugs used for various disorders.

Disorder	Drug class	Report of dry mouth[a] Yes	No
Cardiovascular system Arrhythmias	Antiarrhythmic	Disopyramide, flecainide, mexiletine, propafenone	Amiodarone
Hyperlipidemia	Fibrate		Bezafibrate, ciprofibrate, fenofibrate, gemfibrozil
	Statins		Atorvastatin, fluvastatin, pravastatin, simvastatin
Hypertension and/ or heart failure	ACE inhibitor	Captopril, enalapril, lisinopril, moexepril, perindopril, quinapril, ramipril, trandalopril	Cilazapril, fosinopril
	Angiotensin-2 antagonist	Telmisartan	Candesartan, eprosartan, losartan, olmesartan, valsartan
	Diuretic (loop)	Furosemide, torasemide	Bumetanide
	Diuretic (potassium sparing)	Amiloride	Spironolactone
	Diuretic (thiazide)	Indapamide	Bendroflumethiazide, chlorthalidone, metolazone, xipamide
Hypertension	Alpha-2 agonist	Clonidine	
	Alpha-blocker	Doxazosin, prazosin, terazosin	
	Centrally acting antihypertensive	Methyldopa	
	Beta-blocker	Atenolol, carvedilol, esmolol, metoprolol (isolated cases), nadolol, oxprenolol	Acebutolol, bisoprolol, celiprolol, labetolol, propranolol, pindolol, sotalol, timolol
	Calcium channel blocker	Amlodipine, diltiazem, nifedipine, verapamil	Felodipine, isradipine, lacidipine, lercanidipine, nicardipine, nimodipine, nisoldipine
	Vasodilator	Bosentan	Hydralazine, minoxidil, sitaxenten

61

Table 4.4 *Continued*

Disorder	Drug class	Report of dry mouth[a] Yes	No
Central nervous system			
Alzheimer's	Anticholinesterase inhibitor	Donepezil	Galantamine, rivastigmine
Analgesics	Opioid analgesics	Buprenorphine, codeine, fentanyl, methadone, morphine, pethidine	
Anxiety	Anxiolytic: benzodiazepines, azaspirodecanedione[a]	Diazepam, lorazepam, buspirone[a]	Oxazepam
Depression (or neuropathic pain)	Antidepressant: MAOI	Phenelzine, moclobemide, tranylcypromine	
	Antidepressant: SSRIs, SNRI[a]	Citalopram, fluoxetine, paroxetine, sertraline, venlafaxine[a]	
	Antidepressant: TCA, triazolopyridine[a]	Amitriptyline, clomipramine, dosulepin, imipramine, nortriptyline, trimipramine, trazodone[a]	
Epilepsy (or neuropathic pain)	Anticonvulsant	Carbamazepine, gabapentin, topiramate	Lamotrigine, phenytoin, sodium valproate, vigabatrin
Insomnia	Hypnotic: Benzodiazepine, nonbenzodiazepine[a]	Lormetazepam, temazepam, zopiclone[a]	Nitrazepam, triazolam, zolpidem[a]
Parkinson's disease	Anticholinergic	Benzhexol, benztropine, orphenadrine, procyclidine	
	Antiparkinson agent	Amantadine	
	Levodopa combination	Levodopa/carbidopa	Levodopa/benserazide
	COMT inhibitor	Entacapone	Tolcapone
	Dopamine agonist	Bromocriptine, rotigotine	Cabergoline, pergolide, pramipexole, ropinirole,
	MAOB inhibitor	Selegiline	

Table 4.4 *Continued*

Disorder	Drug class	Report of dry mouth[o] Yes	No
Psychosis	Atypical antipsychotic	Amisulpiride, clozapine, olanzapine, quetiapine, risperidone	
	Typical antipsychotic	Chlorpromazine, flupenthixol, haloperidol, levomepromazine, zuclopenthixol	
Eye			
Glaucoma	Beta-blocker	(Eye drops) timolol	(Eye drops) betaxolol, carteolol, levobunolol, metipranolol
	Alpha-2 agonist	(Eye drops) brimonidine	(Eye drops) dipivefrine
	Prostaglandin analogue		(Eye drops) bimatoprost, latanoprost, travoprost
	Carbonic anhydrase inhibitors	(Eye drops) brinzolamide, dorzolamide	(Tablets) acetazolamide
Gastrointestinal system			
Inflammatory bowel disease	Aminosalicylate	Olsalazine	Mesalazine
Diarrhea	Antidiarrheal	Codeine, loperamide	
Nausea/vomiting	Antiemetic	Cyclizine	Metoclopramide, ondansetron
Irritable bowel	Antispasmodic	Dicyclomine, hyoscine n-butylbromide, propantheline	
Peptic ulcer/GORD	H-2 antagonist	Famotidine	Nizatidine, ranitidine
	Proton pump inhibitor	Lansoprazole, omeprazole	
	Sucrose sulfate aluminium complex	Sucralfate	
Genitourinary system			
Benign prostatic hypertrophy (BPH)	Alpha-blocker 5α-reductase inhibitor[a]	Alfuzosin, doxazosin, prazosin, tamsulosin, terazosin	Finasteride[a]

Table 4.4 *Continued*

Disorder	Drug class	Report of dry mouth[a] Yes	No
Urge incontinence	Anticholinergic	Oxybutynin, propiverine, tolterodine, trospium	
Musculoskeletal system			
Muscle spasm	Muscle relaxants	Baclofen	Dantrolene
Rheumatic disease	NSAIDs	Ketoprofen, nabumetone, piroxicam	Diclofenac, etodolac, ibuprofen, indomethacin, mefenamic acid, meloxicam, naproxen
	COX-2 inhibitors	Celecoxib, etoricoxib	
Respiratory system			
Allergic conditions	Antihistamines	Chlorpheniramine, cyproheptadine, desloratidine, diphenhydramine, fexofenadine, hydroxyzine, loratidine, promethazine, trimeprazine	Phenylephrine, triprolidine
Asthma and COPD	Anticholinergic	Ipratropium, tiotropium	
	Beta-2 agonist, long-acting beta-2 agonist[a]		Salbutamol, terbutaline, formoterol[a], salmeterol[a]
	Corticosteroid (nasal sprays)	Dry nose and throat: beclomethasone nasal spray, budesonide nasal spray, fluticasone nasal spray	
	Methylxanthines		Aminophylline, theophylline
Skin			
Psoriasis	Retinoid	Acitretin	(Phototherapy)

[a]Electronic Medicines Compendium, available at www.emc.medicines.org.uk/ (accessed July 5, 2008), or Medsafe data sheets, available at www.medsafe.govt.nz/profs/datasheet/dsform.asp (accessed July 5, 2008).
SNRI, serotonin–norepinephrine reuptake inhibitor; MAOI, monoamine oxidase inhibitor; TCA, tricyclic antidepressant; COMT, catechol-O-methyl transferase; MAOB, monoamine oxidase type B; GORD, gastroesophageal reflux disease; NSAID, nonsteroidal anti-inflammatory drug; COX-2, cyclo-oxygenase-2; COPD, chronic obstructive pulmonary disease.

Table 4.5 Medications consumed by Mr. Tom Swift (clinical scenario 1).

Medication	Reason for taking	Duration
Timolol eye drops	Glaucoma	3 months
Omeprazole capsules	Heartburn	Several years
Metoprolol tablets	Blood pressure, angina	
Enalapril tablets	Blood pressure	
Isosorbide mononitrate tablets	Angina	
Glyceryl trinitrate spray	Angina	
Simvastatin tablets	High cholesterol	
Aspirin tablets	Prevent heart attacks	

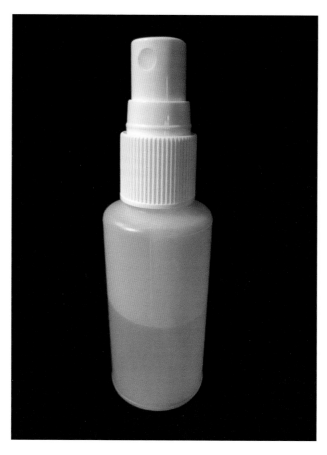

Figure 4.3 Atomizer bottle with water to relieve discomfort from a dry mouth.

PREVALENCE OF DRY MOUTH IN OLDER PEOPLE

The prevalence of xerostomia in representative samples of older populations ranges from 12% to 39%, whereas SGH ranges from 5% to 47%
(Thomson, 2005). The large range in prevalence is due to the different
approaches and case definitions used to identify the disorders in the
various studies.

There have been only a few studies of dry mouth among frail
older people in residential care (Johnson et al., 1984; Thomson et al.,
1993; Van der Putten et al., 2003); however, the greater extent of
polypharmacy among frail elders supports the contention that it is very
prevalent.

MANAGEMENT OF DRY MOUTH IN RESIDENTIAL CARE FACILITIES

Relief of symptoms

The impact of a dry mouth on quality of life dictates that the relief of
symptoms is foremost among the practical issues to be addressed by a
dentist caring for frail elders (Ikebe et al., 2005). The simplest and most
cost-effective way to provide relief is to prescribe a small atomizer bottle
filled with water (Figure 4.3). Elders with severe arthritis may find it
awkward to aim and use, in which case an occupational therapist can
advise on appropriate modifications. Proprietary products on the market
also provide relief, with the addition of constituents, such as xylitol and
antibacterial enzymes, to assist in preventing dental caries. However,
unlike water, the taste and consistency of some proprietary products can
upset patients.

Changes in the quantity and quality of saliva can severely compromise
a denture-wearer's ability to retain an upper denture or to tolerate a lower
denture (Ikebe et al., 2005). Denture adhesives can help some patients
(Ship, 2004), while pharmacological stimulation of salivation, with pilocar-
pine, for example, will help others (Niedermeier and Kramer, 1992). When
natural teeth are supporting the dentures, there is the added problem of
caries, gingivitis, and to a lesser extent, periodontitis (Thomson, 2004).
These serious complications can be reduced by ensuring that dentures are
removed from the mouth, cleaned thoroughly, and allowed to dry overnight. Bacterial and fungal contamination of dentures is much less if the
dentures are dry when not in use (Stafford et al., 1986). Apparently, a wet
environment promotes bacterial and fungal growth, while long-held concerns about the distortion of acrylic resin when allowed to dry are of no
clinical concern.

Clinical scenario 2

Mrs. Mary Windjammer (aged 79) lives with her husband in a retirement village. She has suffered from Parkinson's disease for 4 years, suffering mainly rigidity and slowness of movement. She has recently had "accidents" as she finds it hard to get to the bathroom on time when feeling the urge to empty her bladder. On visiting her dentist, Dr. Hearty, Mary tells her she has had difficulty tasting her food, her mouth feels quite sore, and she has noticed bleeding sometimes when using her electric toothbrush. She bought a proprietary atomizer spray from a pharmacy but finds it hard to use. Dr. Hearty, during the clinical examination, finds inflamed areas of gum that bleed easily, and so she is concerned about the potential for infection. She asks Mary about her medicines, and together they compile a list (Table 4.6).

Her dentist recommends more frequent use of the mouth spray (perhaps with help from her husband) and a softer head for the toothbrush. She also prescribes an anti-inflammatory mouth spray for use each night before Mary goes to bed, and asks to see her again in 2 weeks' time. In the meantime, she checks the medicines against a list (Table 4.4) of those associated with dry mouth and discusses Mary's medication with a clinical pharmacist.

The pharmacist advises Mary's physician to review the dose of oxybutinin, as this commonly causes dry mouth and the effects appear to be dose related. If a reduced dose does not help, then tolterodine might be an alternative for Mary's "accidents" because the xerogenic effects should be less severe. He suggests reviewing the use of amitriptyline if Mary's mouth problems continue. Amlodipine and indapamide may also need to be reviewed, as they are sometimes associated with a dry mouth, and felodipine and bendrofluazide might be possible substitutes. The levodopa combination is essential for Mary's Parkinson's disease and would be reviewed regularly by her physician. Dr. Hearty, at this point, decides that she would write to Mary's physician with these suggestions if the problem continued.

Outcome.

Two weeks later, Mary's mouth is still dry and only a little less sore and inflamed. The dentist writes to Mary's physician, who reviews the medicines as suggested. Before changes to the medication are considered, Mary is referred to a continence advisor for bladder training, and is soon able to stop taking oxybutinin. As Mary's mouth is still a bit sore, she is prescribed a selective serotonin reuptake inhibitor (SSRI) antidepressant (citalopram) rather than amitriptyline, as citalopram might be less xerogenic. Subsequently, Mary continues on her new medication, uses her mouth spray regularly, and sees Dr. Hearty regularly to check on her oral health.

Table 4.6 Medications consumed by Mrs. Mary Windjammer (clinical scenario 2).

Medication	Reason for taking	Duration
Oxybutinin	Bladder "accidents"	2 months
Levodopa/carbidopa	Parkinson's disease	4 years
Amlodipine	High blood pressure	Several years
Indapamide		
Amitriptyline	Depression	

Control of caries is more complicated, but essentially, the daily use of fluoride mouthwash and fluoride toothpaste, together with a nutritious diet with limited intake of cariogenic foods, is the practical approach to controlling caries for people with dry mouth (Wyatt and MacEntee, 1998; Chalmers et al., 2002; Wyatt and MacEntee, 2004).

The incidence of caries among frail elders in residential care is twice as high as the incidence of elders who are not institutionalized, and it is twice as high again if they are demented (Chalmers et al., 2002). Natural teeth should be carefully and thoroughly brushed using a soft toothbrush covered with fluoride toothpaste after breakfast and again after supper. After the evening brushing, which should be the last act before going to bed for the night, nothing but water should go into the mouth until the next morning. This gives the fluoride from the toothpaste time to promote the remineralization or "hardening" of incipient carious lesions in the teeth. Dental floss, interdental brushes, or wooden toothpicks also help clean surfaces that are inaccessible to the toothbrush. This daily routine should be maintained because it is less likely to be forgotten if it is performed at the same time every day.

Dentists should routinely ask about dry mouth when interviewing older patients, especially those who are frail and taking multiple medications. In addition, they should inquire about possible side effects at a follow-up appointment after a new medication is prescribed by either a dentist or a physician. Community pharmacists have an important role in this monitoring process by advising their patients about the likelihood of dryness, loose dentures, and mouth sores when dispensing potentially xerogenic drugs. Moreover, inquiries about dry mouth should be included in the standard medication history recorded by medical staff when admitting an older person to a nursing home or hospital.

CONCLUSIONS

Dry mouth is a serious problem among frail elders as xerostomia and SGH can contribute to a rapid onset of dental caries, mucositis, intolerable dentures, and a very disturbed quality of life. The association between dry mouth and the number and composition of medications taken by older people, particularly as they become frailer, is reasonably clear. Therefore, healthcare professionals who manage the care of this expanding population must be aware of these potential problems and ask older people about their symptoms of dry mouth. When the problem occurs, there are practical measures that can alleviate symptoms and contribute to slowing the rate of frailty by stabilizing physical and psychological well-being.

REFERENCES

Aps JK and Martens LC. 2005. Review: The physiology of saliva and transfer of drugs into saliva. *Forensic Sci Int* 150:119–31.

Atkinson JC and Wu AJ. 1994. Salivary gland dysfunction: Causes, symptoms, treatment. *J Am Dent Assoc* 125:409–16.

Bots CP, Brand HS, Veerman ECI, Korevaar JC, Valentijn-Benz M, Bezemer PD, Valentijn RM, Vos PF, Bijlsma JA, ter Wee PM, Van Amerongen BM, and Nieuw Amerongen AV. 2005. Chewing gum and a saliva substitute alleviate thirst and xerostomia in patients on haemodialysis. *Nephrol Dial Transplant* 20:578–84.

Cassolato SF and Turnbull RS. 2003. Xerostomia: Clinical aspects and treatment. *Gerodontology* 20:64–77.

Chalmers JM, Carter KD, and Spencer AJ. 2002. Caries incidence and increments in community-living older adults with and without dementia. *Gerodontology* 19:80–94.

Chew ML, Mulsant BH, Pollock BG, Lehman ME, Greenspan A, Mahmoud RA, Kirshner MA, Sorisio DA, Bies RR, and Gharabawi G. 2008. Anticholinergic activity of 107 medications commonly used by older adults. *J Am Geriatr Soc* 56:1333–41.

Dawes C. 1972. Circadian rhythms in human salivary flow rate and composition. *J Physiol* 220:529–45.

Dawes C. 2004. Factors influencing salivary flow rate and composition. In: Edgar WM, Dawes C, and O'Mullane DM (eds.), *Saliva and Dental Health*, 3rd edn. London: British Dental Association, pp. 32–49.

Dirix P, Nuyts S, and Van den Bogaert W. 2006. Radiation-induced xerostomia in patients with head and neck cancer: A literature review. *Cancer* 107:2525–34.

Edgar M, Dawes C, O'Mullane D, Edgar M, Dawes C, and O'Mullane DM. 2004. *Saliva and Oral Health*. London: British Dental Association.

Epstein JB, Emerton S, Kolbinson DA, Le ND, Phillips N, Stevenson-Moore P, and Osoba D. 1999. Quality of life and oral function following radiotherapy for head and neck cancer. *Head Neck* 21:1–11.

Fox PC, Busch KA, and Baum BJ. 1987. Subjective reports of xerostomia and objective measures of salivary gland performance. *J Am Dent Assoc* 115:581–4.

Grad H, Grushka M, and Yanover L. 1985. Drug induced xerostomia: The effects and treatment. *J Can Dent Assoc* 4:296–300.

Gupta A, Epstein JB, and Sroussi H. 2006. Hyposalivation in elderly patients. *J Can Dent Assoc* 72:841–6.

Hamlet S, Faull J, Klein B, Aref A, Fontanesi J, Stachler R, Shamsa F, Jones L, and Simpson M. 1997. Mastication and swallowing in patients with postirradiation xerostomia. *Int J Radiat Oncol Biol Phys* 37:789–96.

Handelman SL, Baric JM, Espeland MA, and Berglund KL. 1986. Prevalence of drugs causing hyposalivation in an institutionalized geriatric population. *Oral Surg Oral Med Oral Pathol* 62:26–31.

Ikebe K, Morii K, Kashiwagi J, Nokubi T, and Ettinger RL. 2005. Impact of dry mouth on oral symptoms and function in removable denture wearers in Japan. *Oral Surg Oral Med Oral Pathol Oral Radiol Endod* 99:704–10.

Ikebe K, Matsuda K, Morii K, Wada M, Hazeyama T, Nokubi T, and Ettinger RL. 2007. Impact of dry mouth and hyposalivation on oral health-related quality of life of elderly Japanese. *Oral Surg Oral Med Oral Pathol Oral Radiol Endod* 103:216–22.

Johnson G, Barenthin I, and Westphal P. 1984. Mouthdryness among patients in long-term hospitals. *Gerodontology* 3:197–203.

Johnstone PAS, Peng YP, May BC, Inouye WS, and Niemtzow RC. 2001. Acupuncture for pilocarpine-resistant xerostomia following radiotherapy for head and neck malignancies. *Int J Radiat Oncol Biol Phys* 50:353–7.

Last JM. 2001. *A Dictionary of Epidemiology*. New York: Oxford University Press.

Locker D. 1993. Subjective reports of oral dryness in an older adult population. *Community Dent Oral Epidemiol* 21:165–8.

Loesche WJ, Bromberg J, Terpenning MS, Bretz WA, Dominguez BL, Grossman NS, and Langmore SE. 1995. Xerostomia, xerogenic medications and food avoidances in selected geriatric groups. *J Am Geriatr Soc* 43:401–7.

Logemann JA, Pauloski BR, Rademaker AW, Lazarus CL, Mittal B, Gaziano J, and Stachowiak L (2003). Xerostomia: 12-month changes in saliva production and its relationship to perception and performance of swallow function, oral intake, and diet after chemoradiation. *Head Neck* 25:432–7.

Mandel ID. 1987. The functions of saliva. *J Dent Res* 66:623–7.

Mandel ID. 1990. The diagnostic uses of saliva. *J Oral Pathol Med* 19:119–25.

Mese H and Matsuo R. 2007. Salivary secretion, taste and hyposalivation. *J Oral Rehabil* 34:711–23.

Navazesh M. 1993. Methods for collecting saliva. *Ann N Y Acad Sci* 694:72–7.

Navazesh M and Christensen CM. 1982. A comparison of whole mouth resting and stimulated salivary measurement procedures. *J Dent Res* 61:1158–62.

Nederfors T, Isaksson R, Mörnstad H, and Dahlöf C. 1997. Prevalence of perceived symptoms of dry mouth in an adult Swedish population-relation to age, sex and pharmacotherapy. *Community Dent Oral Epidemiol* 25:211–6.

Niedermeier WH and Kramer R. 1992. Salivary secretion and denture retention. *J Prosthet Dent* 67:211–6.

Pai S, Ghezzi EM, and Ship JA. 2001. Development of a Visual Analogue Scale questionnaire for subjective assessment of salivary dysfunction. *Oral Surg Oral Med Oral Pathol* 91:311–6.

Ship JA. 2004. Xerostomia: Aetiology, diagnosis, management and clinical implications. In: Edgar WM, Dawes C, and O'Mullane DM (eds.), *Saliva and Oral Health*. London: British Dental Association, pp. 50–70.

Ship JA, Pillemer SR, and Baum BJ. 2002. Xerostomia and the geriatric patient. *J Am Geriatr Soc* 50:535–43.

Sreebny LM and Broich G. 1987. Xerostomia (dry mouth) In: Sreebny LM (ed.), *The Salivary System*. Boca Raton, FL: CRC Press, pp. 184–5.

Sreebny LM and Schwartz SS. 1997. A reference guide to drugs and dry mouth—2nd edition. *Gerodontology* 14:33–47.

Sreebny LM and Valdini A. 1988. Xerostomia. Part I: Relationship to other oral symptoms and salivary gland hypofunction. *Oral Surg Oral Med Oral Pathol* 66:451–8.

Stafford GD, Arendorf T, and Huggett R. 1986. The effect of overnight drying and water immersion on candidal colonization and properties of complete dentures. *J Dent* 14:52–6.

Tabak LA, Levine MJ, Mandel ID, and Ellison SA. 1982. Role of salivary mucins in the protection of the oral cavity. *J Oral Pathol* 11:1–17.

Thomson WM. 2004. Dental caries experience in older people over time: What can the large cohort studies tell us? *Br Dent J* 196: 89–92.

Thomson WM. 2005. Issues in the epidemiological investigation of dry mouth. *Gerodontology* 22:65–76.

Thomson WM. 2007. Measuring change in dry-mouth symptoms over time using the Xerostomia Inventory. *Gerodontology* 24:30–5.

Thomson WM and Williams SM. 2000. Further testing of the Xerostomia Inventory. *Oral Surg Oral Med Oral Pathol Oral Radiol Endod* 89:46–50.

Thomson WM, Brown RH, and Williams SM. 1993. Medication and perception of dry mouth in a population of institutionalised elderly people. *N Z Med J* 106:219–21.

Thomson WM, Chalmers JM, Spencer AJ, and Ketabi M. 1999a. The occurrence of xerostomia and salivary gland hypofunction in a population-based sample of older South Australians. *Spec Care Dentist* 19:20–3.

Thomson WM, Chalmers JM, Spencer AJ, and Williams SM. 1999b. The Xerostomia Inventory: A multi-item approach to measuring dry mouth. *Community Dent Health* 16:12–7.

Turner MD and Ship JA. 2007. Dry mouth and its effects on the oral health of elderly people. *J Am Dent Assoc* 138(Suppl.):15S–20S.

Van der Putten GJ, Brand HS, Bots CP, and van Nieuw Amerongen A. 2003. Prevalence of xerostomia and hyposalivation in the nursing home and the relation with number of prescribed medication. *Tijdschr Gerontol Geriatr* 34:30–6.

Whelton H. 2004. Introduction: the anatomy and physiology of salivary glands. In: Edgar M, Dawes C, O'Mullane D, Edgar M, and Dawes C (eds.), *Saliva and Oral Health*. London: British Dental Association, pp. 1–13.

Wyatt CCL and MacEntee MI. 1998. Dental caries in chronically disabled elders. *Spec Care Dentist* 17:196–202.

Wyatt CCL and MacEntee MI. 2004. Caries management for institutionalized elders using fluoride and chlorhexidine mouthrinses. *Community Dent Oral Epidemiol* 32:1–7.

Yoshinaka M, Yoshinaka MF, Ikebe K, Shimanuki Y, and Nokubi T (2007). Factors associated with taste dissatisfaction in the elderly. *J Oral Rehabil* 34:497–502.

Dietary consequences of oral health in frail elders

Paula Moynihan, Jane Bradbury, and Frauke Müller

INTRODUCTION

This chapter focuses on the etiology and consequences of undernutrition and nutritional deficiencies in frail elders, and the interrelationship of this with oral health. An overview of how nutritional needs change with advancing age is presented. This is followed by a discussion of evidence for a relationship between loss of teeth, prosthodontics, quality of life, and nutritional well-being, including how nutritional status is assessed in geriatric populations. Finally, we offer practical suggestions for appropriate foods for older people who are frail and have oral health-related eating problems.

THE IMPORTANCE OF GOOD NUTRITION FOR FRAIL ELDERS

Nutrition and diet are key factors in healthy aging. Undernutrition and micronutrient deficiencies are common among older people, but they are not inevitable consequences of being old. Indeed, prevention of dietary inadequacy helps promote good general and oral health, and promotion of good oral health can impact on dietary adequacy and nutritional well-being.

Oral Healthcare and the Frail Elder: A Clinical Perspective.
Edited by Michael I. MacEntee © 2011 Blackwell Publishing Ltd.

NUTRITIONAL NEEDS OF OLDER PEOPLE

A healthy and balanced diet low in saturated fat and free sugars but high in fruits, vegetables, wholegrain foods, and fiber plays a key role in preventing a number of chronic diseases, including dental caries, diabetes, cardiovascular disease, and some cancers (World Health Organization, 2003). Continuing a healthy balanced diet maintains this protection into old age. Elders who consume 5–10 portions of fruits and vegetables daily when compared with elders who consume less can reduce by one-third their risk of atherosclerotic disease (Liu et al., 2000). In addition, a healthy balanced diet will also help prevent constipation, optimize immune function, and maintain a healthy body weight. Constipation is a chronic problem for many older adults due to reduced peristaltic strength, which is often coupled with an inadequate intake of dietary fiber. Obesity is a risk factor for disability, and a sedentary lifestyle is a risk factor for obesity. Together they contribute to a vicious cycle. Indeed, obesity is associated with functional decline even among community-dwelling elders who are relatively active and healthy (Jensen and Friedman, 2002). The immune response declines with age, and intake of nutrients has an important role in optimizing the function of the immune system in later life.

Energy requirements in old age

Energy requirements decrease due to loss of lean body mass and, in some, a more sedentary lifestyle as we get old (Fujita and Volpi, 2004). They are reduced by approximately 10%–16% in people aged 75 years and over (Institute of Medicine of the National Academies, 2005). To put this into context, the average daily energy requirement of a typically active 70-kg man aged 39–59 years is around 10.5 megajoules (MJ), whereas for a man of similar weight aged 75 years or over it is 8.8 MJ (Department of Health, 1991). Energy intakes, despite this, often fail to meet energy requirements (McDowell et al., 1994; Liu et al., 2000). The U.K. National Diet and Nutrition Survey (NDNS) of people aged 65 years and over indicated that about 1 in 20 (4% of men; 6% of women) aged 75–84 years living in the community were underweight, but the prevalence rose to as high as 1 in 5 older men living in residential care (Finch et al., 1998). Data from the United States suggest that approximately half of long-term care residents are malnourished (Neel, 2001), and 6 out of 10 older people in acute care hospitals in the United Kingdom are at risk of malnutrition (Age Concern, 2006).

Importance of dietary protein in old age

A diet adequate in protein is important to minimize loss of lean body tissue that tends to occur after age 70 years. Protein energy malnutrition (PEM) in older people is associated with reduced lean body tissue, reduced bone mass, impaired cognitive function, poor wound healing, reduced immune response, and increased morbidity and mortality (MacIntosh et al., 2000). Weight loss in later life is often disproportionately due to a loss of lean muscle tissue rather than adipose tissue. This loss of lean body tissue will impact body strength and mobility and, if marked, increases the risk of falls (Gariballa and Sinclair, 2005). Protein requirements in adults are approximately 1 g/kg body weight/day (Department of Health, 1991), but it has been suggested that the level of intake of protein should be increased to ~1.25 g/kg/day for elders (Fujita and Volpi, 2004).

Changes in requirements for micronutrients in old age

Despite a lower requirement for energy, the requirement for many vitamins and minerals does not decrease with age, and can increase due to reduced absorptive capacity of later life. This means that a diet that is nutrient dense is advocated.

Iron

Adequate intake of iron is important for prevention of anemia in later life (Eisenstaedt et al., 2006), for optimum immune function (Ahluwalia, 2004), and for wound healing. Absorptive capacity for iron is often reduced in later life. Vitamin C promotes iron absorption; therefore, concurrent consumption of foods containing iron and vitamin C should be encouraged to maximize the absorption of dietary iron. However, concurrent consumption of tea should be discouraged since it can bind with iron in the gut, reducing absorption further.

Calcium

Calcium is required to maintain bone mass and lower the risk of osteoporosis. However, dietary intakes by elders often fall short of requirements. It has been suggested that an intake of 1,500 mg/day may be required, but usually dietary intakes fail to reach 1,000 mg/day (Finch et al., 1998).

Zinc

Zinc has a role in many enzymes and proteins, and it impacts on gene expression and on immune function. Moderate zinc deficiency is often observed in old age (Blumberg, 1997) probably due to marginal intake coupled with reduced absorptive capacity. The U.S. National Health and Nutrition Examination Survey showed that more than half (57%) of the U.S. population over 70 years had less than adequate intake of zinc (Briefel et al., 2000). Several factors may interfere with its absorption, such as a high intake of phytates or grains. Malabsorption, physiological stress, and trauma reduce zinc status, which dampens the immune response, disturbs taste perception (Meunier et al., 2005), impairs wound healing (Haase et al.,

2006), reduces appetite (Little et al., 1989), and can contribute to age-related osteoporosis (Heaney, 1986). Low concentration of serum zinc is also associated with reduced cognitive function in old age (Ortega et al., 1997).

Vitamin D

Vitamin D has an important role in maintaining bone mineralization, and an adequate intake is required to minimize age-related reduction in bone density (Thomas, 2001) and thereby to prevent osteoporosis (Schneider, 2008). Younger people get most of their requirements entirely by the action of the sun on the skin; however, elders need to consume about 10 μg/day (found in approximately five sardines!) because of the reduced ability of the kidneys to hydroxylate vitamin D to its active form.

Elders, especially if frail and housebound, are also at increased risk of vitamin D deficiency because the precursor to the vitamin in the skin decreases with age, and older people frequently lack exposure to the synthesizing effect of sunlight on vitamin D through the skin (Thomas, 2001). It is difficult to maintain adequate serum vitamin D levels through diet alone (Dawson-Hughes, 2008); therefore, supplements of vitamin D and calcium might help prevent fractures of older bones (Schneider, 2008).

Vitamins B_{12} and folate

Adequate vitamin B status, particularly folate and B_{12}, might be important in preventing dementia (Brachet et al., 2004). Consumption of foods rich in vitamin B_{12} tends to be reduced in old age (Wakimoto and Block, 2001). Animal protein foods provide the richest sources, but they can be expensive and difficult to chew (Chernoff, 2005). Digestion of vitamin B_{12} requires that it be released from protein complexes in the gut; however, age-related achlorhydria and other gastrointestinal disorders reduce the ability to disassociate these complexes (Hurwitz et al., 1997). B_{12} helps the nervous system to function; therefore, there are hopes that dietary supplements of B_{12} might delay the onset of dementia (Bourre, 2006).

Folate is an important vitamin for older people and subclinical deficiency has been associated with depression and cognitive decline, including Alzheimer's disease and other forms of dementia (D'Anci and Rosenberg 2004). It might protect against cognitive decline in older people (McNulty and Scott, 2008). Folate and vitamin B_{12} are needed for transmethylation of neuroactive substances, and this process may be altered if the vitamins are deficient, causing depression and/or dementia—the so-called "hypomethylation hypothesis" (Wolters et al., 2004). A low folate status is associated with increased levels of homocysteine, which contributes to vascular disease, dementia, and Alzheimer's disease.

It is not yet certain that cognitive impairment can be reduced by nutritional intervention to lower homocysteine levels, but the possibility is being investigated. An insufficiency of folate may occur in older people due to low intake, reduced absorptive capacity, or consumption of medications that alter folate status. Therefore, adequate dietary intake of folate is important for frail elders.

Vitamin C

Synthesis of collagen requires vitamin C, which has an important role in wound healing and vascular integrity. It is a powerful antioxidant that protects against age-related oxidative damage. Adequate vitamin C status is also required for optimal immune function.

Achieving a diet that is nutrient-dense with adequate micronutrients can be difficult at any age, but even more so for frail elders due to eating difficulties.

Older adults living in residential and nursing care homes

Malnutrition is common in older people living in residential care facilities, and it contributes to morbidity and mortality, but typically, it impacts negatively on general well-being and quality of life (Crogan and Shultz, 2000; Neel, 2001). There is little information available on the prevalence of malnutrition among frail elders living in residential care. A survey of nutritional status on admission to a care home in the United Kingdom, for example, found malnutrition in approximately one in three residents: Prevalence was higher if they had transferred from an acute-care hospital and other care homes, whereas malnutrition was less prevalent (about one in four) if the residents came directly from their own homes (Russell and Elia, 2008). Similar information has surfaced from Belgium, France, and Spain (Lamy et al., 1999; Dion et al., 2007; Gil-Montoya et al., 2008), with as many as half of the residents of care homes at risk of malnutrition. In the United States, between 50% and 85% of the residential care population is malnourished (Crogan et al., 2001; Neel, 2001).

Causes of malnutrition in older people

A complexity of problems including social, financial, and functional barriers to achieving adequate food intake contributes to malnutrition in older people. Illness, reduced appetite and/or disease-related anorexia, depression, loss of mental capacity, loss of ability to shop and cook, along with chewing and swallowing problems all contribute to the development of malnutrition (Moynihan, 2007).

Socioeconomic factors and disease have a greater impact than advancing age on nutritional status (Gariballa and Sinclair, 2005). Anorexia is common in old age due to age-related early satiety (MacIntosh et al., 2000), diminished taste and sensory perceptions (Mioche et al., 2004), and use of medications that depress appetite and sometimes taste sensation (Morley,

1997). Older people consume smaller meals and eat more slowly, with few snacks between meals (Morley, 1997). Therefore, oral health is just one of many factors impacting on how older people choose and eat food.

Diagnosis of nutritional deficiencies in all older adults is difficult, and symptoms are often unseen until there are clinical signs of advanced nutritional deficiency (Gariballa and Sinclair, 2005). Early signs of micro-nutrient deficiencies are often seen initially in the mouth, and therefore, the dentist has an important role in early diagnosis of deficiencies (Mioche et al., 2004).

There are numerous instruments available for assessing the presence and severity of undernutrition in frail elders, but not all have been adequately validated (Green and Watson, 2005, 2006). The Malnutrition Universal Screening Tool (MUST) established by the British Association for Parenteral and Enteral Nutrition is the preferred instrument for nutritional screening for older persons in the United Kingdom (Elia, 2003), while the Mini Nutritional Assessment (MNA®) developed by Nestlé Nutrition in the 1990s is popular in North America (Bauer et al., 2008). Both measures are used for assessing and screening older populations (Green and Watson, 2005, 2006).

DOES MASTICATORY ABILITY PLAY A ROLE IN ACHIEVING GOOD NUTRITION AMONG FRAIL ELDERS?

Association between dentition and nutrition

The number of natural teeth and their position as opposing pairs are related to chewing ability, and people without teeth or even with dentures tend to chew less effectively compared with people with healthy natural teeth. A reduced ability to chew possibly impacts on selection of food and intake of nutrients, which puts older people at risk of malnutrition. The evidence for a causal relationship between chewing ability and dietary intake is, however, equivocal.

Both masticatory ability and nutrition can be assessed using a variety of measures. Masticatory ability can been assessed using dentition as a proxy measure of chewing ability, clinical measures, and subjective perceptions of chewing ability and oral health-related quality of life (OHRQoL). Nutrition is assessed using dietary assessment methods (food and/or nutrient intakes); anthropometric measurements of height and weight from which body mass index (BMI) is calculated; nutritional screening/assessment tools, such as the MNA; and biological markers such as serum albumin. Variations in the definition of "dentate" and grouping study participants by the status of their dentitions, along with varying methods of assessing nutritional status and inadequacies in reporting these dietary studies, makes it difficult to compare results and limit the conclusions that can be drawn. Moreover, the vast majority of research studies in this area have a cross-sectional design, which seriously restricts inferences or conclusions about whether tooth loss changes diet.

There are two possible scenarios associated with a compromised dentition and nutritional status. Eating difficulties may reduce food intake because it is uncomfortable to chew, leading to a lower energy intake, greater risk of malnutrition, and a lower BMI. Alternatively, they may lead to selection of softer processed foods that may be less nutrient dense but higher in energy, leading to a greater risk of malnutrition and a higher BMI.

Complete denture-wearers can experience difficulties eating some foods, particularly foods that are hard, sticky, or with seeds, such as steak, apples, raw carrots, tomatoes, fresh bread, and toffees (Ettinger, 1973; Sheiham and Steele, 2001). Hard foods might also be avoided by people with few natural teeth, particularly older people who are frail (Sheiham and Steele, 2001). People with ≥20 natural teeth, when compared with denture-wearers, do eat more fruits and vegetables, although the difference is relatively small (Johansson et al., 1994; Joshipura et al., 1996; Sahyoun et al., 2003; Hung et al., 2005; Ervin and Dye, 2009). It is unclear yet whether a higher or lower energy intake is associated with dental status; however, edentulous people have lower intakes of nutrients associated with fruits and vegetables, that is, dietary fiber, vitamin C, carotenes, and folate, although again these differences are small (Joshipura et al., 1996; Krall et al., 1998; Sheiham et al., 2001; Marshall et al., 2002; Hung et al., 2005; Ervin and Dye, 2009).

BMI may be used as an indicator of malnutrition, with a BMI <18.5 defined as underweight and BMI ≥25.0 as overweight (World Health Organization, 2006). In the absence of illness, a low BMI suggests that energy intake does not meet energy expenditure, whereas a high BMI suggests that energy intake exceeds energy expenditure. The relationship between the status of a dentition and BMI is complex, but the pattern emerging is that a higher BMI is associated with a compromised dentition. In other words, people who are edentate and who wear one or no denture, and people without a functionally natural dentition or with many missing natural teeth without a denture, are more likely to be overweight or obese (Sheiham et al., 2001; Rauen et al., 2006; Mack et al., 2008; Hilgert et al., 2009). The pattern might be different with frailer elders living in an institution where residents with a dysfunctional dentition have a significantly lower BMI than elders with better function (Mojon et al., 1999). The likelihood of malnutrition, as defined by the MNA, is higher in those with fewer teeth or no dental prosthesis (Lamy et al., 1999; Dion et al., 2007; De Marchi et al., 2008). Plasma albumin has been used widely as a biochemical indicator of nutritional status to assess the risk associated with dentition (Lamy et al., 1999; Musacchio et al., 2007; Sadamori et al., 2008). However, it is too insensitive and nonspecific to make a good indicator of nutritional status (Crook, 2009).

Diet and masticatory ability

We have seen that the dentition is associated with diet and with risk of malnutrition in frail elders, but are these differences due to a decreased chewing ability, or is a compromised dentition a marker for other factors associated with an inadequate intake of nutrients?

Masticatory ability has little impact on intakes of fruits and vegetables, energy and nutrients, or risk of malnutrition in older adults (Krall et al., 1998; Lamy et al., 1999; Marshall et al., 2002; Shinkai et al., 2001, 2002; Bartali et al., 2003; Chen and Huang, 2003; Liedberg et al., 2007; Bradbury et al., 2008; Gil-Montoya et al., 2008). Factors such as attitude to healthier eating, increasing age, difficulties swallowing, cognitive decline, death of a spouse, living in an institution, in addition to physical limitations associated with age, such as difficulty carrying a shopping bag, are equally or even more important than compromised masticatory ability (Bartali et al., 2003; Chen and Huang, 2003; Dion et al., 2007; Musacchio et al., 2007; Bradbury et al., 2008; Gil-Montoya et al., 2008).

EFFECT OF PROSTHODONTICS ON DIET AND NUTRITIONAL STATUS

There is reasonable evidence of an association between the dentition and nutrition. However, the association between chewing difficulties and compensatory alterations to diet is weak and inconclusive, probably because frailty in old age is itself associated usually with few teeth, chewing difficulties, and malnutrition. Consequently, it is almost impossible to separate the affect of one association from the others.

Loss of teeth and a poor diet have many risk factors in common, such as low socioeconomic status, poor education, and tobacco smoking. The unhealthy diets of those with relatively few teeth, rather than being a consequence of tooth loss, probably contributed to the loss of teeth. Eating habits and diet in childhood and adolescence typically continue into old age, so that children who eat healthy diets are likely to eat healthy diets as adults (Maynard et al., 2005; Mikkilä et al., 2005; Newby et al., 2006).

Impact of prosthodontics on dietary intake

Masticatory efficiency is improved dramatically by implant-supported dentures (van Kampen et al., 2004). However, improved masticatory efficiency does not necessarily lead to improvements in intake of nutrients. Comparison of diet between patients fitted with different types of prostheses, whether implant-supported or conventional, removable, or fixed, show no nutritionally meaningful differences (Sebring et al., 1995; Moynihan et al., 2000; Hamada et al., 2001; Roumanas et al., 2002).

Impact of prosthodontics on nutritional status

The difficulty of measuring nutritional status, and especially changes in nutritional status over time, casts doubt on claims of improved nutritional status after replacing clinically faulty dentures for frail elders. This is especially so when using multiple tests (Morais et al., 2003), or using the MNA, which is a screening instrument that is not sensitive to short-term changes in nutritional status (Wöstmann et al., 2008).

In summary, to improve nutritional status, patients should receive customized dietary advice when receiving new fixed or removable dentures to promote favorable changes to their dietary habits (Bradbury et al., 2006).

IMPACT OF COMPROMISED CHEWING ABILITY, TOOTH LOSS, AND DENTURES ON EATING-RELATED QUALITY OF LIFE

Food provides nourishment for the "soul" as well as for the body, yet despite a wealth of information about the impact on the diet of tooth loss, edentulousness, and prosthodontics, much less attention has focused on the impact of oral health on enjoyment of food and the social aspects of eating-related quality of life (ERQoL). The feelings and experiences of patients are important considerations in the assessment of oral health and the success of prosthodontics (MacEntee et al., 1997; Fiske et al., 1998; Locker, 1998) and nutritional intervention. In elders who are very frail, enjoyment of food and mealtimes can be as important to health and well-being as the nutritional benefits of the food. In contrast, poor eating experiences can lead to loss of interest in food and social interactions, and subsequently contribute to poor nutritional status and further ill health.

Elders who have problems chewing and swallowing specific food are also more likely to perceive problems eating in front of others (Gil-Montoya et al., 2008). OHRQoL questionnaires typically ask several questions about eating and enjoyment of food (Slade, 1997; Brondani and MacEntee, 2007), and the responses of people without natural teeth generally reveal discomfort on eating, difficulty chewing, food avoidance, diminished taste, interruption to meals, and social withdrawal (Table 5.1).

Dental function is not only an important determinant of ERQoL among elders who are able, and loss of teeth can have a very disturbing affect on the pleasure of eating, especially among frail elders in residential care (Lamy et al., 1999). Certainly some people avoid eating in the company of others for fear that their denture will loosen or fall out, while others speak of being "socially reborn" when a removable prosthesis is replaced by a fixed partial denture (Trulsson et al., 2002).

Denture-wearers can find food less tasty and appetizing, which can lead to a loss of interest in food. Therefore, it is important to provide dietary advice that promotes flavorsome, texturally appealing, and nutritious foods.

Table 5.1 Percentage of elders aged 60+ years (*n* = 1,217) who reported impacts on quality of life within the preceding 12 months because of oral health-related problems (adapted from Slade and Spencer, 1994a).

	Edentate		Dentate	
	Often	Occasionally	Often	Occasionally
Uncomfortable to eat foods	14.7	39.2	6.6	22.2
Difficulty chewing all foods	14.3	37.3	6.4	22.5
Avoided some foods	11.5	37.6	5.4	15.5
Less flavor in foods	6.2	10.5	1.9	5.1
Sense of taste has worsened	5.4	11.0	2.1	7.7
Had to interrupt meals	4.7	25.0	1.9	8.9

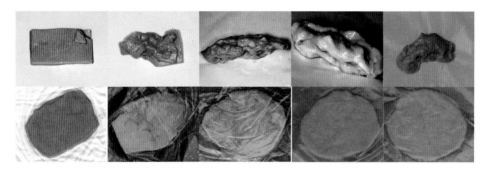

Figure 5.1 Chewing efficiency measured with two colors of gum mixed together by chewing for a set period of time (top row) and compared with five standard mixes (bottom row). (Adapted from Schimmel et al., 2007.)

SCREENING FOR CHEWING DEFICIENCIES IN FRAIL ELDERS

Chewing can influence dietary intake in frail elders; therefore, screening for chewing deficiencies in frail elders in residential care should be considered because it may highlight those who are particularly at nutrition risk. Electronic systems enhance registration and analysis of masticatory movements and efficiency (Müller et al., 2002), but the gold standard for chewing efficiency is the "sieving method" in which subjects chew peanuts or cubes of silicone for 20 cycles, and spit the bolus into a stack of sieves with decreasing seizes of mesh to estimate the effectiveness of mastication (van Kampen et al., 2004). Similar tests are available with fresh carrots, but they are difficult to analyze, as they cannot be easily sieved (Wöstmann et al., 2008). More feasible tests analyze photographs of multicolored chewing gum (Figure 5.1) after it has been chewed like a bolus of food (Prinz, 1999; Schimmel et al., 2007).

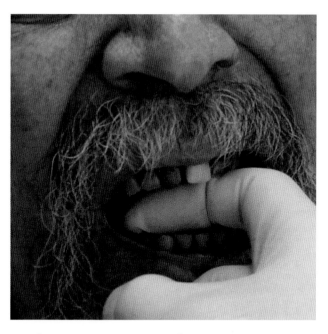

Figure 5.2 If a patient can create a small impression on the examiner's finger, the chewing efficiency is usually sufficient for eating a normal diet.

Indeed, the most straightforward test to screen for chewing deficiencies is the "finger test" for which the patient is asked to bite as hard as possible on the examiners finger (Heath, 1982). Chewing force as a consequence of frailty and tooth loss is usually around 2–3 kg and sufficient for chewing food of normal consistency if the patient can leave small indentations of the cuspid teeth on the examiner's finger (Figure 5.2). Patients are usually amused by this simple test, no special equipment or test food is necessary, and the biting pressure usually is insufficient to hurt the examiner.

Clinical scenario

Madam Guesette is 84 years old, and despite severe arthritis, she lives alone in her own home with regular help from a social worker who attends to her "official" well-being, and a neighbor who does her grocery shopping and "looks after her." She has no children or siblings, and her husband died 3 years previously. She lost all of her natural teeth many years ago because, as she explains, she grew up in a poor family where the quality of food was poor and there was little concern about oral hygiene.

She received her first set of complete dentures before she got married—it saved her husband the cost of dental treatment—so she has learned over the years to tolerate and manage the difficulties of chewing hard and tough foods.

Mostly, she selects and prepares food so that it will be easy to chew. Her dentures were replaced once over the years, but recently, the upper denture broke when she dropped it into the sink. A dental technician who she knew nearby repaired the denture, but when he returned the denture he noticed the poor fit of both dentures and he offered to make her a new set at home so she would not have the inconvenience of traveling to a dentist. Madam Guesette was pleased with this arrangement, but when the new dentures were delivered by the technician, she was very disappointed by the fit of the lower denture. It moved about in her mouth "like a fish." Twice, the dental technician returned to adjust the dentures until he announced that he could do no more because her lower jaw was too flat to stabilize the denture. Sadly, Madam Guesette explained to her neighbor that she would accept her "destiny" without further complaint—it was, she said, "just another part of growing old."

In the following months, she became increasingly frailer and moving around the house became even more difficult for her. One day, she overlooked the edge of a carpet and fell and broke the neck of her right femur. When she was hospitalized, she weighed only 47 kg. A geriatrician examined her and told her that her "BMI" was 18.5, which meant that she was suffering from "undernutrition." She felt relieved to hear this because she believed it was always good when the doctor knows what is wrong. So, despite her broken hip, she was able to enjoy the "lively" environment of the hospital.

As her hip healed, she joined the other patients to eat her meals but she was immediately discouraged by the instability of her dentures. She was sure that everyone noticed the lower denture "flopping around" and "making noises," and she was particularly embarrassed by the fact that she was always the last person to leave the table. The older nurse who she now considered as a friend suggested that she should eat alone in her room to avoid this embarrassment, but Madam Guesette refused to be isolated like this and asked if she could visit a dentist.

Dr. Grim, the hospital's dentist, was summoned and, as part of her examination, she tested Madam Guesette's ability to bite firmly on her finger. Immediately, she saw that the dentures were dislodged. Further examination revealed that the occlusal vertical dimension of the dentures prevented Madam Guesette from closing her lips competently without effort. Moreover, the upper denture was loose because of a faulty peripheral seal, and the periphery of the lower denture was overextended.

Dr. Grim immediately reduced the flanges of the lower denture, relined the upper denture, and adjusted the vertical height of occlusion, which, to Madam Guesette's amazement, made the dentures feel "so much better—almost a part of me like my old set." Gradually, with the help of a dietician and the nursing staff, she was able to modify her diet to include more fresh vegetables and whole fruits, in addition to meats that were firmer. And so, she reduced her reliance on soft breads and sweets to satisfy her appetite. She found also that she enjoyed eating in the company of others as her confidence grew and she realized that she could control the lower denture to finish her meals with everyone else.

Her hip healed satisfactorily and as she prepared to leave the hospital, her doctor informed her that she had gained weight. The dietician explained to her what her correct weight should be, and although she was grateful for this advice, when alone at home there just was not the same incentives to eat as in the hospital. After all, who cared now how long it took to eat, and it was difficult to get the fresh vegetables, fruits, and meats that she received in the hospital without being too demanding of her neighbor. Gradually, she slipped into her old ways of relying on bread and jam, with the occasional bowl of soup. Although the dentures after Dr. Grim's adjustments were so much better than before, they still hurt when she chewed on harder varieties of vegetables and fruits, especially when seeds lodged under the denture. These were new problems, or so it seemed to Madam Guesette, and it all became too much of a bother. Slowly, she isolated herself from her neighbor and anyone else who came to her door. Her appetite began to fade again, which she incorrectly took to mean that her body no longer needed much food. It was all too depressing— she had no energy, no friends, and no future.

After a week or so of near starvation, Madam Guesette began to have dizzy spells that frightened her greatly. She dreaded another fall and broken hip because she had heard that old people died when their hips broke. Eventually, she mustered the courage to summon her neighbor by phone, and the social worker was called immediately. Subsequently, the local community nurse determined that Madam Guesette's physical and psychological health was deteriorating rapidly, and with help from the local health authority, she was assigned a place in a residential care facility nearby. Initially, Madam Guesette resisted the idea of moving from her home again, but with carefully rendered advice and reassurance from her neighbor and the social worker, she accepted with some relief that it was time to make "the move."

Madam Guesette settled into the care facility with ease, and found that eating in company was much more pleasant than eating alone, especially since the cook knew how to prepare the meat and vegetables so that she could enjoy eating again with her dentures. And yes, she began quite quickly to see that there was enjoyment in food and in the company that came with it.

SCREENING FOR UNDERNUTRITION IN FRAIL ELDERS

Regular nutritional screening of frail people in a residential care facility should be part of routine health. Nutritional screening allows for early intervention if needed. For example, extra personal care to provide encouragement at meal times, snacks between meals, or referral to a dietician for a more comprehensive nutritional assessment if needed (Coull, 2003). Standard 15.9 of the Welsh National Minimum Standards for Care Homes for Older People, and Standard 8.9 of the English version, state that "nutritional screening is undertaken on admission and re-assessed periodically; a record is maintained of nutrition, including weight gain or loss, and appropriate action is taken" (Department of Health, 2003).

People with dementia are at particular risk of undernutrition; therefore, they need regular screening and monitoring because they often have low body weight, refuse to eat or drink, or have behavioral or physiological problems that result in reduced intake of food (Hargreaves, 2008). Stanner

(2007) offers good practical advice on coping with eating difficulties, while the Edinburgh Feeding Evaluation in Dementia (EdFED) scale is available specifically for people with dementia (Watson and Dreary, 1997), with an online video available to demonstrate how it is used (*American Journal of Nursing*, 2010).

FOOD FOR FRAIL ELDERS WITH ORAL HEALTH PROBLEMS

Current global dietary goals promote a diet that is low in fat, especially saturated fat, and free sugars, and high in fiber and fruits and vegetables. Nutritional advice should consider the level of dental impairment, limitation, and difficulty confronting edentulous elders. Practical guidance for eating well are available for older people (Caroline Walker Trust, 2004) and their carers (Food Standards Agency, 2007), and for people with dementia (VOICES, 1998), with emphasis on choice and enjoyment of food.

Fruits and vegetables

Most edentulous elders find whole fresh apples, celery, and raw carrots difficult to eat, but many other fruits and vegetables require little mastication. Moreover, raw vegetables can be grated for salads or juiced. Generally, cooked vegetables are softer and if chewing is severely compromised, the vegetables can be pureed or used as a main ingredient for soups. Diced vegetables and fruits for elders should be avoided because there is risk of choking. A glass of fresh fruit juice is a useful way to obtain a daily portion of fruits, while fresh fruits can be liquidized with either milk or fresh juice to make a "smoothie." Stewed fruits also require little mastication and can be used as the base for many desserts, while soft fruits, such as bananas and avocado, can be mashed. Seeds from tomatoes and other fruits or vegetables can be very bothersome underneath a removable denture, so they should be removed by a sieve when necessary.

Fiber

Foods that are high in dietary fiber usually, but not always, require considerable mastication, and food can be prepared to reduce the need for chewing if this is a problem. Softer varieties of wholegrain breads can be promoted, and wholegrain bread may also be used in desserts, such as bread pudding where it is softened in milk, or summer pudding when softened in fruit juice. Oats are also a rich source of fiber and wholegrains, which can be made into porridge or Swiss muesli (oats soaked in juice or milk with dried fruits). High-fiber breakfast cereals can be softened with milk. The fiber in pulses (peas, beans, and lentils) can be obtained in soups and purees, such as dahl, pea puree, and lentil pates, or in stews and casseroles that are easy to masticate and swallow.

Meat and other sources of protein

Some cuts of meat, such as steak, are tough for the denture-wearers and may be difficult for elders who have no teeth to eat (Millwood and Heath, 2000). Fortunately, minced meat and poultry can be used in a wide range of recipes. Meat-based pates require little mastication, although they can be very high in saturated fat. Fish generally requires less mastication and is easier to digest than red meat and has the added benefit of being low in saturated fat. Good vegetarian sources of protein include pulses and nuts, which if necessary can be ground for some recipes. Lacto-vegetarians (and carnivores) will also obtain dietary protein from milk and dairy products.

SUMMARY AND CONCLUSIONS

This chapter has considered issues relating to the nutritional requirements of frail elders and the factors contributing to malnutrition in older people, in particular the potential impact of tooth loss on diet and nutritional well-being, and the limited role of prosthodontics on diet and nutritional status.

Our concluding advice is that

- older people require a diet that is nutrient dense to provide a rich source of micronutrients and protein, with adequate energy to maintain an ideal weight;
- a diet low in saturated fat and free sugars and high in fruits, vegetables, and fiber is likely to prevent obesity and chronic diseases, and it might also protect against disorders found commonly with increasing frailty, such as constipation and decline in immune function;
- socioeconomic factors, mobility, illness, depression, and cognitive and physical impairment are all barriers to achieving a healthier diet and nutritional well-being;
- impaired chewing function through tooth loss is one factor among many that can impact on choice of food and nutritional status;
- edentulous elders compared with elders with natural teeth consume less fiber, fruits, and vegetables and more fat;
- the relationship between dental status and nutrition is unclear;
- frail elders should be screened routinely for risk of undernutrition and inadequate chewing function;
- prosthodontic treatment should be accompanied with dietary counseling to change dietary behavior if necessary;
- tooth loss disturbs enjoyment of food and ERQoL; and

- food has a very significant social as well as nutritional role in all societies.

REFERENCES

Age Concern. 2006. *Hungry to be Heard. The Scandal of Malnourished Older People in Hospital*. London: Age Concern. Available at www.ageconcern.org.uk/AgeConcern/Documents/Hungry_to_be_Heard_August_2006.pdf (accessed October 31, 2009).

Ahluwalia N. 2004. Aging, nutrition and immune function. *J Nutr Health Aging* 8:2–6.

American Journal of Nursing. 2010. *How to Try This Series: The Edinburgh Feeding Evaluation in Persons with Dementia*. Available at http://links.lww.com/A281 (accessed February 2, 2010).

Bartali B, Salvini S, Turrini A, Lauretani F, Russo CR, Corsi AM, Bandinelli S, D'Amicis A, Palli D, Guralnik JM, and Ferrucci L. 2003. Age and disability affect dietary intake. *J Nutr* 133:2868–73.

Bauer JM, Kaiser MJ, Anthony P, Guigoz Y, and Sieber CC. 2008. The Mini Nutritional Assessment®—Its history, today's practice, and future perspectives. *Nutr Clin Pract* 23:388–96

Blumberg J. 1997. Nutritional needs of seniors. *J Am Coll Nutr* 16:517–23.

Bourre JM. 2006. Effects of nutrients (in foods) on the structure and function of the nervous system: Update of dietary requirements for the brain. Part one: Micronutrients. *J Nutr Health Aging* 10:377–85.

Brachet P, Chanson A, Demigné C, Batifoulier F, Alexandre-Gouabau M-C, Tyssandier V, and Rock E. 2004. Age-associated B vitamin deficiency as a determinant of chronic diseases. *Nutr Res Rev* 17:55–68.

Bradbury J, Thomason JM, Jepson NJA, Walls AWG, Allen PF, and Moynihan PJ. 2006. Nutrition counseling increases fruit and vegetable intake in the edentulous. *J Dent Res* 85:463–8.

Bradbury J, Thomason JM, Jepson NJA, Walls AWG, Mulvaney CE, Allen PF, and Moynihan PJ. 2008. Perceived chewing ability and intake of fruit and vegetables. *J Dent Res* 87:720–5.

Briefel RR, Bialostosky K, Kennedy-Stephenson J, McDowell MA, Ervin RB, and Wright JD. 2000. Zinc intake of the U.S. population: Findings from the third National Health and Nutrition Examination Survey 1988–1994. *J Nutr* 130(Suppl. 5S):13667S–73S.

Brondani MA and MacEntee MI. 2007. The concept of validity in sociodental indicators and oral health-related quality-of-life measures. *Community Dent Oral Epidemiol* 35:472–8.

Caroline Walker Trust. 2004. *Eating Well for Older People*. London: The Caroline Walker Trust. Available at www.cwt.org.uk (accessed November 1, 2009).

Chen HL and Huang YC. 2003. Fiber intake and food selection of the elderly in Taiwan. *Nutrition* 19:332–6.

Chernoff R. 2005. Micronutrient requirements in older women. *Am J Clin Nutr* 81(Suppl.):1240S–5S.

Coull Y. 2003. The importance of nutritional screening in care homes. *Nurs Residential Care* 5:521–4.

Crogan NL and Shultz JA. 2000. Nursing assistants' perceptions of barriers to nutrition care for residents in long-term care facilities. *J Nurses Staff Dev* 16:216–21.

Crogan NL, Schultz JA, Adams CE, and Massey LK. 2001. Barriers to nutrition care for nursing home residents. *J Gerontol Nurs* 27:25–31.

Crook MA. 2009. Hypoalbuminemia: The importance of correct interpretation. *Nutrition* 25:1006–10.

D'Anci KE and Rosenberg IH. 2004. Folate and brain function in the elderly. *Curr Opin Clin Nutr Metab Care* 7:659–64.

Dawson-Hughes B. 2008. Serum 25-hydroxyvitamin D and functional outcomes in the elderly. *Am J Clin Nutr* 88(Suppl.):537S–40S.

De Marchi RJ, Hugo FN, Hilgert JB, and Padilha DMP. 2008. Association between oral health status and nutritional status in south Brazilian independent-living older people. *Nutrition* 24:546–53

Department of Health. 1991. *Dietary Reference Values for Food Energy and Nutrients in the United Kingdom.* Report on Health and Social Subjects No 41. London: HMSO.

Department of Health. 2003. *Care Homes for Older People. National Minimum Standards and the Care Homes Regulations 2001*, 3rd edn. London: TSO. Available at www.dh.gov.uk/en/Publicationsandstatistics/Publications/PublicationsPolicyAndGuidance/DH_4005819 (accessed January 24, 2010).

Dion N, Cotart J-L, and Rabilloud M. 2007. Correction of nutrition test errors for more accurate quantification of the link between dental health and malnutrition. *Nutrition* 23:301–7.

Eisenstaedt R, Penninx BWJH, and Woodman RC. 2006. Anaemia in the elderly: current understanding and emerging concepts. *Blood Rev* 20:213–26.

Elia M. 2003. *The 'MUST' Report. Nutritional Screening of Adults: A Multidisciplinary Responsibility.* Malnutrition Advisory Group, British Association of Parenteral and Enteral Nutrition. Available at www.bapen.org.uk/must_tool.html (accessed December 4, 2009).

Ervin RB and Dye BA. 2009. The effect of functional dentition on Health Eating Index scores and nutrient intakes in a nationally representative sample of older adults. *J Public Health Dent* 69:207–16.

Ettinger RL. 1973. Diet, nutrition, and masticatory ability in a group of elderly edentulous patients. *Aust Dent J* 18:12–9.

Finch S, Doyle W, Lowe C, Bates CJ, Prentice A, Smithers G, and Clarke PC. 1998. *National Diet and Nutrition Survey: People Aged 65 Years and Over, Volume 1: Report of the Diet and Nutrition Survey.* London: TSO.

Fiske J, Davis DM, Frances C, and Gelbier S. 1998. The emotional effects of tooth loss in edentulous people. *Br Dent J* 184:90–3.

Food Standards Agency. 2007. *Guidance on Food Served to Older People in Residential Care.* Available at www.food.gov.uk/multimedia/pdfs/olderresident.pdf (accessed December 4, 2009).

Fujita S and Volpi E. 2004. Nutrition and sarcopenia of ageing. *Nutr Res Rev* 17:69–76.

Gariballa S and Sinclair A. 2005. Ageing and older people. In: Geissler CA and Powers HJ (eds.), *Human Nutrition*, 11th edn. Edinburgh: Elsevier Churchill Livingstone, pp. 319–34.

Gil-Montoya JA, Subirá C, Ramón JM, and González-Moles MA. 2008. Oral health-related quality of life and nutritional status. *J Public Health Dent* 68:88–93.

Green SM and Watson R. 2005. Nutritional screening and assessment tools for use by nurses: Literature review. *J Adv Nurs* 50:69–83.

Green SM and Watson R. 2006. Nutritional screening and assessment tools for older adults: Literature review. *J Adv Nurs* 54:477–90.

Haase H, Mocchegiani E, and Rink L. 2006. Correlation between zinc status and immune function in the elderly. *Biogerontology* 7:421–8.

Hamada MO, Garrett NR, Roumanas ED, Kapur KK, Freymiller E, Han T, Diener RM, Chen T, and Levin S. 2001. A randomized clinical trial comparing the efficacy of mandibular implant-supported overdentures and conventional dentures in diabetic patients. Part IV: Comparisons of dietary intake. *J Prosthet Dent* 85:53–60.

Hargreaves T. 2008. Nutrition: Issues for people with dementia. *Nurs Residential Care* 10:118–22.

Heaney RP. 1986. Calcium, bone health and osteoporosis. In: Peck W (ed.), *Bone and Mineral Research*, Vol. 4. New York: Elsevier, pp. 255–301.

Heath MR. 1982. The effect of maximum biting force and bone loss upon masticatory function and dietary selection of the elderly. *Int Dent J* 32:345–56.

Hilgert JB, Hugo FN, de Sousa MdLR, and Bozzetti MC. 2009. Oral status and its association with obesity in Southern Brazilian older people. *Gerodontology* 26:46–52.

Hung HC, Colditz G, and Joshipura KJ. 2005. The association between tooth loss and the self-reported intake of selected CVD-related nutrients and foods among US women. *Community Dent Oral Epidemiol* 33:167–73.

Hurwitz A, Brady DA, Schaal SE, Samloff IM, Dedon J, and Ruhl CE. 1997. Gastric acidity in older adults. *J Am Med Assoc* 278:659–62.

Institute of Medicine of the National Academies. 2005. *Dietary Reference Intakes for Energy, Carbohydrate, Fiber, Fat, Fatty Acids, Cholesterol, Protein and Amino Acids*. Food and Nutrition Board, Institute of Medicine of the National Academies. Washington DC: National Academies Press.

Jensen GL and Friedman J. 2002. Obesity is associated with functional decline among community-dwelling older persons. *J Am Geriatr Soc* 50:918–23.

Johansson I, Tidehag P, Lundberg V, and Hallmans G. 1994. Dental status, diet and cardiovascular risk-factors in middle-aged people in northern Sweden. *Community Dent Oral Epidemiol* 22:431–6.

Joshipura KJ, Willett W, and Douglass CW. 1996. The impact of edentulousness on food and nutrient intake. *J Am Dent Assoc* 127:459–67.

Krall E, Hayes C, and Garcia R. 1998. How dentition status and masticatory function affect nutrient intake. *J Am Dent Assoc* 129:1261–9.

Lamy M, Mojon P, Kalykakis G, Legrand R, and Butz-Jorgensen E. 1999. Oral status and nutrition in the institutionalized elderly. *J Dent* 27:443–8.

Liedberg B, Stoltze K, Norlén P, and Öwall B. 2007. 'Inadequate' dietary habits and mastication in elderly men. *Gerodontology* 24:41–6.

Little KY, Castellanos X, Humphries LL, and Austin J. 1989. Altered zinc metabolism in mood disorder patients. *Biol Psychiatry* 26:646–8.

Liu S, Manson JE, Lee I-M, Cole SR, Hennekens CH, Willett WC, and Buring JE. 2000. Fruit and vegetable intake and risk of cardiovascular disease: The Women's Health Study. *Am J Clin Nutr* 72:922–8.

Locker D. 1998. Patient-based assessment of the outcomes of implant therapy: A review of the literature. *Int J Prosthodont* 11:453–61.

MacEntee MI, Hole R, and Stolar E. 1997. The significance of the mouth in old age. *Soc Sci Med* 45:1449–58.

MacIntosh C, Morley JE, and Chapman IM. 2000. The anorexia of ageing. *Nutrition* 16:983–95.

Mack F, Abeygunawardhana N, Mundt T, Schwahn C, Proff P, Spassov A, Kocher T, and Biffar R. 2008. The factors associated with body mass index in adults from the Study of Health in Pomerania (SHIP-0), Germany. *J Physiol Pharmacol* 59:5–16.

Marshall TA, Warren JJ, Hand JS, Xie X-J, and Stumbo PJ. 2002. Oral health, nutrient intake and dietary quality in the very old. *J Am Dent Assoc* 133:1369–79.

Maynard M, Gunnell D, Ness AR, Abraham L, Bates CJ, and Blane D. 2005. What influences diet in early old age? Prospective and cross-sectional analyses of the Boyd Orr cohort. *Eur J Public Health* 16:315–23.

McDowell MA, Briefel RR, Alaimo K, Bischof AM, Caughman CR, Carroll MD, Loria CM, and Johnson CL. 1994. Energy and macronutrient intakes of persons ages 2 months and over in the United States: Third National Health and Nutrition Examination Survey, Phase 1, 1988–91. In *Vital and Health Statistics of the Centers for Disease Control and Prevention*, No. 255. Hyattsville, MD: National Centre for Health Statistics.

McNulty H and Scott JM. 2008. Intake and status of folate and related B-vitamins: Considerations and challenges in achieving optimal status. *Br J Nutr* 99(Suppl. 3):S48–54.

Meunier N, O'Connor JM, Maiani G, Cashman KD, Secker DL, Ferry M, Roussel AM, and Coudray C. 2005. Importance of zinc in the elderly: the ZENITH study. *Eur J Clin Nutr* 59(Suppl. 2):S1–4.

Mikkilä V, Räsänen L, Raitakari OT, Pietinen P, and Viikari J. 2005. Consistent dietary patterns identified from childhood to adulthood: The Cardiovascular Risk in Young Finns Study. *Br J Nutr* 93:923–31.

Millwood J and Heath MR. 2000. Food choice by older people: The use of semi-structured interviews with open and closed questions. *Gerodontology* 17:25–32.

Mioche L, Bourdiol P, and Peyron M-A. 2004. Influence of age on mastication: Effects on eating behaviour. *Nutr Res Rev* 17:43–54.

Mojon P, Budtz-Jørgensen E, and Rapin C-H. 1999. Relationship between oral health and nutrition in very old people. *Age Ageing* 28:463–8.

Morais JA, Heydecke G, Pawliuk J, Lund JP, and Feine JS. 2003. The effects of mandibular two-implant overdentures on nutrition in elderly edentulous individuals. *J Dent Res* 82:53–8.

Morley JE. 1997. Anorexia of aging: physiologic and pathologic. *Am J Clin Nutr* 66:760–73.

Moynihan PJ. 2007. The relationship between nutrition and systemic and oral well-being in older people. *J Am Dent Assoc* 138:493–7.

Moynihan PJ, Butler TJ, Thomason JM, and Jepson NJA. 2000. Nutrient intake in partially dentate patients: The effect of prosthetic rehabilitation. *J Dent* 28:557–63.

Müller F, Heath MR, Ferman AM, and Davis GR. 2002. Modulation of mastication during experimental loosening of complete dentures. *Int J Prosthodont* 15:553–8.

Musacchio E, Perissinotto E, Binotto P, Sartori L, Silva-Netto F, Zambon S, Manzato E, Corti MC, Baggio G, and Crepaldi G. 2007. Tooth loss in the elderly and its association with nutritional status, socio-economic and lifestyle factors. *Acta Odontol Scand* 65:78–86.

Neel AB. 2001. Malnutrition in the elderly: Interactions with drug therapy. *Ann Longterm Care* 9:24–34.

Newby PK, Weismayer C, Åkesson A, Tucker KL, and Wolk A. 2006. Long-term stability of food patterns identified by use of factor analysis among Swedish women. *J Nutr* 136:626–33.

Ortega RM, Requejo AM, Andres P, Lopez-Sobaler AM, Quintas ME, Redondo MR, Navia B, and Rivas T. 1997. Dietary intake and cognitive function in a group of elderly people. *Am J Clin Nutr* 66:803–9.

Prinz JF. 1999. Quantitative evaluation of the effect of bolus size and number of chewing strokes on the intra-oral mixing of a two-colour chewing gum. *J Oral Rehabil* 26:243–7.

Rauen MS, Moreira EAM, Calvo MCM, and Lobo AS. 2006. Oral condition and its relationship to nutritional status in the institutionalized elderly population. *J Am Diet Assoc* 106:1112–4.

Roumanas ED, Garrett NR, Hamada MO, Diener RM, and Kapur KK. 2002. A randomized clinical trial comparing the efficacy of mandibular implant-supported overdentures and conventional dentures in diabetic patients. Part V: Food preference comparisons. *J Prosthet Dent* 87:62–73.

Russell CA and Elia M. 2008. *Nutrition Screening Survey in the UK in 2007.* Redditch: BAPEN. Available at www.bapen.org.uk/pdfs/nsw/nsw07_report.pdf (accessed July 23, 2009).

Sadamori S, Hayashi S, and Hamada T. 2008. The relationships between oral status, physical and mental health, nutritional status and diet type in elderly Japanese women with dementia. *Gerodontology* 25:205–9.

Sahyoun NR, Lin C-L, and Krall E. 2003. Nutritional status of the older adult is associated with dentition status. *J Am Diet Assoc* 103:61–6.

Schimmel M, Christou P, Herrmann F, and Müller F. 2007. A two-colour chewing gum test for masticatory efficiency: Development of different assessment methods. *J Oral Rehabil* 34:671–8.

Schneider DL. 2008. Management of osteoporosis in geriatric populations. *Curr Osteoporos Rep* 6:100–7.

Sebring NG, Guckes AD, Li S-H, and McCarthy GR. 1995. Nutritional adequacy of reported intake of edentulous subjects treated with new conventional or implant-supported mandibular dentures. *J Prosthet Dent* 74:358–63.

Sheiham A and Steele J. 2001. Does the condition of the mouth and teeth affect the ability to eat certain foods, nutrient and dietary intake and nutritional status amongst older people? *Public Health Nutr* 4:797–803.

Sheiham A, Steele JG, Marcenes W, Lowe C, Finch S, Bates CJ, Prentice A, and Walls AWG. 2001. The relationship among dental status, nutrient intake, and nutritional status in older people. *J Dent Res* 80:408–13.

Shinkai RSA, Hatch JP, Sakai S, Mobley CC, Saunders MJ, and Rugh JD. 2001. Oral function and diet quality in a community-based sample. *J Dent Res* 80:1625–30.

Shinkai RSA, Hatch JP, Rugh JD, Sakai S, Mobley CC, and Saunders MJ. 2002. Dietary intake in edentulous subjects with good and poor quality complete dentures. *J Prosthet Dent* 87:490–8.

Slade GD. 1997. *Measuring Oral Health and Quality of Life*. Chapel Hill: University of North Carolina, Dental Ecology.

Slade GD and Spencer AJ. 1994a. Development and evaluation of the Oral Health Impact Profile. *Community Dent Health* 11:3–11.

Slade GD and Spencer AJ. 1994b. Social impact of oral conditions among older adults. *Aust Dent J* 39:358–64.

Stanner S. 2007. Older people with dementia: Eating and drinking healthily. *Nurs Residential Care* 9:18–21.

Thomas B. 2001. *Manual of Dietetic Practice*, 3rd edn. Oxford: Blackwell Science Ltd.

Tolson D, Schofield I, Booth J, and Ramsay R. 2002. Nutrition for physically frail older people. *Nurs Times* 98:38–40.

Trulsson U, Engstrand P, Berggren U, Nannmark U, and Brånemark P-I. 2002. Edentulousness and oral rehabilitation: Experiences from the patients' perspective. *Eur J Oral Sci* 110:417–24.

van Kampen FMC, van der Bilt A, Cune MS, Fontijn-Tekamp FA, and Bosman F. 2004. Masticatory function with implant-supported overdentures. *J Dent Res* 83:708–11.

VOICES. 1998. Eating well for older people with dementia. Hertfordshire: VOICES. Available at www.cwt.org.uk/pdfs/Dementia%20Report.pdf (accessed January 24, 2010).

Wakimoto P and Block G. 2001. Dietary intake, dietary patterns, and changes with age: an epidemiological perspective. *J Gerontol A Biol Sci Med Sci* 56A(Special Issue II):65–80.

Watson R and Dreary IJ. 1997. A longitudinal study of feeding difficulty and nursing intervention in elderly patients with dementia. *J Adv Nurs* 26:25–32.

Wolters M, Strohle A, and Hahn A. 2004. Age-associated changes in the metabolism of vitamin B12 and folic acid: Prevalence, aetiopathogenesis and pathophysiological consequences. *Z Gerontol Geriatr* 37:109–35.

World Health Organization. 2006. *Global Database on Body Mass Index. BMI Classification.* Available at http://apps.who.int/bmi/index.jsp?introPage=intro_3.html (accessed July 7, 2009).

World Health Organization. 2003. *Diet, Nutrition and the Prevention of Chronic Diseases.* Technical Report Series 916. Geneva: WHO.

Wöstmann B, Michel K, Brinkert B, Melchheier-Weskott A, Rehmann P, and Balkenhol M. 2008. Influence of denture improvement on the nutritional status and quality of life of geriatric patients. *J Dent* 36:816–21.

Management of periodontal and gingival diseases and other oral disorders in frail elders with cardiovascular disease or diabetes

6

Jim Yuan Lai, H.C. Tenenbaum, and Michael B. Goldberg

INTRODUCTION: THE ORAL-SYSTEMIC CONTINUUM

A clinical challenge

Mr. Yafnaro is 75 years of age. He had periodontal disease that was treated successfully over the past 20 years. However, on his latest clinical examination, his gingival tissues were swollen, they bled on probing, and the periodontal pockets had increased significantly since the previous recording 6 months prior. Now, most of the pockets are deeper than 5 mm, and yet his oral hygiene regimen is moderately effective as before. However, his general health is obviously frailer than previously, and he advises you that he is a "borderline" diabetic. Nonetheless, he reports with enthusiasm that he selects his diet carefully to control the diabetes, and his weight is now closer to the weight he proudly carried as a young man!

What do you think is happening to Mr. Yafnaro, and how do you care for him?

Periodontitis

Periodontitis is a mixed bacterial infection, predominantly caused by gram-negative anaerobic species, resulting from the deposition of plaque and calculus both above and below the gingiva. If left undisturbed, bacterial toxins and other cell-associated products can induce an inflammatory response systemically and within periodontal tissues. The local inflamma-

---

Oral Healthcare and the Frail Elder: A Clinical Perspective.
Edited by Michael I. MacEntee © 2011 Blackwell Publishing Ltd.

tory processes lead to the breakdown of the periodontium, and tooth loss can ensue if left untreated. The goal of periodontal treatment for frail elders is to establish and maintain oral comfort and prevent tooth loss. Consequently, frail people and their carers should know about the importance of oral care and hygiene (Kornman et al., 1994). Treatments of gingivitis and periodontitis should be rendered with minimal stress and control of potential complications. Moreover, dentists occasionally are the first to see signs of diabetes and other systemic diseases that warrant referral to a physician.

Treatment of the early stages of periodontitis consists of scaling and root planing, and in many cases, the response will be a reduction in clinical signs of tissue inflammation, such as erythema, bleeding, and pain on probing, accompanied by reductions in probing depths and tooth mobility. However, in more severe cases, surgery produces a better environment for long-term maintenance of the periodontium. Either way, if periodontal health deteriorates, systemic antibiotic treatment (e.g., metronidazole, metronidazole plus amoxicillin, doxycycline) with or without local antimicrobial therapy (e.g., doxycycline hyclate, minocycline hydrochloride, tetracycline hydrochloride) might be required.

Optimal treatments for younger patients may not necessarily be suitable for frail patients. Nonsurgical treatments supported by good daily oral care, for example, are generally preferable for patients with comorbid systemic illnesses such as cardiovascular diseases (CVDs). Indeed, teeth with quite severe periodontal disease can function quite successfully for several years if managed with a combination of debridement augmented by short-term applications of antimicrobial agents (e.g., metronidazole, doxycycline) for 5–7 days (Loesche et al., 2005).

Periodontitis and systemic disease

The relationship between oral health, diabetes, CVD, and other diseases in elders is complex. Periodontal treatment reduces the levels of risk markers for CVD by decreasing, for instance, serum levels of C-reactive protein and increasing carotid elasticity (Tonetti et al., 2007; Paraskevas et al., 2008). However, despite several untested models or theories, there is no *direct* evidence showing that periodontitis causes CVD. It is important nonetheless to recognize the increased clinical risk of CVD, and the potential of good periodontal care to reduce the risk of CVD, especially in people who are frail. Consequently, the American Academy of Periodontology and the American College of Cardiology jointly recommend that dentists refer patients for a cardiovascular assessment when periodontitis is diagnosed (Friedewald et al., 2009).

In the United States, about one in four newly diagnosed diabetics have overt signs of CVD, while diabetes or glucose intolerance is present in about one-third of the older (>65 years) population (Wilson and Kannel, 2002). People with diabetes are at particular risk to periodontitis, and conversely, periodontal infections increase the severity of diabetes (Grossi and Genco, 1998). Although periodontitis does not necessarily coexist with diabetes in older people (Persson et al., 2003), it does interfere with glucose tolerance and glucose metabolism (Saito et al., 2004; Bullon et al., 2009).

FRAIL ELDERS WITH CVD

Clinical management of frail elders with CVD

Coronary heart disease, congestive heart failure, cerebrovascular disease, peripheral arterial disease, rheumatic heart disease caused by streptococcal infection, congenital heart disease, deep vein thrombosis, and pulmonary embolism are all disorders of the heart and blood vessels (WHO, 2009). Dental treatment, if not managed properly, is associated with pain, anxiety, and discomfort (Vassend, 1993) and may be perceived as a stressful experience. Changes in concentrations of adrenaline and noradrenaline occur in plasma and urine after preparing, restoring, or extracting teeth (Brand et al., 1995a). Furthermore, changes in heart rate and mean systolic and diastolic blood pressure (BP) are induced not only by dental treatment but also by the patient's *anticipation* of the treatment (Brand and Braham-Inpijn, 1996). Hypertensive and borderline hypertensive patients have a systolic BP of >140 mmHg and/or a diastolic BP of >90 mmHg, and their systolic pressure increases by about 5 mmHg when invited merely to describe dental problems (Brand et al., 1995a). The systolic BP in hypertensive patients increases much more markedly than in normotensive patients during scaling and root planing (Singer et al., 1983), administration of local anesthetic (Brand et al., 1995b), and oral surgery (Meiller et al., 1983). The consequences in frail patients with CVD could be serious.

It is wise therefore to provide short appointments with minimal pain or stress. Many dental procedures, including scaling and root planing, require local anesthetic with a vasoconstrictor, at least until inflammation has been reduced. Vasoconstrictors do not always increase BP (Silvestre et al., 2001), but from a clinical perspective, it is prudent to avoid epinephrine altogether or reduce it as much as possible in patients with CVD (Vernale, 1960).

Management of patients on cardiovascular drugs

Some drugs used in the treatment or prevention of CVDs increase the risk of bleeding. Anticoagulants, such as warfarin, are used widely to prevent blood clots in patients at risk of atrial fibrillation or other thromboembolic diseases, but they can cause serious bleeding when scaling teeth, especially if gingival inflammation is severe. Similarly, excessive bleeding causing hypovolemic shock can occur anytime up to 12h after scaling teeth for patients on antiplatelet agents, such as acetylsalicylic acid (ASA), ticlopidine, clopidogrel, or dipyridamole (Elad et al., 2008). Indeed, posttreatment bleeding is more likely to occur after scaling and root planing than after surgery, particularly in patients on anticoagulants.

Typically, 81 mg/day of ASA is the preventive dose for patients with CVD, and it would make sense to reduce the dose in frail elderly to somewhere in the range of 50 mg/day, but there is no empirical evidence to support this practice.

Management of patients on antiplatelet or anticoagulant therapy is best conducted with local hemostatic methods, such as sutures and direct packing of surgical sites with gauze, resorbable gelatin sponge, oxidized cellulose, or microfibrillar collagen (Brennan et al., 2007), and in some cases it is necessary to use a surgical stent (Figure 6.1) to retain a dressing on a periodontal wound.

Systemic antibiotics will reduce gingival bleeding and the depth of periodontal pockets in healthy patients with moderate to severe periodontitis (Kornman et al., 1994). Consequently, frail patients can be treated similarly with a combination of systemic and/or locally applied antimicrobial tetra-

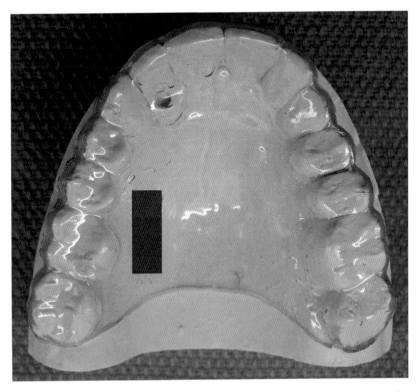

Figure 6.1 A surgical stent made with clear acrylic resin on a cast to cover the site of the planned surgical wound (shown in red).

cycline derivatives, such as minocycline hydrochloride (e.g., Arestin® [OraPharm Inc., Warminster, PA]/minocycline spheres, or Atridox® [Tolmar Inc., Fort Collins, CO]/doxycycline gel) about 2–3 weeks prior to scaling, root planing, or other surgery. They will reduce postscaling bleeding and infection, permit more efficient surgery, and shorten the length of the surgery. However, some antibiotics, in particular metronidazole, will alter warfarin metabolism and increase bleeding by increasing the international normalized ratio (INR). Therefore INR should be monitored more closely while the patient is taking metronidazole. If the patient is taking metronidazole concurrently with scaling or surgery, INR and possibly bleeding time should be determined before scaling and surgery to control and avoid dangerous postsurgical bleeds (Wood and Deeble, 1993). There is some evidence that posttreatment bleeding is not increased when patients are on antihemostatic medications (Napeñas et al., 2009), but there is also at least one report of a very severe postoperative bleed from a patient who was taking a low-dose ASA (Elad et al., 2008). To err on the side of caution though, it is not a good idea to cease anticoagulant treatment prior to invasive dental treatment, but it is always a good idea to consult with the patient's physician in case severe bleeding becomes a problem.

Drug-induced periodontal disorders

About one in five people on calcium channel-blocking medications such as nifedipine or amlodipine for coronary artery spasm can get gingival hyperplasia, particularly elders with poor oral hygiene and severe gingivitis (Miranda et al., 2001; Eslami et al., 2004; Lafzi et al., 2006).

MANAGEMENT OF OTHER ORAL DISORDERS IN FRAIL PATIENTS WITH CVDs

Oral infectious diseases as risk factors for CVDs

The link between dental surgery and bacterial endocarditis is well established (Lacassin et al., 1995; Li et al., 2000). Periodontitis increases the risk of CVD by at least 19%, presumably by increasing the risks for vascular calcification and hypertension (Yalda et al., 1994; Grossi 2001; Mercado et al., 2001; Glurich et al., 2002; Janket et al., 2003; Bahekar et al., 2007; Persson and Persson, 2008; Eddington et al., 2009).

CLINICAL MANAGEMENT OF THE FRAIL ELDERS WITH DIABETES

Diabetes is characterized by hyperglycemia due to an absolute or relative deficiency of insulin. It is categorized as type 1 or insulin dependent, which occurs at a young age, and type 2 or noninsulin dependent, which is much more prevalent and occurs typically in old age when insulin fails to promote the metabolic ingestion of glucose (Lalla and D'Ambrosio, 2001; Moore et al., 2003).

Typically, the management of type 2 diabetes combines diet, exercise, weight reduction, and medication, and dentists usually consult the patient's physician for blood levels of glycated hemoglobin (HbA1c), which should be <7% if the sugar levels in the blood are under control (Mealey, 2008). However, only about one-third of type 2 diabetics attain an HbA1c of <7% (Koro et al., 2004), so sugar control is likely to be even poorer among frail elders.

In general, diabetic patients fair better in the morning when higher cortisol levels increase blood sugar (Hucklebridge et al., 1999). A serum assay of the fasting glucose level in the blood is possible (e.g., in a hospital-based practice, or if request by dentist that MD order such a test on the day of treatment) and all but emergency treatment should be postponed if the level is above 6 mmol/L (Alexander, 1999). Normally, antibiotic prophylaxis is unnecessary for diabetic patients unless emergency surgery is required when the glucose level is high (Alexander 1999; Tong and Rothwell, 2000).

Hypoglycemia during dental treatment is an additional concern with the frail patient who has diminished responses of glucagon, and epinephrine to hypoglycemia, particularly if cognitively impaired and unaware of their weakened condition (Meneilly et al., 1994; Chau and Edelman, 2001). Vasoconstrictors, such as epinephrine, and ASA are best avoided during treatment because of risky hyperglycemic effects (Gerich et al., 1976; Lalla & D'Ambrosio, 2001). If a glycemic episode, which typically mimics syncope, is suspected, dental treatment should be terminated and a fast-acting oral carbohydrate (e.g., orange juice) should be administered immediately (Lalla & D'Ambrosio, 2001).

MANAGEMENT OF PERIODONTAL CONDITIONS IN FRAIL ELDERS WITH DIABETES

Diabetics in general are prone to severe gingivitis and periodontitis as the "sixth complication of diabetes" (Loe, 1993; Taylor et al., 1996), but effective management of the periodontitis helps control glycemic levels (Mealey and Oates, 2006). Frail patients with poorly controlled diabetes will have increased infection and slow healing of wounds; therefore, it is prudent, when possible, to avoid surgery (Galili et al., 1994). Of course they will need good oral hygiene, supplemented by dental scaling, to prevent gingival and periodontal diseases. The diabetic patient who smokes tobacco is at even greater risk of periodontitis and tooth loss, but unfortunately, their nicotine addiction is very difficult to overcome (Hays et al., 2001).

MANAGEMENT OF OTHER ORAL CONDITIONS IN THE ELDERLY FRAIL PATIENT WITH DIABETES

Acute periodontal abscess

Multiple periodontal abscesses are a sign of uncontrolled diabetes. Systemic antimicrobial therapy including medications such as metronidazole, doxy-cycline, or clindamycin in combination with local debridement of the affected area, preferably without raising a surgical flap, should help relieve the acute problem after consulting the patient's physician to control the diabetes.

Fungal infections

Diabetic patients, especially with complete or partial dentures, nicotine addiction, and salivary hypofunction, are predisposed to denture stomatitis, angular cheilitis, median rhomboid glossitis, and other mycotic infections (Guggenheimer et al., 2000; Vernillo, 2003). Topical agents, such as nystatin, or systemic agents, such as fluconazole and ketoconazole, are helpful, but avoid clotrimazole troches because they contain sugar (Vernillo, 2003). Nystatin is the safest antimycotic agent (Figure 6.2). It is not absorbed systemically through the mucosa, so it can also be swallowed if pharyngeal candidal growth is suspected.

Lichen planus

Lichen planus of unknown cause is an intense mucocutaneous rash that occasionally occurs in frail patients with diabetes (Lundstrom, 1983). It can be controlled with topical corticosteroids, such as betamethasone ointment (Figure 6.3). Do not use a cream because it dissolves quickly in the mouth.

> RX: Nystatin 100,000 unit/ml suspension
>
> Dispense: 1 litre
> Label: Rinse with 15 ml for 30 seconds and expectorate q4-6 hours for 1-2 weeks.
>
>   Dr. Gram Goodgum DMD

Figure 6.2   A prescription for candidiasis.

RX: Betamethasone ointment 0.1% combined with mycostatin ointment (ratio of 70% betamethasone to 30% mycostatin).

Dispense: 20 grams
Label: Apply ointment to mouth sores 3-4 times daily for 2 weeks.

Dr. Gram Goodgum DMD

Figure 6.3   A prescription for lichen planus.

RX: 3-4% Hydrocortisone; 250 ml Benadryl elixir; 250 ml Distilled water, and 50 ml Mycostatin suspension.

Dispense: 1 bottle
Label: Shake well, and rinse with 15 ml for 30 seconds and expectorate TID.

Dr. Gram Goodgum DMD

Figure 6.4   A prescription for painful erosive lichen planus.

Pain can persist as a consequence of neuropathy, and topical corticosteroid must be used cautiously in diabetic patients because the steroid is absorbed systemically. The dose should be reduced if fluid retention is suspected based on a patient's description of weight gain or swelling of the ankles, other extremities, or of the face.

A mouthrinse containing 3%–4% hydrocortisone, 250 mL of benadryl elixir, 250 mL of distilled water, and 50 mL of mycostatin suspension is more effective for managing mucocutaneous lesions such as erosive lichen planus that are painful (Figure 6.4). The mouthrinse is used more or less permanently to manage the erosive lichen planus. Since it is expectorated, the systemic effects should be minimal to none. However, brittle diabetics must be told to monitor their blood sugars more frequently when using the rinse because excess absorption of hydrocortisone, albeit unanticipated, can increase glucose levels.

BIDIRECTIONAL ASSOCIATION BETWEEN DIABETES AND GINGIVOPERIODONTITIS

The presence of diabetes can lead to a two- to threefold increase in the risk for periodontitis, while there is a sixfold increase in the risk of poor glycemic control in diabetic patients with severe periodontitis (Taylor et al., 1996). So, there is mounting evidence that the presence of periodontitis indicates that a patient is at risk for diabetes (Demmer et al., 2008). Explanations for the association between periodontal disease and diabetes include decreased collagen production, reduced polymorphonuclear neutrophil function, and the accumulation of advanced glycation end products (AGEs) in the periodontium (Perrino, 2007). Increased immunoreactivity for AGEs does occur in the gingiva of diabetics (Schmidt et al., 1996). The AGEs bind to a receptor on the surface of endothelial cells and monocytes to increase the level of inflammatory mediators such as tumor necrosis factor (TNF)-alpha, interleukin-1 (IL1), and interleukin-6 (IL6). This leads to a state of enhanced oxidant stress, which is a potential explanation for accelerated tissue injury and destruction (Schmidt et al., 1996; Lalla et al., 2001; Perrino, 2007). TNF-alpha, IL1, and IL6 are involved in insulin resistance (Nishimura et al., 2003; Tilg and Moschen, 2008), as are acute and possibly chronic infections of the gingiva and periodontium (Sammalkorpi, 1989; Yki-Jarvinen et al., 1989). Therefore, there is probably a bidirectional association between gingivoperiodontitis and diabetes where exacerbation of one disease can exacerbate the other (Grossi and Genco, 1998; Mealey and Oates, 2006; Mealey, 2008).

Furthermore, when periodontitis is reduced in diabetic patients, so too is the HbA1c (Janket et al., 2005; Kiran et al., 2005). However, reduced HbA1c will not predict improved periodontal health, and the extent of the relationship needs further explanation (Aldridge et al., 1995; Grossi et al., 1997; Christgau et al., 1998). Nevertheless, the important point is that periodontal health can deteriorate rapidly in patients with poor metabolic control, and if placed on a maintenance program for strict plaque control at 3-month intervals, the initial healing appears to be maintained in the long term (Gustke, 1999). The most important factor is that patients with diabetes should be managed carefully to maintain optimal gingival and periodontal health. Moreover, when a frail patient presents with severe periodontitis, the presence of diabetes must be considered seriously.

THE FUTURE

We now understand that AGEs, such as HbA1c produced in diabetics, exacerbate inflammation and participate in the disease process rather than

Table 6.1 Target range[a] for glycemic control.

Range at time of test	
Before meals	2h after a meal
4–7 mmol/L	5–10 mmol/L

[a]Imran and Ross (2008).

Clinical scenario (action)

It is very likely that Mr. Yafnaro is not controlling his diet or his diabetes adequately. He should be asked whether he tests his glucose levels daily, and if so, what the results are. If his blood glucose levels are elevated (e.g., 9 mM from time to time), he should be referred back to his physician for additional assessment and management. Even if his glucose readings are within normal limits (Table 6.1), Mr. Yafnaro should return to his MD for reevaluation.

Do not refer Mr. Yafnaro to his physician with the general request for a "workup." This is nonspecific and the physician might misinterpret the referral as a request for general management of the disease rather than a professionally informed concern about the current status of Mr. Yafnaro's diabetes. It is wiser to inform the physician that Mr. Yafnaro's periodontal disease, which was well controlled, is again unstable without any obvious changes in his oral hygiene or dental management regimen. Consequently, the referral should state explicitly that the diabetes is probably out of control.

It is appropriate also to request that random and fasting glucose levels be assayed along with a test for HbA1c.

Presuming abnormal results are found, and Mr. Yafnaro, with help from his physician, has managed to regain control of his diabetes by adjusting medications and/or more assiduous dietary control, his periodontal status should improve noticeably within a few weeks. At the same time, given the bidirectional relationship between diabetes and periodontitis, he should receive more frequent scaling and probably a prescription for a 0.12% chlorhexidine mouthrinse (Figure 6.5) until both the diabetes and periodontitis are fully control, and Mr. Yafnaro can return to a more carefully monitored regimen by both his physician and his dentist who should continue to work together to maintain Mr. Yafnaro's health and reduce his frailty.

merely being indicators of the disease. Similarly, these products increase periodontal inflammation and alter collagen metabolism, all of which can worsen periodontal disease (Chong et al., 2007) It is possible in the future that synthetic analogues of AGEs, used therapeutically, can replace the natural AGEs without precipitating the negative associations between periodontal diseases and diabetes (Lalla et al., 2000). Indeed, the existence of these complex interrelationships hints at the possibility of periodontitis as a syndromic disorder associated with a wide array of disorders ranging from diabetes to CVD.

RX: 0.12% Chlorhexidine.

Dispense: 1 bottle
Label: Shake well, and
rinse with 15 ml for 30
seconds and expectorate
TID.

Dr. Gram Goodgum DMD

Figure 6.5   A prescription for gingivitis and periodontitis.

CONCLUSIONS

Maintenance of oral health and management of periodontal and oral diseases for frail elders should reduce the risk for CVD and diabetes. Management of frail people is often limited to palliative care by the fear that they might not tolerate periodontal treatment. However, elderly people are frequently more robust physically and psychologically—even if frail—than many clinicians recognize. Consequently, we recommend that periodontal diseases can and should be managed quite aggressively in frail elders, with the aim of reducing the risk of more serious diseases and their complications. Frail patients should be maintained for as long as possible to insure an acceptable quality of life free of oral discomfort and distress.

REFERENCES

Aldridge JP, Lester V, Watts TL, Collins A, Viberti G, and Wilson RF. 1995. Single-blind studies of the effects of improved periodontal health on metabolic control in type 1 diabetes mellitus. *J Clin Periodontol* 22:271–5.

Alexander RE. 1999. Routine prophylactic antibiotic use in diabetic dental patients. *J Calif Dent Assoc* 8:611–8.

Bahekar AA, Singh S, Saha S, Molnar J, and Arora R. 2007. The prevalence and incidence of coronary heart disease is significantly increased in periodontitis: A meta-analysis. *Am Heart J* 154:830–6.

Brand HS and Braham-Inpijn L. 1996. Cardiovascular responses induced by dental treatment. *Eur J Oral Sci* 104:245–52.

Brand HS, Gortzak RA, and Braham-Inpijn L. 1995a. Anxiety and heart rate correlation prior to dental checkup. *Int Dent J* 45:347–51.

Brand HS, Gortzak RA, Palmer-Bouva CC, Abraham RE, and Braham-Inpijn L. 1995b. Cardiovascular and neuroendocrine responses during acute stress induced by different types of dental treatment. *Int Dent J* 45:45–8.

Brennan MT, Wynn RL, and Miller CS. 2007. Aspirin and bleeding in dentistry: An update and recommendations. *Oral Surg Oral Med Oral Pathol Oral Radiol Endod* 104:316–23.

Bullon P, Morillo JM, Ramirez-Tortosa MC, Quiles JL, Newman HN, and Battino M. 2009. Metabolic syndrome and periodontitis: Is oxidative stress a common link? *J Dent Res* 88:503–18.

Chau D and Edelman SV. 2001. Clinical management of diabetes in the elderly. *Clin Diabetes* 19:172–5.

Christgau M, Palitzsch KD, Schmalz G, Kreiner U, and Frenzel S. 1998. Healing response to non-surgical periodontal therapy in patients with diabetes mellitus: Clinical, microbiological, and immunologic results. *J Clin Periodontol* 25:112–24.

Chong SAC, Lee W, Arora PD, Laschinger C, Young EWK, Simmons CA, Manolson M, Sodek J, and McCulloch CA. 2007. Methylglyoxal inhibits the binding step of collagen phagocytosis. *J Biol Chem* 282:8510–20.

Demmer RT, Jacobs DR Jr., and Desvarieux M. 2008. Periodontal disease and incident type 2 diabetes: Results from the First National Health and Nutrition Examination Survey and its epidemiologic follow-up study. *Diabetes Care* 31:1373–9.

Eddington H, Sinha S, Li E, Hegarty J, Ting J, Lane B, Chrysochou C, Foley R, O'Donoghue D, Kalra PA, and Middleton R. 2009. Factors associated with vascular stiffness: Cross-sectional analysis from the chronic renal insufficiency standards implementation study. *Nephron Clin Pract* 112:c190–8.

Elad S, Chackartchi T, Shapira L, and Findler M. 2008. A critically severe gingival bleeding following non-surgical periodontal treatment in patients medicated with anti-platelet. *J Clin Periodontol* 35:342–5.

Eslami M, Baghaii F, and Nadery J. 2004. An investigation on gingival hyperplasia induced by nifedipine. *J Dent* 1:33–6.

Friedewald VE, Kornman KS, Beck JD, Genco R, Goldfine A, Libby P, Offenbacher S, Ridker PM, Van Dyke TE, and Roberts WC. 2009. *The American Journal of Cardiology* and *Journal of Periodontology* editors' consensus: Periodontitis and atherosclerotic cardiovascular disease. *J Periodontol* 80:1021–32.

Galili D, Findler M, and Garfunkel AA. 1994. Oral and dental complications associated with diabetes and their treatment. *Compendium* 15:496,498,500–9.

Gerich JE, Lorenzi M, Tsalikian E, and Karam JH. 1976. Studies on the mechanism of epinephrine-induced hyperglycemia in man. Evidence for participation of pancreatic glucagon secretion. *Diabetes* 25:65–71.

Glurich I, Glurich I, Grossi S, Albini B, Ho A, Shah R, Zeid M, Baumann H, Genco RJ, and De Nardin E. 2002. Systemic inflammation in cardiovascular and periodontal disease: Comparative study. *Clin Diagn Lab Immunol* 9:425–32.

Grossi SG. 2001. Treatment of periodontal disease and control of diabetes: An assessment of the evidence and need for future research. *Ann Periodontol* 6:138–45.

Grossi SG and Genco RJ. 1998. Periodontal disease and diabetes mellitus: A two-way relationship. *Ann Periodontol* 3:51–61.

Grossi SG, Skrepcinski FB, DeCaro T, Robertson DC, Ho AW, Dunford RG, and Genco RJ. 1997. Treatment of periodontal disease in diabetics reduces glycated hemoglobin. *J Periodontol* 68:713–9.

Guggenheimer J, Moore PA, Rossie K, Myers D, Mongelluzzo MB, Block HM, Weyant R, and Orchard T. 2000. Insulin-dependent diabetes mellitus and oral soft tissue pathologies: II. Prevalence and characteristics of candida and candidal lesions. *Oral Surg Oral Med Oral Pathol Oral Radiol Endod* 89:570–6.

Gustke CJ. 1999. Treatment of periodontitis in the diabetic patient. A critical review. *J Clin Periodontol* 26:133–6.

Hays JT, Hurt RD, Rigotti NA, Niaura R, Gonzales D, Durcan MJ, Sachs DP, Wolter TD, Buist AS, Johnston JA, and White JD. 2001. Sustained-release bupropion for pharmacologic relapse prevention after smoking cessation. A randomized, controlled trial. *Ann Intern Med* 135:423–33.

Hucklebridge FH, Clow A, Abeyguneratne T, Huezo-Diaz P, and Evans P.1999. The awakening cortisol response and blood glucose levels. *Life Sci* 64:931–6.

Imran SA and Ross SA. 2008. Targets for glycemic control. In Canadian Diabetes Association Clinical Practice Guidelines Expert Committee. Canadian Diabetes Association 2008 clinical practice guidelines for the pre-vention and management of diabetes in Canada. *Can J Diabetes* 32(Suppl. 1):S29–31.

Janket SJ, Baird AE, Chuang SK, and Jones JA. 2003. Meta-analysis of periodon-tal disease and risk of coronary heart disease and stroke. *Oral Surg Oral Med Oral Pathol Oral Radiol Endod* 95:559–69.

Janket SJ, Wightman A, Baird AE, Van Dyke TE, and Jones JA. 2005. Does periodontal treatment improve glycemic control in diabetic patients? A meta-analysis of intervention studies. *J Dent Res* 84:1154–9.

Kiran M, Arpak N, Unsal E, and Erdogan MF. 2005. The effect of improved periodontal health on metabolic control in type 2 diabetes mellitus. *J Clin Periodontol* 32:266–72.

Kornman KS, Newman MG, Moore DJ, and Singer RE. 1994. The influence of supragingival plaque control on clinical and microbial outcomes following the use of antibiotics for the treatment of periodontitis. *J Periodontol* 65:848–54.

Koro CE, Bowlin SJ, Bourgeois N, and Fedder DO. 2004. Glycemic control from 1988 to 2000 among U.S. adults diagnosed with type 2 diabetes: A prelimi-nary report. *Diabetes Care* 27:17–20.

Lacassin F, Hoen B, Leport C, Selton-Suty C, Delahaye F, Goulet V, Etienne J, and Briançon S. 1995. Procedures associated with infective endocarditis in adults. A case control study. *Eur Heart J* 16:1968–74.

Lafzi A, Farahani RM, and Shoja MA. 2006. Amlodipine-induced gingival hyperplasia. *Med Oral Patol Oral Cir Bucal* 11:E480–2.

Lalla RV and D'Ambrosio JA. 2001. Dental management considerations for the patient with diabetes mellitus. *J Am Dent Assoc* 132:1425–32.

Lalla E, Lamster IB, Feit M, Huang L, Spessot A, Qu W, Kislinger T, Lu Y, Stern DM, and Schmidt AM. 2000. Blockade of RAGE suppresses periodontitis associated bone loss in diabetic mice. *J Clin Invest* 105:1117–24.

Lalla E, Lamster IB, Stern DM, and Schmidt AM. 2001. Receptor for advanced glycation end products, inflammation, and accelerated periodontal disease in diabetes: Mechanisms and insights into therapeutic modalities. *Ann Periodontol* 6:113–8.

Li X, Kolltveit KM, Tronstad L, and Olsen I. 2000. Systemic diseases caused by oral infection. *Clin Microbiol Rev* 13:547–58.

Loe H. 1993. Periodontal disease. The sixth complication of diabetes mellitus. *Diabetes Care* 16:329–34.

Loesche WJ, Giordano JR, Soehren S, and Kaciroti N. 2005. The nonsurgical treatment of patients with periodontal disease: Results after 6.4 years. *Gen Dent* 53:298–306.

Lundstrom IM. 1983. Incidence of diabetes mellitus in patients with oral lichen planus. *Int J Oral Surg* 12:147–52.

Mealey BL. 2008. The interactions between physicians and dentists in managing the care of patients with diabetes mellitus. *J Am Dent Assoc* 139(Suppl.):4S–7S.

Mealey BL and Oates TW. 2006. Diabetes mellitus and periodontal diseases. *J Periodontol* 77:1289–303.

Meiller TF, Overholser CD, Kutcher MJ, and Bennett R. 1983. Blood pressure fluctuations in hypertensive patients during oral surgery. *J Oral Maxillofac Surg* 41:715–8.

Meneilly GS, Cheung E, and Tuokko H. 1994. Altered responses to hypoglycemia of healthy elderly people. *J Clin Endocrinol Metab* 78:1341–8.

Mercado FB, Marshall RI, Klestov AC, and Bartold PM. 2001. Relationship between rheumatoid arthritis and periodontitis. *J Periodontol* 72:779–86.

Miranda J, Brunet L, Roset P, Berini L, Farre M, and Mendieta C. 2001. Prevalence and risk of gingival enlargement in patients treated with nifedipine. *J Periodontol* 72:605–11.

Moore PA, Zgibor JC, and Dasanayake AP. 2003. Diabetes: A growing epidemic of all ages. *J Am Dent Assoc* 134(Spec No):11S–15S.

Napeñas JJ, Hong CH, Brennan MT, Furney SL, Fox PC, and Lockhart PB. 2009. The frequency of bleeding complications after invasive dental treatment in patients receiving single and dual antiplatelet therapy. *J Am Dent Assoc* 140:690–5.

Nishimura F, Iwamoto Y, Mineshiba J, Shimizu A, Soga Y, and Murayama Y. 2003. Periodontal disease and diabetes mellitus: The role of tumor necrosis factor-alpha in a 2-way relationship. *J Periodontol* 74:97–102.

Paraskevas S, Huizinga JD, and Loos BG. 2008. A systematic review and meta-analyses on C-reactive protein in relation to periodontitis. *J Clin Periodontol* 35:277–90.

Perrino MA. 2007. Diabetes and periodontal disease: An example of an oral/systemic relationship. *N Y State Dent J* 73:38–41.

Persson GR and Persson RE. 2008. Cardiovascular disease and periodontitis: An update on the associations and risk. *J Clin Periodontol* 35(Suppl. 8):362–79.

Persson RE, Hollender LG, MacEntee MI, Wyatt CC, Kiyak HA, and Persson GR. 2003. Assessment of periodontal conditions and systemic disease in older subjects. *J Clin Periodontol* 30:207–13.

Saito T, Shimazaki Y, Kiyohara Y, Kato I, Kubo M, Iida M, and Koga T. 2004. The severity of periodontal disease is associated with the development of glucose intolerance in non-diabetics: The Hisayama study. *J Dent Res* 83:485–90.

Sammalkorpi K. 1989. Glucose intolerance in acute infections. *J Intern Med* 225:15–9.

Schmidt AM, Weidman E, Lalla E, Yan SD, Hori O, Cao R, Brett JG, and Lamster IB. 1996. Advanced glycation endproducts (AGEs) induce oxidant stress in the gingiva: A potential mechanism underlying accelerated periodontal disease associated with diabetes. *J Periodontal Res* 31:508–15.

Silvestre FJ, Verdu MJ, Sanchis JM, Grau D, and Penarrocha M. 2001. Effects of vasoconstrictors in dentistry upon systolic and diastolic arterial pressure. *Med Oral* 6:57–63.

Singer J, Meiller TF, and Rubinstein L. 1983. Blood pressure fluctuations during dental hygiene treatment. *Dent Hyg* 57:24–6,28.

Taylor GW, Burt BA, Becker MP, Genco RJ, Shlossman M, Knowler WC, and Pettitt DJ. 1996. Severe periodontitis and risk for poor glycemic control in patients with non-insulin-dependent diabetes mellitus. *J Periodontol* 67(Suppl. 10):1085–93.

Tilg H and Moschen AR. 2008. Inflammatory mechanisms in the regulation of insulin resistance. *Mol Med* 14:222–31.

Tonetti MS, D'Aiuto F, Nibali L, Donald A, Storry C, Parkar M, Suvan J, Hingorani AD, Vallance P, and Deanfield J. 2007. Treatment of periodontitis and endothelial function. *N Engl J Med* 356:911–20.

Tong DC and Rothwell BR. 2000. Antibiotic prophylaxis in dentistry: A review and practice recommendations. *J Am Dent Assoc* 131:366–74.

Vassend O. 1993. Anxiety, pain and discomfort associated with dental treatment. *Behav Res Ther* 31:659–66.

Vernale CA. 1960. Cardiovascular responses to local dental anesthesia with epinephrine in normotensive and hypertensive subjects. *Oral Surg Oral Med Oral Pathol* 13:942–52.

Vernillo AT. 2003. Dental considerations for the treatment of patients with diabetes mellitus. *J Am Dent Assoc* 134:24S–33S.

Wilson PW and Kannel WB. 2002. Obesity, diabetes, and risk of cardiovascular disease in the elderly. *Am J Geriatr Cardiol* 11:119–23,125.

Wood GD and Deeble T. 1993. Warfarin: Dangers with antibiotics. *Dent Update* 20:350,352–3.

WHO. 2009. *Cardiovascular Diseases*. Geneva: World Health Organization. Available at www.who.int/mediacentre/factsheets/fs317/en/index.html (accessed November 4, 2009)

Yalda B, Offenbacher S, and Collins JG. 1994. Diabetes as a modifier of periodontal disease expression. *Periodontol 2000* 6:37–49.

Yki-Jarvinen H, Sammalkorpi K, Koivisto VA, and Nikkila EA. 1989. Severity, duration, and mechanisms of insulin resistance during acute infections. *J Clin Endocrinol Metab* 69:317–23.

Oral health, dysphagia, and aspiration pneumonia

Marcia Carr, Lynda McKeown, and Michael I. MacEntee

INTRODUCTION

Dysphagia is a condition in which there is difficulty swallowing (Logemann, 1998). It occurs in less than 10% of the general population, and in at least half of the elderly population in long-term care facilities (Achem and Devault, 2005). Indeed, most people who are frail have difficulties at meal-times not only because of dysphagia but also because of postural difficulties, defective hand-to-mouth coordination, cognitive–behavioral problems, and defective dentures (Steele et al., 1997). The aims of this chapter are to describe how oral ill health and dysphagia are associated with aspiration pneumonia, and explain how interdisciplinary and patient-centered care can sustain oral health and prevent aspiration pneumonia.

The mouth is a portal through which air passes with oxygen to the lungs and food and drink pass with sustenance and pleasure to the stomach. However, the mouth can also harbor great distress when bacterial and viral infections upset general health and comfort, and inhibit our ability to thrive, especially if we are frail (MacEntee et al., 1997). Bacteria proliferate in food debris that accumulates in the mouth when oral hygiene is neglected. They infect the biofilm of the oral mucosa, gingiva, periodontium, and teeth to precipitate mucositis, gingivitis, periodontitis, and caries. However, many of these bacteria have been isolated also from the lungs with pneumonia, which leads to an assumption that accumulations of oral bacteria are significant risk factors for pneumonia (Mojon and Bourbeau, 2003; Sumi et al., 2006; Yoon and Steele, 2007; Abe et al., 2008; Weed, 2009). The risk is magnified even further when an elderly person has dysphagia and the

Oral Healthcare and the Frail Elder: A Clinical Perspective.
Edited by Michael I. MacEntee © 2011 Blackwell Publishing Ltd.

laryngeal valve is defective. Dentists, dental hygienists, and other health-care professionals who are aware of dysphagia can help reduce the risks associated with this disorder by managing the daily routines of oral hygiene and by maintaining the dentition as frailty increases.

DYSPHAGIA, ASPIRATION PNEUMONIA, AND ORAL HEALTH

Swallowing and dysphagia

We rarely think about swallowing until something goes wrong, and there is an unsettling feeling that something "went down the wrong way." Usually, when this happens, we cough and retch until the misdirected food or drink is retrieved from the airway. It can be transient from postsurgical weakness or sedation, or persistent from degenerative disorders—such as Parkinson's disease, stroke, advanced dementia, or kyphotic curves from osteoporosis in the spine—all disorders associated with frailty and a weak-ening of one or more of the 26 muscle groups involved in swallowing (Buettner et al., 2001). Consequently, in an effort to avoid the distress of dysphagia, the risk of dehydration and malnutrition increases as control over swallowing weakens.

DYSPHAGIA IN FOUR STAGES

Swallowing is a four-stage process from initial placement of food in the mouth to the entry of the food into the stomach (Ertekin and Aydogdu, 2003; Paik, 2008). Difficulties at each stage can shunt food, fluid, and saliva into the trachea rather than the esophagus, and if the mouth is infected with excessive numbers of pathogenic bacteria, the risk for aspiration pneumonia is high (Shay et al., 2005; Awano et al., 2008).

Presentation of food

People who have difficulty swallowing tend to decrease their consumption of food and drink. Occasionally, they will change the texture and consis-tency of food by overcooking or liquefying it, but mashed or pureed foods looks unappetizing and unpleasant.

Posture for optimal swallowing and oral hygiene

Receiving and swallowing food and drink is easiest when the trunk of the body upright, in midline position, and the head and chin slightly flexed downward (Trombly and Radomski, 2002). An appropriate posture to straighten the oesophagus, preferably seated at a table (Figure 7.1a) or

(a) Seated at a table

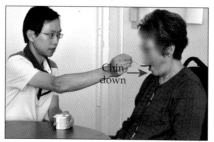

(c) Support for knees and pelvis

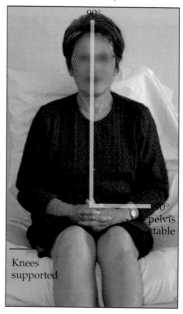

(b) Propped up in bed

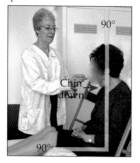

Figure 7.1 Optimal seating posture for swallowing.

propped up in bed (Figure 7.1b) will ease the passage of food and drink into the esophagus and the stomach.

This posture is easily obtained by sitting upright with feet on the floor or on the foot pedals of a wheelchair, and arms on the arm rests. Similarly, eating and swallowing is easier in bed when the back and sides are supported by pillows or by adjusting the bed to produce the same comfortable orientation of the head and neck to the rest of the body. A roll placed under the knees helps also to remain stabile in this flexed position (Figure 7.1c).

Elders with neuromusculoskeletal deficiencies from a stroke or other disorders that cause difficulty with upright posture frequently require special supports or positioning devices to achieve and maintain head and neck alignment (Paik, 2008). The chin, when preparing to swallow, can be lowered in the "chin down" position to allow food to move down the throat while protecting the airway. Alternatively, retraction of the mandible in the "chin tuck" position reduces the space between the tongue and the posterior wall of the pharynx, which increases pressure to propel the food bolus through pharynx past a narrowed entrance to the airway. Either postural support should remain in place for at least 30 min, and preferably 2 h, after the meal to reduce the possibility of gastroesophageal reflux and aspiration (Wolf and Glass, 1992).

The optimal posture of the head and neck for oral hygiene is the same as for swallowing to prevent aspiration of water or toothpaste. Special toothbrushes (e.g., Plak-Vac®, Trademark Medical, St. Louis, MO) or other suction devices also help to reduce the possibility of aspirating fluids into the airway.

Preparing to swallow

A water spray or moist towel will ease the discomfort of dry lips and a dry mouth while food that looks and smells appealingly will serve as a stimulant to the appetite and to the flow of saliva. The natural teeth and dentures along with the tongue, gingival, and all of the oral mucosa should be brushed frequently—preferably twice daily—to remove microbial plaque. This will lessen the numbers of bacteria and the taste of stale food, and it will go a long way toward reducing the risk of aspirating bacteria into the airway and lungs. Loose dentures complicate swallowing even further, so if necessary, an adhesive powder or cream will help to hold a denture in place (Grasso, 2004). There are no serious side effects to denture adhesives other than the residue that is difficult to clean off the dentures and supporting mucosa.

When food or liquid is placed in the mouth, the lips and tongue move it onto the occlusal tooth surfaces for chewing before it is propelled to the pharynx. The lips should form a good seal to keep the food and liquid in the mouth. Loose and unstable dentures or abnormally protruding teeth interfere with the lips, and can cause drooling or dribbling. It is important to know that drinking through a straw poses a difficult challenge for incompetent lips; therefore, it best avoided by people who cannot form a good lip seal around the straw or who cannot coordinate the sucking and swallowing action. Similarly, the muscles of the tongue and pharynx should form a good seal posteriorly to allow breathing through the nose, larynx, and pharynx when chewing, and to prevent fluids dribbling down the throat before the swallowing begins.

It is difficult to swallow solid foods that have not been chewed adequately and moistened or broken down by saliva. Fatty sauces will help lubricate food, whereas broths and other low-fat sauces only moisten the food. Sticky or thick liquids, such as puddings and milkshakes, when compared with thin liquids are easier to contain in the mouth and to swallow, although some people find them more difficult to swallow. Nonetheless, liquids thickened to various consistencies with nectar, honey, or pudding gels should prevent aspiration and ease the swallow. The sensory information emitted by the muscles, jaw joints, and mucosa of the mouth and lips prevent biting, enhance enjoyment of the texture and temperature of food, and generally provide the guidance needed to eat comfortably and safely.

Frailty is accompanied by weakened and uncoordinated muscles so that eating becomes difficult and inefficient while the preparatory phase of swallowing is elongated. Consequently, people as they grow frail will increase the number of chewing cycles to compensate for the chewing inefficiency (Mioche et al., 2004). Their preference is for soft foods, especially when their teeth are defective.

Oral phase of swallowing

The oral phase of swallowing occurs when the food is chewed, mixed with saliva, and ready to be swallowed. The moistened bolus of food is moved to the back of the mouth as the tongue rolls backward, forming a "chute" into the throat. Again, there are multiple muscles involved in this movement, and weakness in any of them can disturb the action. If the lips are weak, the soft foods and liquids can dribble or drool when food is not propelled backwards. Similarly, sticky food may stick to the roof of the mouth if the tongue is weak. The cheek muscles help keep the bolus on the teeth and out of the lateral vestibule, while the soft palate lowers during all of this activity to allow nasal breathing.

The oral phase of swallowing ends by triggering the pharyngeal phase, which often slows down in old age, and liquid trickles into the throat before the pharyngeal swallow is triggered (Marik and Kaplan, 2003).

Pharyngeal phase of swallowing

Food or liquid is moved through the pharynx to the esophagus during this third phase. The larynx and hyoid bone move upward and forward to allow the epiglottis to close off the airway and to open the cricopharyngeal sphincter at the top of the esophagus. The vocal folds close to prevent anything entering the trachea. Weakness of muscles, typically from respiratory diseases or general fatigue, prevents complete closure of the airway and allows leakage or aspiration of fluids (and bacteria) into the lungs. It is also very distressing when the normal rhythm of breathing is delayed because of a prolonged swallow (Logemann, 1998; Vaiman et al., 2005).

Esophageal phase of swallowing

When the food enters the esophagus, the walls contract in a reflexive movement of peristalsis to push the food down to the stomach. The muscles in the walls along with the sphincter muscle at the top of the stomach keep the food and gastric fluids in the stomach. However, with frailty, the peristalsis lessens, muscles weaken, and gastric acid can seep into the esophagus and upward to the pharynx and larynx (Achem and Devault, 2005). Consequently, the mucosa may become inflamed and swollen, which impedes swallowing even further.

SCREENING FOR SWALLOWING DIFFICULTIES

There are a number of clinical signs of dysphagia, but none definitely indicates the problem because they are associated also with other problems. However, the "red alerts" are drooling, choking, and coughing after drinking fluids or eating, along with dental plaque and residues of food around the mouth (Table 7.1).

Dehydration disturbs swallowing and nutrition, and increases dependency on others for eating, which is probably the most significant risk factor for aspiration pneumonia in bedbound elderly individuals (Rigney, 2006).

People over 65 years typically need to drink about 30 mL of fluid per kilogram of body weight to maintain hydration and good health. Hence, a 55-kg (101-lb) person should consume about 1,680 mL of fluid per day (Table 7.2).

A decline in thirst sensation, for example, can upset hydration and electrolyte balance, particularly for frail elders who drink large volumes of tea, coffee, or alcohol, all with strong diuretic affects. The fluid loss from fever, vomiting, or diarrhea will have a similar outcome, as will the dry mouth and salivary gland hypofunction caused by the copious supply of medications consumed by elderly people. Assessment of past medical history and current health status offer clues to current nutritional and hydration status. The nutritional profile requires background information on the usual and current consumption of food, fluid, medications, along with the domestic arrangements, personal temperament, and general mood of the elder individual. However, unintentional weight loss is probably the best indicator of poor nutritional status and should be investigated

Table 7.1   Clinical alerts to dysphagia and risk for aspiration.

Alerts	Significance
Reduced alertness	Eating requires responsiveness
Drooling or dribbling	Muscular weakness and dysphagia
Dental plaque and food residue in the mouth	High numbers of bacteria.
Sticky mucous in the mouth and pharynx	Salivary deficiency
Neurological disorders	Disturbed swallow
Dementia, delirium, or depression	Needs help to eat or drink
Chronic obstructive pulmonary disease (e.g., inhaling immediately before or after swallow)	Disturbs coordination between breathing and swallowing
Difficulty coughing	Loss of protective reflex
Gastroesophageal reflux disease	Irritation of larynx and pharynx
Repeated chest infections	Dysphagia and aspiration
Frailty	Prolonged swallow with reduced peristalsis, muscular tension, taste sensitivity, and smell
Weight loss, dehydration, or complaints of difficulty swallowing	Dysphagia

Table 7.2   A healthy intake of fluid per day for a 55-kg woman at age 65 years.

Drink	Quantity	Volume mL	oz	Meal
Juice	1 glass	120	4	Breakfast
Milk	2 glasses	360	12	At or between meals or at bedtime
Soup	1 bowl	120	6	Lunch or dinner
Decaffeinated coffee	3 cups	720	24	At or between meals
Water	2 glasses	360	12	With medications
Total		1,680	58	

for underlying pathoses, including neurodegenerative decline or psychological disorders such as depression.

INCREASED RISK FOR DYSPHAGIA AND ASPIRATION

The usual acute and chronic diseases associate with dysphagia and aspiration are stroke, Parkinson's disease, dementia, and osteoporosis of the spine.

Acute and chronic cardiovascular accidents

Large proportions (28%–45%) of patients who have had a stroke suffer from dysphagia, but fortunately, about one in five will regain their ability to swallow normally within a few weeks following the stroke (Murray, 1999). A dysphagia that does not resolve is likely to cause chest infections, malnutrition, dehydration, and even death. Furthermore, the common side effects of stroke, such as apraxia, extremity weakness, and hemiplegia, limit a person's ability to feed themselves.

Parkinson's disease

The tremor, rigidity, postural instability, and bradykinesia associated with Parkinson's disease disturb the ability to eat independently. Nearly everyone with the disease will have dysphagia due to multiple prepharyngeal, pharyngeal, and esophageal abnormalities (Murray, 1999).

Dementia

Decreased food and fluid intake in elders with dementia occurs usually because (1) they are unaware of hunger and thirst, or they cannot recognize food or how to use eating utensils; (2) their sense of smell and taste has declined; (3) they cannot swallow or communicate their needs and wishes;

(4) they refuse to eat; or (5) they are depressed (Tilly and Reed, 2006). Indeed, the vast majority (>90%) of people with dementia cannot swallow normally, and eventually, they lose this ability altogether (Murry and Carrau, 2001). Death occurs usually within 3–6 months after dysphagia begins.

Osteoporosis

Spinal kyphosis from progressive osteoporosis gradually compresses the diaphragm and stomach, and increases the risk for aspiration because it is necessary to turn the head to the side when eating or drinking. There is also a tendency to protrude the chin, which interferes with the closure of the trachea. It is also very difficult to reach the posterior teeth when the neck if bent downward.

ASPIRATION

The gagging reflex is not directly associated with the ability to swallow. About 1 in 10 adults do not gag, but this has no effect on their ability to eat or drink comfortably (Rigney, 2006). Indeed, aspiration occurs silently without coughing or gagging in about 40% of elders (Morley and Silver, 1995); nonetheless, there are several indicators to reduce the possibility of serious consequences when aspiration does occur (Table 7.3).

Oral health-related risks for aspiration pneumonia

The most significant risk indicator for aspiration pneumonia, as mentioned before, is dependency on others for feeding. There are numerous other factors that increase the risk of pneumonia, including caries and periodontal disease (Shay et al., 2005). Clearly, if general health and independence are compromised, leading to frailty, there is a higher chance of developing pneumonia when aspirating food or fluids. Good oral health and hygiene helps considerably to avoid chest infections by reducing the number of oral bacteria for aspiration (Langmore et al., 1998; Azarpazhooh and Leake, 2006; Sumi et al., 2006; Abe et al., 2008; Sjogren et al., 2008; Weed, 2009).

MANAGING DYSPHAGIA AND ASPIRATION

Frail elderly patients who cannot swallow safely may not be fed by mouth, although some might take ice chips or sips of water to satisfy their need for pleasurable oral stimulation and hydration. In this situation, with little movement of food through the mouth, the oral muscles are less active and self-cleaning of the oral cavity is reduced (Figure 7.2). Consequently, a

Table 7.3 Indicators for aspiration.

Indicators	Significance
Repeated coughing or clearing of the throat	Insensitive reflex or weak muscles
Choking, cyanosis or teary eyes	Respiratory distress
Constant swallows during a meal	Residue from food or liquid in the mouth or throat
Change in respirations	Inhaling food
Gurgling voice	Food or liquid (including saliva) in the larynx
Food pocketing in the mouth	Reduced awareness of food in the mouth
Food stuck in the throat after swallowing	Food in the pharynx
Drink or food from the nose	The soft palate is incompetent
Missing teeth or poorly fitting dentures	Food is inadequately chewed and moistened

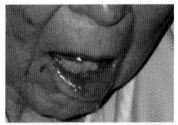
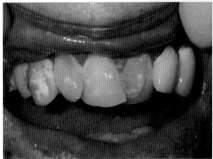
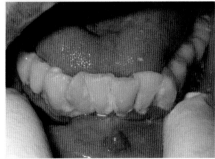

Figure 7.2 Dental plaque, food residue, and drooling in a patient with moderate dementia. (Photographs courtesy of L. Donnelly.)

thick biofilm of microbial plaque forms on the teeth and mucosa, and food residue lingers around the mouth (Awano et al., 2008; Sona et al., 2009).

A 0.12% chlorhexidine mouthrinse applied with a soft toothbrush on a suction tube (Suction Toothbrush System, Sage Products, Cary, IL) to suction off saliva and excess mouthrinse will clean the mouth and teeth without increasing the risk of aspiration (Figure 7.3).

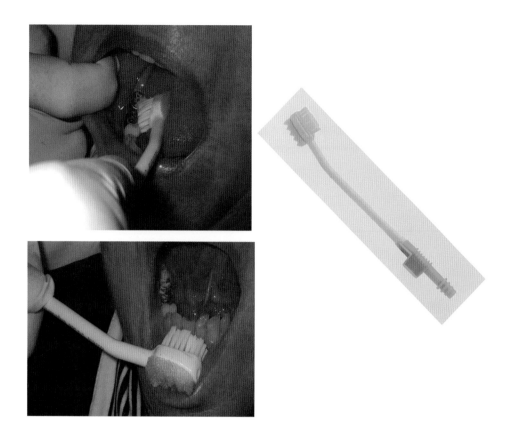

Figure 7.3   "Suction toothbrush" (Sage Products, Cary, IL) to reduce the risk of aspiration. (Photos [a] and [b] courtesy of L. Donnelly. Photo [c] by Michael I. MacEntee.)

Dysphagia and oral health

Mildred and Frank McDuff have been married for 60 years. Mildred is 78 years old and Frank is 80 years. Frank has Parkinson's disease diagnosed 10 years ago, but he tries hard to maintain his independence. A home-support worker helps him bathe twice a week, but he is unable to clean his teeth adequately due to his impaired mobility and hand tremors. Nonetheless, with Mildred's help, they have been managing to live a reasonably full life until this year.

Over the past year, Mildred had become increasingly alarmed at Frank's loss of weight and episodes of choking. He also uses at least three paper napkins during meals because of drooling, which he finds embarrassing. He has not finished a full meal in 3 months and has been choking at least once per meal. On prompting, Frank admitted that he also coughs frequently when drinking liquids and so he avoids fluids as much as possible. As a result, his hydration and nutritional balance are compromised. His home-support worker mentioned that Frank's dentures "clack around," which makes Frank's speech difficult to understand. Frank no longer enjoys going with his family for Sunday brunch at a restaurant because he is embarrassed about his choking, drooling, and loose dentures.

Recently, Frank became despondent and was looking pale and ill, so Mildred called their daughter to take him to their family physician. On examination, the physician noted that Frank had a congested-sounding chest with and his oral cavity had a heavy accumulation of dental plaque. The physician ordered blood tests, urinalysis, a chest X-ray, and referred Frank for a swallowing assessment. He suggested that Frank see his dentist. Frank refused, saying that there was no need to fuss about dentures when he was not eating anything that he would have to chew, so "why pay for stuff that I don't need?"

Frank's children noticed his decline over the next month. They tried to talk to their parents about this, but both Frank and Mildred kept repeating that this is just part of his Parkinson's disease and his age. During a family gathering, Frank had a terrible choking episode with soup, and Mildred finally admitted to the children that she knew he was afraid to eat anything because of choking and drooling. They had never seen their father look so anxious, and insisted that Frank return to his physician.

The physician, through a series of tests, diagnosed microcytic anemia, iron deficiency, low albumin, low vitamin B12, malnutrition, and mild renal insufficiency consistent with dehydration. In addition, a chest X-ray confirmed a right basal pneumonia consistent with aspiration pneumonia.

The physician arranged for Frank to see a speech language pathologist, an occupational therapist, a physiotherapist, and a dietitian. The speech pathologist assessed Frank's swallowing and recommended a change of foods to include nectar thick liquids (such as tomato juice and milkshakes) along with moist, easy-to-chew foods, and to avoid foods that are difficult to swallow, such as mixed consistencies and crumbly items. She also emphasized the need for Frank to brush his teeth—or have them brushed—before and after every meal. The occupational therapist advised him to sit upright at the table when eating and provided modified cutlery and dishes to help him feel less embarrassed when eating. She also provided a toothbrush with a handle that he could hold more easily. The physiotherapist provided Frank with mobility aids that would improve his ability to get around with minimal help from Mildred, while the occupational therapist and physiotherapist counseled him on ways to conserve his energy so that he could care for himself and eat with less difficulty.

The dietitian met with Mildred and complimented her on her cooking and other efforts to help Frank's nutrition. She recommended six small meals or snacks throughout the day rather than three large meals to help reduce Frank's fatigue and increase his calories.

A week later, Frank's son accompanied him to a dentist, who identified an abscessed lower molar tooth that was severely decayed and fractured. The dentist found also that Frank's gingiva bled easily on probing, and his lower incisors were loose because of advanced periodontitis. The dentist explained that the upper denture was loose probably because it had not been relined or adjusted form many years, and possibly because of Frank's recent weight loss. She recommended that the abscessed tooth be extracted, emphasized even more the speech pathologist's advice about oral hygiene, and offered to reline the upper complete denture. She indicated that the lower incisors would probably improve when the periodontitis resolved after thorough cleaning and subgingival curettage to resolve the inflammation and stabilize the gingival attachment.

Frank went to the dental hygienist as recommended and was able to develop an oral care regime that was feasible with some help from his family.

Mildred was so preoccupied with Frank's care that she frequently forgot to take her medication for high blood pressure. One Friday morning, Frank called his daughter, saying in a panic that Mildred's speech was slurred and that she was unable to get out of bed. Her daughter came immediately. She found her mother with her face drooping on one side, and called an ambulance immediately. Mildred was taken to the hospital, where she was diagnosed with an ischemic stroke.

Over the weekend, as they watched Mildred's progress, the nurses cleaned Mildred's teeth and mouth, and kept her sitting upright to reduce the risk of aspiration. They used a toothbrush with a suction attachment to clean her teeth without increasing the risk of aspiration further (Figure 7.3). The nurses explained to the family that they must not give Mildred food or drink by mouth.

The speech language pathologist assessed Mildred's swallowing and noted severe oral weakness, delayed swallowing reflex, and poor cough sensitivity. He found aspiration to be a risk on all consistencies and recommended that Mildred receive only small ice chips by mouth. The family was informed that Mildred's swallow might improve in the early days after the stroke; however, they were told that her dysphagia is severe and that it is also possible that her swallowing might deteriorate.

The stroke had paralyzed Mildred's right side. Consequently, her balance has been significantly compromised and she was unable to sit up unsupported or to feed herself. The physician, following a family conference, ordered feeding through a nasogastric tube with appropriate nutrition. The dietitian closely assessed and monitored her nutritional intake, and the nursing staff cleaned her teeth and mouth regularly to prevent aspiration, which can occur even when a feeding tube is present.

During the next week, Mildred continually mimed motions of eating or drinking. The family were very upset by this because they knew how much food means to their mother and how proud she was with her cooking skills. In fact, Mildred believed that good food would cure all ills!

Mildred had another more extensive stroke, which left her even more debilitated with an even greater risk of aspiration. Frank and the children recognized that her mime was a plea for food and drink by mouth, so they decided that she should be fed orally in compliance with her wish, and despite the magnified risk of aspiration. The care team decided to remove the feeding tube after Mildred had purposely pulled it out several times. Subsequently, Mildred became visibly more settled and happier.

The children asked if they could help with their mother's care and offered to provide daily mouthcare. So, with guidance from a dental hygienist, they cleaned Mildred's teeth and mouth daily, and Mildred responded well to her family's help.

Mildred had frequent choking episodes when eating. The nursing staff reduced this distress by suctioning excess saliva and fluids from her mouth.

However, she seemed happier and more settled when she had something to eat. Despite the attentive and competent oral care, within a few weeks, she developed aspiration pneumonia and died peacefully with her family present.

Following Mildred's death, Frank and his children told the social worker that it was heartening to them that they could help in Mildred's care to the end and that they appreciated the team's collaboration to ensure a dignified and respectful final journey for Mildred.

SUMMARY

When inadequate oral care and dysphagia are combined, the risk of aspiration pneumonia is very high. Consequently, dentists and dental hygienists have a significant role on the healthcare team of frail elders to identify early signs of dysphagia and to reduce the number of pathogenic organisms in the mouth.

REFERENCES

Abe S, Ishihara K, Adachi M, and Okuda K. 2008. Tongue-coating as risk indicator for aspiration pneumonia in edentate elderly. *Arch Gerontol Geriatr* 47:267–75.

Azarpazhooh A and Leake JL. 2006. Systematic review of the association between respiratory diseases and oral health. *J Periodontol* 77:1465–82.

Achem SR and Devault KR. 2005. Dysphagia in aging. *J Clin Gastroenterol* 39:357–71.

Awano S, Ansai T, Takata Y, Soh I, Akifusa S, Hamasaki T, Yoshida A, Sonoki K, Fujisawa K, and Takehara T. 2008. Oral health and mortality risk from pneumonia in the elderly. *J Dent Res* 87:334–9.

Buettner A, Beer A, Hannig C, and Settles M. 2001. Observation of the swallowing process by application of videofluoroscopy and real-time magnetic resonance imaging—Consequences for retronasal aroma stimulation. *Chem Senses* 26:1211–9.

Ertekin C and Aydogdu I. 2003. Neurophysiology of swallowing. *Clin Neurophysiol* 114:2226–44.

Grasso JE. 2004. Denture adhesives. *Dent Clin North Am* 48:721–33.

Langmore SE, Terpenning MS, Schork A, Chen Y, Murray JT, Lopatin D, and Loesche WJ. 1998. Predictors of aspiration pneumonia: How important is dysphagia? *Dysphagia* 13:69–81.

Logemann JA. 1998. *Evaluation and Treatment of Swallowing Disorders*, 2nd edn. Austin, TX: PRO-ED.

MacEntee MI, Hole R, and Stolar E. 1997. The significance of the mouth in old age. *Soc Sci Med* 45:1449–58.

Marik PE and Kaplan D. 2003. Aspiration pneumonia and dysphagia in the elderly. *Chest* 124:328–36.

Mioche L, Bourdiol P, Monier S, Martin JF, and Cormier D. 2004. Changes in jaw muscle activity with age: Effects of food bolus properties. *Physiol Behav* 82:621–7.

Mojon P and Bourbeau J. 2003. Respiratory infection: How important is oral health? *Curr Opin Pulm Med* 9:166–70.

Morley JE and Silver AJ. 1995. Nutritional issues in nursing home care. *Ann Intern Med* 123:850–9.

Murray J. 1999. Medical record review and patient interview. In: J. Murray (ed.), *Manual of Dysphagia Assessment in Adults*. San Diego, CA: Singular Publishing Group, Inc., pp. 1–35.

Murry T and Carrau RL. 2001. *Clinical Manual for Swallowing Disorders*. San Diego, CA: Singular Publishing Group, Inc., pp. 1–11.

Paik NJ. 2008. *Dysphagia: eMedicine Physical Medicine and Rehabilitation*. Available at http://emedicine.medscape.com/article/324096-overview (accessed December 18, 2009).

Rigney TS. 2006. Delirium in the hospitalized elder and recommendations for practice. *Geriatr Nurs* 27:151–7.

Shay K, Scannapieco FA, Terpenning MS, Smith BJ, and Taylor GW. 2005. Nosocomial pneumonia and oral health. *Spec Care Dentist* 25:179–87.

Sjogren P, Nilsson E, Forsell M, Johansson O, and Hoogstraate J. 2008. A systematic review of the preventive effect of oral hygiene on pneumonia and respiratory tract infection in elderly people in hospitals and nursing homes: Effect estimates and methodological quality of randomized controlled trials. *J Am Geriatr Soc* 56:2124–30.

Sona CS, Zack JE, Schallom ME, McSweeney M, McMullen K, Thomas J, Coopersmith CM, Boyle WA, Buchman TG, Mazuski JE, and Schuerer DJ. 2009. The impact of a simple, low-cost oral care protocol on ventilator-associated pneumonia rates in a surgical intensive care unit. *Intensive Care Med* 24:54–62.

Steele CM, Greenwood C, Ens I, Robertson C, Seidman-Carlson R. 1997. Mealtime difficulties in a home for the aged: Not just dysphagia. *Dysphagia* 12:43–50, discussion 51.

Sumi Y, Miura H, Nagaya M, Michiwaki Y, and Uematsu H. 2006. Colonisation on the tongue surface by respiratory pathogens in residents of a nursing home—A pilot study. *Gerodontology* 23:55–9.

Tilly J and Reed P (eds.). 2006. *Dementia Care Practice Recommendations for Assisted Living Residences and Nursing Homes*. Chicago, IL: Alzheimer's Association. Available at: http:// www.alz.org/national/documents/brochure_DCPRphases1n2.pdf (accessed August 4, 2010).

Trombly CA and Radomski MV (eds.). 2002. *Occupational Therapy for Physical Dysfunction*, 5th edn. Baltimore: Lippincott Williams & Wilkins.

Vaiman M, Gabriel C, Eviatar E, and Segal S. 2005. Surface electromyography of continuous drinking in healthy adults. *Laryngoscope* 115:68–73.

Weed HG. 2009. Review: Enhanced oral hygiene prevents respiratory infection in older persons in hospitals and nursing homes. *ACP J Club* 150:JC3–7.

Wolf LS and Glass RP. 1992. *Feeding and Swallowing Disorders in Infancy*. Tucson, AZ: Therapy Skill Builders, pp. 335–47.

Yoon MN and Steele CM. 2007. The oral care imperative: The link between oral hygiene and aspiration pneumonia. *Top Geriatr Rehabil* 23:280–8.

Periodontal diseases in frail elders

G. Rutger Persson

INTRODUCTION

This chapter will address (1) how the definitions of periodontal conditions apply to frail people; (2) the available evidence on the prevalence of gingivitis and periodontitis in older populations; (3) social and perceptual factors influencing periodontal health in frail elders; (4) frailty and periodontal infection; and (5) periodontal treatments for frail patients.

Clinical scenario

Mr. Erikson is 76 years old with a medical record of arthritis, phytoin-controlled epilepsy, and a heart attack at age 74. He is overweight, uses a wheelchair to move around, and resides in a long-term care facility. He smoked tobacco for more than 30 years but stopped after the heart attack. Now he takes 100 mg/day of aspirin.

Clinical examination of his mouth 3 years ago found 24 teeth. He had previously lost four teeth—two in a car accident and two from failed endodontic treatments. He had buccal or interproximal gingival recession at most teeth (Figure 8.1). Several teeth were restored with large intracoronal restorations, and others had prosthetic crowns with exposed margins. His oral hygiene was good. A periodontal examination revealed that 18 teeth had periodontal pockets ≥6 mm, while 12 had pockets >7 mm, and three teeth were noticeably (Class II) mobile (Table 8.1).

Intraoral radiographs show advanced alveolar bone loss at most teeth with a distance between the CEJ to bone of ≥4 mm at >40% of sites, and osteitis at the root apices of teeth #16 and #46 (Figure 8.2).

Mr. Erikson's dentist, Dr. Smith concluded that the upper anterior teeth could not be saved and also that the lower right first and second molars should be extracted and implants placed to restore function. In addition scaling and root planing would be performed.

Oral Healthcare and the Frail Elder: A Clinical Perspective.
Edited by Michael I. MacEntee © 2011 Blackwell Publishing Ltd.

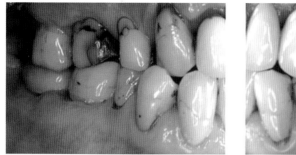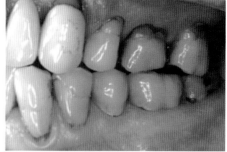

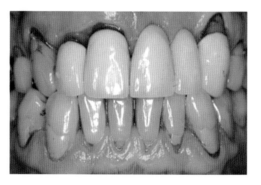

Figure 8.1   Mr. Erikson's teeth before his recent heart attack.

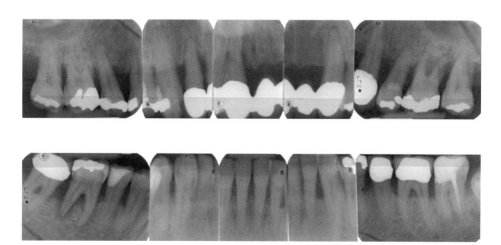

Figure 8.2   Radiographs of Mr. Erikson's teeth before extraction.

Table 8.1 Classification of mobility (Mo) and depth (in millimeters) of periodontal pockets (PP) recorded for each tooth.

Tooth #		17	16	15	14	13	12	11	21	22	23	24	25	26	27
Mo		1	1	1		0	2	2			2		1	1	1
PP	**Bu**	636	738	728		627	757	735			639		437	728	346
	Pa	626	627	639		767	678	878			739		437	826	877
PP	**Li**	369	1088	635	663	323	423	323	313	324	523	333	324	738	659
	Bu	379	1236	424	723	325	623	316	513	223	316	313	323	328	776
Mo		1	1	0	0	0	0	0	0	0	0	0	0	0	0
Tooth #		47	46	45	44	43	42	41	31	32	33	34	35	36	37

Bu, buccal; Pa, palatal; Li, lingual.

GOALS OF PERIODONTAL THERAPY

The goal of periodontal therapy is to prevent and manage periodontal disease and to preserve a functional dentition for life (Wennström, 1998). Most of our knowledge about periodontal interventions relate to young and relatively healthy adults, and we know that the periodontium can remain reasonably stable throughout life. However, the assumption that people with little or no signs of periodontal disease in midlife will remain immune to it in old age is questionable. Successful periodontal therapy depends on good oral hygiene, which is not a common finding among frail elders (Kay and Locker 1996; Söderpalm et al., 2006). Consequently, two fundamental questions arise: (1) does periodontal debridement control periodontitis for frail elders, and (2) does periodontitis with associated bacteremia constitute a serious risk to the general health of frail elders?

The social and physical changes of natural aging disturb the periodontium as they disturb other organs, even in people who are seemingly robust. Altered immunity, for example, changes gingival cells (Zavala and Cavicchia, 2006), which can lead to gingival recession (De Rossi and Slaughter, 2007). Moreover, osteoporosis and deep (≥5 mm) periodontal pockets increase the risk of further periodontal bone loss in people of Caucasian or African descent as they age (Swoboda et al., 2008). Similarly, genes, lifestyle, healthcare, and the other physical insults of life take their toll on the periodontium (Petersen and Yamamoto, 2005).

The periodontium is constantly exposed to microbiota that induce inflammation. Loss of teeth reduces the bacterial burden and inflammation in the mouth, which is an association that prompted Benjamin Rush in the 1820s to propose extracting all natural teeth to cure rheumatoid arthritis. Consequently, until the mid-20th century, it was widely believed that extraction of teeth would reduce the risk of focal infection. This belief resurfaced recently to reduce counts of serum nonspecific markers of inflammation (Taylor et al., 2006; Ellis et al., 2007). Indeed, this might be appropriate treatment for people with severe periodontitis who are medically compromised because information on the prevention and treatment of periodontitis in older people is limited (Renvert and Persson, 2002, 2004). Nonetheless, the consequences of tooth loss can also be very unhealthy, and inflammation in the jaws can be a serious complication of oral implants (Renvert et al., 2008). In many instances, it may be easier for frail elders with or without assistance to maintain reasonable oral hygiene around teeth than around implants, especially when recovering from a seriously debilitating illness (Figure 8.3).

The mucosa around oral implants in susceptible subjects may become infected with *Staphylococcus aureus*, *Pseudomonas aeruginosa*, and other highly virulent bacteria that we do not know how to eliminate reliably (Harris et al., 2007; Renvert et al., 2008; Salvi et al., 2008; Van de Velde et al., 2009).

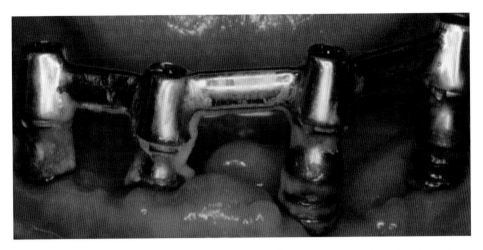

Figure 8.3 Mandibular endosseous implants in a patient 4 weeks after a heart attack.

DEFINITIONS OF GINGIVITIS AND PERIODONTITIS

Gingivitis is a reversible inflammatory condition of the gingiva without loss of clinical attachment, whereas periodontitis is a similar inflammatory condition but complicated by irreversible loss of gingival attachment and periodontal bone. Both conditions can occur at any age, but aggressive periodontitis presents typically in younger adults and in association with other diseases.

Susceptibility to periodontal disease is highly variable and depends on host responses to pathogens (Colonna-Romano et al., 2008; Suvas, 2008). A decline in immune responses, for example, occurs with increased serum levels of immunoglobulin, cytokine, natural killer, and memory T lymphocytes in old age (Percival et al., 1996). Gingivitis, in effect, is a cytokine-related immune response to prevent bacteremia within gingival cells. Periodontitis might be the effects of a humoral (antigen-antibody) driven immune response that continues until the infection is either resolved or teeth are exfoliated or extracted. Moreover, the stress of chronic exposure to bacterial antigens compromises the immune system and overburdens the immune system (Colonna-Romano et al., 2008).

The clinical signs of gingival inflammation are often inconsistent with the quantity of plaque on the teeth of older people, which suggests an inefficient response of the host. Gingival recession, for example, occurs typically at the interproximal and mid-buccal surfaces of teeth (Figure 8.1). Similarly, regular intakes of aspirin, which is a common medication for arthritis and heart problems, will increase tendencies for gingival bleeding (Royzman et al., 2004; Kim et al., 2007).

Good nutrition also helps control periodontal inflammation (Jepsen and Kuchel, 2006; Irish et al., 2008; Baumgartner et al., 2009). Flavonoids and omega-3 are examples of immune boosters that have a significant impact on inflammatory responses to infection, and that educe colonization of the mouth by virulent bacteria (Brüünsgaard and Pedersen, 2003).

In summary, periodontal therapy for frail elders should be adjusted for medical conditions, access to care, and the propensity to self-care. Teeth that are infected beyond control should be extracted with the immediate objective of reducing the burden of infection and stabilizing the level of frailty as quickly as possible (Gill et al., 2002).

PREVALENCE OF PERIODONTITIS AND GINGIVITIS IN FRAIL POPULATIONS

The belief that periodontitis affects entire populations and that the disease progresses with age changed in the 1980s. In fact, severe periodontitis occurs in only a minority (~15%–20%) of the general population in western countries, and it does so independently of age (Borrell et al., 2005; Dye et al., 2007; Hugoson et al., 2008). Partly influenced by geographic and socioeconomic conditions, the prevalence ranges from 27% to 73% of elderly populations (Borges-Yáñez et al., 2006), and there is little doubt that the widely ranging prevalence figures are due to different ways of measuring the disease. Nonetheless, there is an emerging consensus that periodontitis occurs in about half of the relatively robust elderly populations in northern Europe (Holm-Pedersen et al., 2006; Krustrup and Petersen, 2006; Holtfreter et al., 2010). Gingivitis, in contrast, is much more prevalent among frail elders, and in some populations, almost all of the elderly residents in long-term care have severely inflamed gingiva (MacEntee, 2005). There are no reliable data on the prevalence of periodontitis among elderly people who are frail.

Clinical scenario (continued)

Dr. Smith did not feel that it was necessary to consult with Mr. Erikson's physicians because he felt sufficiently experienced to manage any emergencies that might arise during treatment.

Following the reevaluation of the first phase of treatment, Mr. Erikson was offered two follow-up options: (1) extraction of teeth with guarded prognosis, with the aim of leaving at least 20 teeth; or (2) extraction of teeth with a bad prognosis, and restoring the dentition with oral implants and fixed dental prostheses.

After further discussions, Mr. Erikson selected implant treatment and conservative nonsurgical periodontal therapy. Four teeth (#11, #25, #26, #46) were extracted, and implants were placed after 6 months at the sites for teeth #12, #22, #26, #46, and #47. After an additional 6 months, the dentist replaced the old intracaronal restorations with resin composite fillings, and attached single crowns to the posterior (#26, #46, #47) implants, along with a fixed prosthesis with pontics to the implants in the anterior maxilla (Figure 8.4).

Two years later, eight interproximal sites had pocket depths ≥5 mm. A Class III furcation was probed at the lower left first molar, and a Class II furcation at the second molar. Bleeding on probing was seen around three of the implants that had 4-mm probing depths.

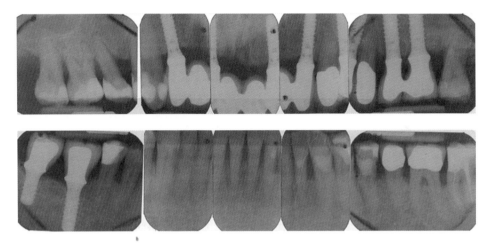

Figure 8.4 Radiographs of Mr. Erikson's teeth after treatment with implants.

SOCIAL FACTORS AND PERCEPTIONS OF PERIODONTAL CONDITIONS

Socioeconomic factors

Socioeconomic factors have been identified as possible risks to elders with periodontitis (Borrell et al., 2008). Retirement with little or no dental insurance, for example, can prevent older people from accessing periodontal care, whereas wholesome nutrition can reduce periodontal inflammation (Jenzsch et al., 2008). However, nutritious foods can be expensive, especially for people on low fixed pensions. There are many foods with anti-inflammatory properties, although methods of production and preparation have a significant influence on their nutritional properties (Table 8.2).

Honey is rich in flavonoids, for instance, whereas diets high in refined sugars are associated with inflammation, obesity, and chronic disease. Therefore, advice on reduction of sugar consumption is important not only to reduce the risk of caries. Moreover, the link between obesity and inflammation is illustrated further by the increased plasma levels of several

Table 8.2 Food items (i.e., omega-3, flavonoids) with high anti-inflammatory properties.

Fish[a]	Meat	Vegetables/ plants	Spices and tea	Nuts (beans)	Berries[a]/fruits/ juices	Oils
Cod	Lamb	Alfalfa seeds	Basil (fresh)	Almonds	Apple	Cranberry oil
Fish roe	Grass-fed beef	Arugula	Black tea leaves	Beans	Apricots	Flaxseed oil (linseed oil)
Flounder		Cabbage	Black tea	Chocolate (dark)	Avocado	Margarine
Herring		Cauliflower	Cloves (ground)	Hazelnuts	Blackberries (fresh)	Olive oil
Mackerel		Cereals	Cinnamon	Macadamia	Blueberries (fresh)	Soybean oil
Pollock		Chard	Green tea leaves	Pecan nuts	Cherries (fresh)	Vegetable oils
Salmon (wild caught)		Green pepper	Green tea	Sunflower seeds	Cranberries	
Sardines		Garlic	Oregano (dried)	Tofu	Guava	
Snapper		Kale	Parsley	Walnut	Kiwi	
Trout		Leeks	Peppermint (fresh)		Oranges (blood)	
Tuna		Olives	Rosemary		Raspberries (fresh)	
Whitefish		Spinach	Spearmint (fresh)		Red wine	
					Strawberries (fresh)	
			Thyme (fresh)			

[a]Properties can vary by processing—wild fish and wild berries are preferable.

proinflammatory markers including cytokines and acute phase proteins such as C-reactive protein (CRP) in obese individuals (Trayhurn and Wood, 2005; Florez et al., 2006).

Risk of periodontitis from tobacco and alcohol

The nicotine in smoking tobacco is associated strongly with frailty (Woods et al., 2005) and with periodontitis (Fardal et al., 2004; Susin et al., 2005; Torrunruang et al., 2005; Bahrami et al., 2006). Hence, advice on the hazards of tobacco is an important target for prevention of periodontal disease and unnecessary frailty (Anonymous, 2008a), although it will not necessarily reduce the severity of periodontitis in old age because it can take 30 years of smoking and 10 years of abstinence from tobacco to benefit the periodontium (Persson et al., 2005).

Information on alcohol consumption and periodontitis in elders is limited and contradictory. Some evidence associates excessive alcohol with damage to the gingival attachment (Tezal et al., 2004), whereas other information suggests that there is no causal link (Torrunruang et al., 2005).

Depression and periodontal disease

Cognitive disability or inadequacies, possibly influenced by social status and education early in life, influence periodontal health (Persson et al., 2004). In general, people understand how previous activities can increase future risks for periodontal disease (Suominen-Taipale et al., 2009; Ekanyaki and Perera, 2005; Mariño et al., 2008; Stewart et al., 2008), but they do not always agree with the advice offered by dentists (Locker and Gibson, 2005). Depression is associated with periodontitis and high concentrations of interleukin-6 in crevicular fluid from the gingiva (Johannsen et al., 2007) and with tooth loss (Persson et al., 2003). Unfortunately, depression can lead also to a general disinterest in personal hygiene, including oral hygiene. Indeed, these physiological and behavioral responses to depression might well explain why elderly people who are single rather than living with a partner are at increased risk for periodontitis (Persson et al., 2004; Airila-Månsson et al., 2007). Elders often have to change their living conditions as they grow frailer, especially when their spouse dies. Consequently, the increased stress can affect the immune functions with an accompanying increase in the severity of chronic diseases (De Martinis et al., 2007; Leng et al., 2007). Depression also predisposes to "quick fix" treatments, such as tooth extraction, as a solution to periodontal disease, particularly when loose teeth are bothersome and compound the feelings of depression (Needleman et al., 2004). This reaction is particularly difficult to contradict when people believe that tooth loss is an inevitable consequence of aging.

FRAILTY AND PERIODONTAL INFECTION

Old mouths carry a large variety of bacteria associated with periodontitis, most commonly *Campylobacter rectus*, *Capnocytophaga* sp., *Eubacterium saburreum*, *Fusobacterium nucleatum*, *Prevotella intermedia*, *Porphyromonas gingivalis*, *Streptococcus sanguinis*, and *Tannerella forsythia* (Könönen et al., 1994; Brennan et al., 2007). Many of these bacteria have also been linked to infections of the endocardium, meninges, mediastinum, vertebrae, hepatobiliary system, prosthetic joints, and lungs (Shay, 2002), which suggests that control of gingivitis, periodontitis, and other oral infections should reduce the risk of untimely death from aspiration pneumonia (Awano et al., 2008). The benefits of routine scaling and root planing for periodontitis are enhanced by a 0.12% chlorhexidine mouthrinse to prevent reinfection from a select group of bacteria, including *P. gingivalis* and *T. forsythia*, prevalent in the periodontal pockets of older people (Persson et al., 2000, 2007; Teles et al., 2008) and recently associated with ventilator-associated aspiration pneumonia (Awano et al., 2008).

Other systemic diseases and periodontitis

Cardiovascular diseases, diabetes mellitus, osteoporosis, and rheumatoid arthritis are all chronic disorders potentially linked to periodontitis. Several studies have assessed the strength of the links (Persson et al., 2002, 2003; Buhlin et al., 2003; Cueto et al., 2005; Lee et al., 2006), and a large number of markers of inflammation have been investigated, including interleukin-6, tumor necrosis factor α, plasminogen activator inhibitor (PAI-1) factor, and serum high sensitivity C-reactive factor. However, no specific etiological factors have been found, which makes it difficult to assess the full impact of periodontitis on frailty (see Chapter 6 for a more extensive discussion of the potential links). Nonetheless, the prevalence of most chronic disorders increase with aging, and most frail elders have several disorders that should be considered as an integral to any periodontal therapy.

CONTROLLING PERIODONTAL DISEASE

Investigation of elderly patients who might have periodontal disease should include (1) assessment of physical and cognitive abilities; (2) exploration for signs or symptoms of xerostomia and salivary gland hypofunction, mucocutaneous lesions, gingival hyperplasia, excessive gingival bleeding, hemorrhage, or other acute and chronic pathoses; and (3) identification of medications, tobacco use, chemical dependency, and psychological or emotional disorders (Anonymous, 2008b). The clinical examination should include assessment of oral hygiene and periodontal pocket depths, even though frailty can increase the difficult of this examination for both the patient and the clinician. Panoramic radiographs provide information on pathoses in the mouth, but they can also show carotid calcification that warrant further investigations by a physician (Figure 8.5). Indeed, the perceived link between periodontitis and cardiovascular diseases suggest that signs of carotid calcification might be highly prevalent among frail elders with advanced chronic periodontitis (Ravon et al., 2003).

Treatment of periodontitis should be adjusted to the patient's level of frailty and propensity for treatment (Mojon and MacEntee, 1994). Most frail elders can tolerate uncomplicated scaling and subgingival debridement without distress. However, extraction of teeth severely affected by periodontitis might be a better option than attempting to maintain teeth that are painful or excessively loose.

Daily mouthrinses with a 0.12%–0.2% chlorhexidine solution can help control gingivitis and nosocomial infections (Figure 8.6), and are indicated

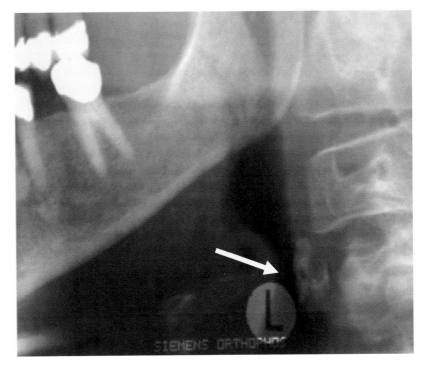

Figure 8.5 Section of a panoramic radiograph showing carotid calcifications (*arrow*).

RX: 0.12% Chlorhexidine.
Dispense: 1 bottle
Label: Rinse with 15 ml for 30
seconds and expectorate TID.

Dr. Gram Goodgum DMD

Figure 8.6 A prescription for chlorhexidine.

RX: Doxycycline
Dispense: 15 tablets 100 mg
Label: Take 2 tablets day one
(every 12 hour), then one
tablet daily

Dr. Gram Goodgum DMD

Figure 8.7 A prescription for doxycline.

strongly for elders who cannot use a standard or electric toothbrush (Segers et al., 2006). (Chlorhexidine solutions can occasionally stain teeth and dentures, but they are easily removed with fine pumice or toothpaste [McCoy et al., 2008].)

The anti-inflammatory properties of systemic doxycycline (Figure 8.7) can be helpful also in managing periodontitis for elders who are very frail (Mohammad et al., 2005; Promsudthi et al., 2005), whereas a 2% minocycline gel on gingiva after scaling and root planing also supports healing by reducing inflammation and controlling bacteria (Jarrold et al., 1997).

Treatment developments

Periodontal and gingival inflammation could be controlled by resolvins and protectins as endogenous compounds made from the omega-3 fatty acid eicosapentaenoic acid (EPA). The newly described EPA-derived resolvin E1 (RvE1) might control neutrophil tissue destruction in periodontal disease (Hasturk et al., 2006), whereas dietary changes to increase intake of natural antioxidants and flavonoids with antifungal, antiviral, and antibacterial properties might enhance natural resistance to inflammation (Cushnie and Lamb, 2005).

Full-mouth periodontal debridement increases the risk of thrombosis by reducing the quantity of thrombomodulin in serum, and thrombomodulin is required to convert thrombin into an anticoagulant (Ushida et al., 2008). Therefore, full-mouth debridement elevates the risk of vascular diseases, including deep venal thrombosis and acute coronary syndrome. Preventive anticoagulants (e.g., aspirin 81 mg daily) might be a helpful approach to controlling this risk (Kim et al., 2007; Yerman et al., 2007).

ORAL SURGERY IN FRAIL PATIENTS

Rarely do extractions of periodontally weak teeth present a problem even for patients on anticoagulant therapies including vitamin K antagonists or antiplatelet drugs, such as aspirin and low-molecular-weight heparin (Carter et al., 2004; Douketis et al., 2008). Simple compression, possibly with sutures across extraction sockets, should be sufficient to control bleeding following extraction of a tooth in subjects on anticoagulants unless the dose is high. According to the Northwest Medicines Information Centre (2007), "[p]atients who have an INR [international normalized ratio] greater than 4.0 should not undergo any form of surgical procedure without consultation with the clinician who is responsible for maintaining their anticoagulation (this may be a physician or pharmacist in primary care or the hospital anticoagulant clinic) ... [and] patients who are maintained with an INR >4.0 or who have very erratic control may need to be referred to a dental hospital or hospital based oral/maxillofacial surgeon."

Open-flap surgery, either with a mechanical scalpel or a laser with careful suturing to stop bleeding, is preferable over gingivectomy if periodontal reconstruction is indicated. In addition, the duration of the surgery should be weighed against the duration of local anesthesia and the need for a vasoconstrictor.

A prophylactic antibiotic should be considered for tooth extractions and periodontal surgery only if there is an underlying systemic concern that is likely to be compromised by bacteremia. The guidelines on antibiotic prophylaxis should be followed as applicable in each country, bearing in mind that there is a global policy to reduce the use of prophylactic antibiotics (ADA Council on Scientific Affairs, 2004; WHO, 2008). Current praxis of prescribing antibiotics as part of "defensive" medicine has resulted in a life-threatening increase in antibiotic resistance. Antibiotics should be used with caution and careful consideration. This may be more important in old and frail patients because many of them have been treated frequently with antibiotics to control serious infections. Therefore, before prescribing antibiotics for dental infections, the history of antibiotic use should be known, which usually requires a consultation with other medical care providers. Interaction between antibiotics and other medications are common. For example, the antibiotic azithromycin, which is used to combat bacterial infections in patients with compromised immune systems, enhances the risk of bleeding in patients who are on anticoagulants. Therefore, antibiotics should not be prescribed for patients who are frail except with the cooperation of their physicians.

Commentary on the clinical scenario

Mr. Erikson's treatment stretched over 18 months. The periodontal and implant surgery was performed despite his history of acute coronary syndrome, epilepsy, and rheumatoid arthritis without the knowledge or approval of his physicians. However, as predicted, no problems occurred during the treatment.

A conventional fixed prosthesis on natural teeth in the anterior maxilla along with acceptance of shortened dental arches in the posterior of both jaws (Armellini and von Fraunhofer, 2004), or removable partial dentures, might have been less invasive.

Mr. Erikson's dental problems relate to several of the issues and concerns raised in this chapter. The treatment committed him to a long-term supportive periodontal program. Already, at the first posttreatment assessment, there is evidence of recurrent gingival inflammation and early signs of mucosal detachment from the implants. If Mr. Erikson becomes frailer and more dependent on others, he will encounter significant difficulties with oral hygiene and other mouthcare.

The more conservative treatment involving shortened dental arches with a fixed prosthesis on the maxillary natural teeth supplemented by daily fluoride mouthrinses would have offered him more flexibility of care and a greater chance of maintaining his oral health, with fewer physical and psychological complications as he grows frailer.

Although the dental treatment was sophisticated, the clinical goal to control periodontitis and peri-implantitis was unsuccessful. Dr. Smith did not consult with Mr. Erikson's physician, and Mr. Erikson's frailty was not considered appropriately.

CONCLUSIONS

- Periodontitis is prevalent in many elders who are frail.
- Social factors and self-perception of oral and periodontal health are important components in periodontal treatments of frail elders.
- Nonsurgical mechanical debridement and oral hygiene reinforcement, possibly with antibacterial mouthrinses, should be performed regularly in frail patients who have periodontitis.
- Teeth that are severely infected should be extracted.
- Clinical depression can predispose to periodontal and medical complications.
- Several systemic diseases have been linked to periodontitis and periodontal treatment.
- Reconstructions to enhance chewing ability and appearance can never compromise good oral hygiene.

REFERENCES

ADA Council on Scientific Affairs. 2004. Combating antibiotic resistance. *J Am Dent Assoc* 135:484–7. Available at http://jada.ada.org/cgi/reprint/135/4/484 (accessed November 12, 2009).

Airila-Månsson S, Bjurshammar N, Yakob M, and Söder B. 2007. Self-reported oral problems, compared with clinical assessment in an epidemiological study. *Int J Dent Hyg* 5:82–6.

Anonymous. 2008a. *CDC Urges Older Adults to Improve Health, Increase Longevity, through Smoking Cessation.* Available at www.chronicdisease.org/files/public/smokingFINAL3_21_08.pdf (accessed August 18, 2008).

Anonymous. 2008b. *American Academy of Periodontology Guidelines.* Available at http://perio.org/resources-products/posppr3-2.html#11 (accessed October 28, 2008).

Armellini D and von Fraunhofer JA. 2004. The shortened dental arch: A review of the literature. *J Prosthet Dent* 92:531–5.

Awano S, Ansai T, Takata Y, Soh I, Akifusa S, Hamasaki T, Yoshida A, Sonoki K, Fujisawa K, and Takehara T. 2008. Oral health and mortality risk from pneumonia in the elderly. *J Dent Res* 87:334–9.

Bahrami G, Wenzel A, Kirkevang LL, Isidor F, and Vaeth M. 2006. Risk indicators for a reduced marginal bone level in the individual. *Oral Health Prev Dent* 4:215–22.

Baumgartner S, Imfeld T, Schicht O, Rath C, Persson RE, and Persson GR. 2009. The impact of stone age diet in the absence of oral hygiene on gingival conditions. *J Periodontol* 80:759–68.

Borges-Yáñez SA, Irigoyen-Camacho ME, and Maupomé G. 2006. Risk factors and prevalence of periodontitis in community-dwelling elders in Mexico. *J Clin Periodontol* 33:184–94.

Borrell LN, Burt BA, and Taylor GW. 2005. Prevalence and trends in periodontitis in the USA: The [corrected] NHANES, 1988 to 2000. *J Dent Res* 84:924–30.

Borrell LN, Burt BA, Neighbors HW, and Taylor GW. 2008. Social factors and periodontitis in an older population. *Am J Public Health* 98(Suppl. 9):S95–101.

Brennan RM, Genco RJ, Wilding GE, Hovey KM, Trevisan M, and Wactawski-Wende J. 2007. Bacterial species in subgingival plaque and oral bone loss in postmenopausal women. *J Periodontol* 78:1051–61.

Brüünsgaard H and Pedersen BK. 2003. Age-related inflammatory cytokines and disease. *Immunol Allergy Clin North Am* 23:15–39.

Buhlin K, Gustafsson A, Ahnve S, Janszky I, Tabrizi F, and Klinge B. 2003. Oral health in women with coronary heart disease. *J Periodontol* 76:544–50.

Carter G, Lee M, McKelvey V, Sourial A, Halliwell R, and Livingston M. 2004. Oral health status and oral treatment needs of dependent elderly people in Christchurch. *N Z Med J* 117:1194.

Colonna-Romano G, Bulati M, Aquino A, Vitello S, Lio D, Candore G, and Caruso C. 2008. B cell immunosenescence in the elderly and in centenarians. *Rejuvenation Res* 11:433–9.

Cueto A, Mesa F, Bravo M, and Ocaña-Riola R. 2005. Periodontitis as risk factor for acute myocardial infarction. A case control study of Spanish adults. *J Periodontal Res* 40:36–42.

Cushnie TP and Lamb AJ. 2005. Antimicrobial activity of flavonoids. *Int J Antimicrob Agents* 5:343–56.

De Martinis FC, Monti D, and Ginaldi L. 2007. Apoptosis remodeling in immunosenescence: Implications for strategies to delay ageing. *Curr Med Chem* 14:1389–97.

De Rossi SS and Slaughter YA. 2007. Oral changes in older patients: A clinician's guide. *Quintessence Int* 38:773–80.

Douketis JD, Berger PB, Dunn AS, Jaffer AK, Spyropoulos AC, Becker RC, and Ansell J. 2008. American College of Chest Physicians. The perioperative management of antithrombotic therapy: American College of Chest Physicians Evidence-Based Clinical Practice Guidelines (8th Edition). *Chest* 133(Suppl. 6):299S–339S.

Dye BA, Tan S, Smith V, Lewis BG, Barker LK, Thornton-Evans G, Eke PI, Beltran-Aguilar ED, Horowitz AM, and Li CH. 2007. Trends in oral health status: United States, 1988–1994 and 1999–2004. *Vital Health Stat 11* 248:1–92.

Ellis JS, Averley PA, Preshaw PM, Steele JG, Seymour RA, and Thomason JM. 2007. Change in cardiovascular risk status after dental clearance. *Br Dent J* 202:543–4.

Ekanyaki L and Perera I. 2005. Perceived need for dental care among dentate older individuals in Sri Lanka. *Spec Care Dentist* 25:199–205.

Fardal O, Johannessen AC, and Linden GJ. 2004. Tooth loss during maintenance following periodontal treatment in a periodontal practice in Norway. *J Clin Periodontol* 31:550–5.

Florez H, Castillo-Florez S, Mendez A, Casanova-Romero P, Larreal-Urdaneta C, and Lee D. 2006. C-reactive protein is elevated in obese patients with the metabolic syndrome. *Diabetes Res Clin Pract* 71:92–100.

Gill TM, Baker DI, Gottschalk M, Peduzzi PN, Allore H, and Byers A. 2002. A program to prevent functional decline in physically frail, elderly persons who live at home. *N Engl J Med* 347:1068–74.

Harris LG, Meredith DO, Eschbach L, and Richards RG. 2007. Staphylococcus aureus adhesion to standard micro-rough and electropolished implant materials. *J Mater Sci Mater Med* 18:1151–6.

Hasturk H, Kantarci A, Ohira T, Arita M, Ebrahimi N, Chiang N, Petasis N, Levy BD, Serhan CN, and Van Dyke TE. 2006. RvE1 protects from local inflammation and osteoclast-mediated bone destruction in periodontitis. *FASEB J* 20:401–3.

Holtfreter B, Kocher T, Hoffmann T, Desvarieux M, and Micheelis W. 2010. Prevalence of periodontal disease and treatment demands based on a German dental survey (DMS IV). *J Clin Periodontol* 37:211–9.

Holm-Pedersen P, Russell SL, Avlund K, Viitanen M, Winblad B, and Katz RV. 2006. Periodontal disease in the oldest-old living in Kungsholmen, Sweden: Findings from the KEOHS project. *J Clin Periodontol* 33:376–84.

Hugoson A, Sjödin B, and Norderyd O. 2008. Trends over thirty years, 1973-2003, in the prevalence and severity of periodontal disease. *J Clin Periodontol* 35:405–14.

Irish J, Carter DA, Blair SE, and Heard TA. 2008. Antibacterial activity of honey from the Australian stingless bee Trigona carbonaria. *Int J Antimicrob Agents* 1:89–90.

Jarrold CR, Allaker RP, Young KA, Heath MR, Hardie JM, and Lynch E. 1997. Clinical and microbiological effects of topical minocycline in the treatment of elderly patients with periodontitis. *Br Dent J* 183:51–6.

Jenzsch A, Eick S, Rassoul F, Purschwitz R, and Jentsch H. 2008. Nutritional intervention in patients with periodontal disease: Clinical, immunological and microbiological variables during 12 months. *Br J Nutr* 20:1–7.

Jepsen R and Kuchel GA. 2006. Nutrition and inflammation: The missing link between periodontal disease and systemic health in the frail elderly? *J Clin Periodontol* 33:309–11.

Johannsen A, Rydmark I, Söder B, and Asberg M. 2007. Gingival inflammation, increased periodontal pocket depth and elevated interleukin-6 in gingival crevicular fluid of depressed women on long-term sick leave. *J Periodontal Res* 42:546–52.

Kay EJ and Locker D. 1996. Is dental health education effective? A systematic review of current evidence. *Community Dent Oral Epidemiol* 24:231–5.

Kim DM, Koszeghy KL, Badovinac RL, Kawai T, Hosokawa I, Howell TH, and Karimbux NY. 2007. The effect of aspirin on gingival crevicular fluid levels of inflammatory and anti-inflammatory mediators in patients with gingivitis. *J Periodontol* 78:1620–6.

Könönen E, Asikainen S, Saarela M, Karjalainen J, and Jousimies-Somer H. 1994. The oral gram-negative anaerobic microflora in young children: Longitudinal changes from edentulous to dentate mouth. *Oral Microbiol Immunol* 9:136–41.

Krustrup U and Petersen E. 2006. Periodontal conditions in 35-44 and 65-74-year-old adults in Denmark. *Acta Odontol Scand* 64:65–73.

Lee HJ, Garcia RI, Janket SJ, Jones JA, Mascarenhas AK, Scott TE, and Nunn ME. 2006. The association between cumulative periodontal disease and stroke history in older adults. *J Periodontol* 77:1744–54.

Leng SX, Xue QL, Tian J, Walston JD, and Fried LP. 2007. Inflammation and frailty in older women. *J Am Geriatr Soc* 55:864–71.

Locker D and Gibson B. 2005. Discrepancies between self-ratings of and satisfaction with oral health in two older adult populations. *Community Dent Oral Epidemiol* 33:280–8.

MacEntee MI. 2005. Caring for elderly long-term care patients: Oral health-related concerns and issues. *Dent Clin North Am* 49:429–43.

Mariño R, Schofield M, Wright C, Calache H, and Minichiello V. 2008. Self-reported and clinically determined oral health status predictors for quality of life in dentate older migrant adults. *Community Dent Oral Epidemiol* 36:85–94.

McCoy LC, Wehler CJ, Rich SE, Garcia RI, Miller DR, and Jones JA. 2008. Adverse events associated with chlorhexidine use: Results from the Department of Veterans Affairs. Dental Diabetes study. *J Am Dent Assoc* 139:178–83.

Mohammad AR, Preshaw PM, Bradshaw MH, Hefti AF, Powala CV, and Romanowicz M. 2005. Adjunctive subantimicrobial dose doxycycline in the management of institutionalised geriatric patients with chronic periodontitis. *Gerodontology* 22:37–43.

Mojon P and MacEntee MI. 1994. Estimates of time and propensity for dental treatment among institutionalized elders. *Gerodontology* 11:99–107.

Needleman I, McGrath C, Floyd P, and Biddle A. 2004. Impact of oral health on the life quality of periodontal patients. *J Clin Periodontol* 31:454–7.

Northwest Medicines Information Centre. 2007. *Surgical Management of the Primary Care Dental Patient on Warfarin*. Liverpool: Pharmacy Practice Unit. Available at www.dundee.ac.uk/tuith/Static/info/warfarin.pdf (accessed February 7, 2010).

Percival DS, Marsh PD, and Challacombe SJ. 1996. Serum antibodies to commensal oral and gut bacteria vary with age. *FEMS Immunol Med Microbiol* 23:846–52.

Persson GR, Schlegel-Bregenzer B, Chung WO, Houston L, Oswald T, and Roberts MC. 2000. Serum antibody titers to Bacteroides forsythus in elderly subjects with gingivitis or periodontitis. *J Clin Periodontol* 27:839–45.

Persson RE, Hollender LG, Powell VL, MacEntee M, Wyatt CC, Kiyak HA, and Persson GR. 2002. Assessment of periodontal conditions and systemic disease in older subjects. II. Focus on cardiovascular diseases. *J Clin Periodontol* 29:803–10.

Persson GR, Ohlsson O, Pettersson T, and Renvert S. 2003. Chronic periodontitis, a significant relationship with acute myocardial infarction. *Eur Heart J* 24:2108–15.

Persson GR, Persson RE, Hollender LG, and Kiyak HA. 2004. The impact of ethnicity, gender, and marital status on periodontal and systemic health of older subjects in the Trials to Enhance Elders' Teeth and Oral Health (TEETH). *J Periodontol* 75:817–23.

Persson RE, Kiyak AH, Wyatt CC, MacEntee M, and Persson GR. 2005. Smoking, a weak predictor of periodontitis in older adults. *J Clin Periodontol* 32:512–7.

Persson GR, Yeates J, Persson RE, Hirschi-Imfeld R, Weibel M, and Kiyak HA. 2007. The impact of a low-frequency chlorhexidine rinsing schedule on the subgingival microbiota (the TEETH clinical trial). *J Periodontol* 78:1751–8.

Petersen PE and Yamamoto T. 2005. Improving the oral health of older people: The approach of the WHO Global Oral Health Programme. *Community Dent Oral Epidemiol* 33:81–92.

Promsudthi A, Pimapansri S, Deerochanawong C, and Kanchanavasita W. 2005. The effect of periodontal therapy on uncontrolled type 2 diabetes mellitus in older subjects. *Oral Dis* 11:293–8.

Ravon NA, Hollender LG, McDonald V, and Persson GR. 2003. Signs of carotid calcification from dental panoramic radiographs are in agreement with Doppler sonography results. *J Clin Periodontol* 30:1084–90.

Renvert S and Persson GR. 2002. A systematic review on the use of residual probing depth, bleeding on probing and furcation status following initial periodontal therapy to predict further attachment and tooth loss. *J Clin Periodontol* 29(Suppl. 3):82–9.

Renvert S and Persson GR. 2004. Supportive periodontal therapy. *Periodontol 2000* 36:179–95.

Renvert S, Roos-Jansåker AM, and Claffey N. 2008. Non-surgical treatment of peri-implant mucositis and peri-implantitis: A literature review. *J Clin Periodontol* 35(Suppl. 8):305–15.

Royzman D, Recio L, Badovinac RL, Fiorellini J, Goodson M, Howell H, and Karimbux N. 2004. The effect of aspirin intake on bleeding on probing in patients with gingivitis. *J Periodontol* 75:679–84.

Salvi GE, Fürst MM, Lang NP, and Persson GR. 2008. One-year bacterial colonization patterns of Staphylococcus aureus and other bacteria at implants and adjacent teeth. *Clin Oral Implants Res* 19:242–8.

Segers P, Speekenbrink RG, Ubbink DT, van Ogtrop ML, and de Mol BA. 2006. Prevention of nosocomial infection in cardiac surgery by decontamination of the nasopharynx and oropharynx with chlorhexidine gluconate: A randomized controlled trial. *JAMA* 296:2460–6.

Shay K. 2002. Infectious complications of dental and periodontal diseases in the elderly population. *Clin Infect Dis* 34:1215–23.

Söderpalm Andersen E, Söderfeldt B, and Kronström M. 2006. Oral health and treatment need among older individuals living in nursing homes in Skaraborg, Västra Götaland, Sweden. *Swed Dent J* 30:109–15.

Stewart R, Sabbah W, Tsakos G, D'Aiuto F, and Watt RG. 2008. Oral health and cognitive function in the Third National Health and Nutrition Examination Survey (NHANES III). *Psychosom Med* 70:936–41.

Suominen-Taipale AL, Mettovaara HL, Uutela A, Härkänen T, Vehkalahti MM, and Knuuttila ML. 2009 Cynical hostility as a determinant of poor oral health status in an adult population. *Eur J Oral Sci* 117:144–53.

Susin C, Valle P, Oppermann RV, Haugejorden O, and Albandar JM. 2005. Occurrence and risk indicators of increased probing depth in an adult Brazilian population. *J Clin Periodontol* 32:123–9.

Suvas S. 2008. Advancing age and immune cell dysfunction: Is it reversible or not? *Expert Opin Biol Ther* 8:657–68.

Swoboda JR, Kiyak HA, Darveau R, and Persson GR. 2008. Correlates of periodontal decline and biologic markers in older adults. *J Periodontol* 79:1920–6.

Taylor BA, Tofler GH, Carey HM, Morel-Kopp MC, Philcox S, Carter TR, Elliott MJ, Kull AD, Ward C, and Schenck K. 2006. Full-mouth tooth extraction lowers systemic inflammatory and thrombotic markers of cardiovascular risk. *J Dent Res* 85:74–8.

Teles RP, Patel M, Socransky SS, and Haffajee AD. 2008. Disease progression in periodontally healthy and maintenance subjects. *J Periodontol* 79:784–94.

Tezal M, Grossi SG, Ho AW, and Genco RJ. 2004. Alcohol consumption and periodontal disease. The Third National Health and Nutrition Examination Survey. *J Clin Periodontol* 31:484–8.

Torrungruang K, Tamsailom S, Rojanasomsith K, Sutdhibhisal S, Nisapakultorn K, Vanichjakvong O, Prapakamol S, Premsirinirund T, Pusiri T, Jaratkulangkoon O, Unkurapinun N, and Sritata P. 2005. Risk indicators of periodontal disease in older Thai adults. *J Periodontol* 76:558–65.

Trayhurn P and Wood IS. 2005. Signalling role of adipose tissue: Adipokines and inflammation in obesity. *Biochem Soc Trans* 33:1078–81.

Ushida Y, Koshy G, Kawashima Y, Kiji M, Umeda M, Nitta H, Nagasawa T, Ishikawa I, and Izumi Y. 2008. Changes in serum interleukin-6, C-reactive protein and thrombomodulin levels under periodontal ultrasonic debridement. *J Clin Periodontol* 35:969–75.

Van de Velde T, Thevissen E, Persson GR, Johansson C, and De Bruyn H. 2009. Two-year outcome with Nobel Direct implants: a retrospective radiographic and microbiologic study in 10 patients. *Clin Implant Dent Relat Res* 11:183–93.

Wennström JL. 1998. Treatment of periodontal disease in older adults. *Periodontol 2000* 16:106–12.

WHO. 2008. *World Alliance for Patient Safety. WHO Guidelines for Safe Surgery.* Geneva: World Health Organization.

Woods NF, LaCroix AZ, Gray SL, Aragaki A, Cochrane BB, Brunner RL, Masaki K, Murray A, and Newman AB. 2005. Frailty: Emergence and consequences in women aged 65 and older in the Women's Health Initiative Observational Study. *J Am Geriatr Soc* 53:1321–30.

Yerman T, Gan WQ, and Sin DD. 2007. The influence of gender on the effects of aspirin in preventing myocardial infarction. *BMC Med Online J* 5:29.

Zavala WD and Cavicchia JC. 2006. Deterioration of the Langerhans cell network of the human gingival epithelium with aging. *Arch Oral Biol* 51:1150–5.

Caries and Frail Elders

Chris Wyatt, Athena S. Papas, and Michael I. MacEntee

INTRODUCTION

Caries, as the primary cause of tooth loss in all age groups (Chestnut et al., 2000; Fure, 2003; Broadbent et al., 2006), places a large biological, sociological, and financial burden on society (Miller, 1978; Gift et al., 1992). Essentially, it is a bacterial infection exacerbated by an array of biological and behavioral interactions that over time weaken and ultimately demolish tooth structure (Figure 9.1).

The risk of infection increases substantially when inadequate oral hygiene permits large numbers of bacteria to accumulate on the teeth, and when frequent ingestions of sugars and refined carbohydrates provide the nourishment for bacteria to produce acids that demineralize, and ultimately, weaken the structural integrity of teeth (Wyatt and MacEntee, 1997).

The infection is particularly prevalent among vulnerable segments of the elderly population who cannot access regular dental care because they are institutionalized or housebound (Wyatt, 2002a, b; Wyatt and MacEntee, 2004; Institute of Medicine, 2009). Indeed, we are at particular risk to caries when old and frail because many of the medications for the usual physical and cognitive disabilities of old age disturb the natural buffering capacity of saliva that, under healthier circumstances, neutralizes the salivary pH induced by acidogenic bacteria (Chew et al., 2008).

The collapse and destruction of the natural dentition as a consequence of this carious process typically leads to chewing difficulties and disfigurement. However, only rarely is it associated with toothache in older teeth, probably because the insulation from secondary dentin deposited over the years allows the structural collapse without the acute sensitivity and pain that emerges from younger teeth (Fejerskov and Nyvad, 1986; Schüpbach

Oral Healthcare and the Frail Elder: A Clinical Perspective.
Edited by Michael I. MacEntee © 2011 Blackwell Publishing Ltd.

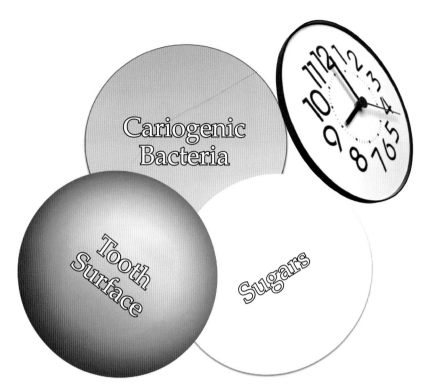

Figure 9.1   Factors interacting to create a cariogenic environment.

et al., 1990; MacEntee, 1994). However, the accumulation of bacteria associated with rampant caries can have a more insidious outcome by increasing the risk of aspiration pneumonia and an untimely death (Taylor et al., 2000).

THE CARIOUS LESION

Streptococcus mutans, *Streptococcus sobrinus*, *Streptococcus cricetus*, *Lactobacilli*, and possibly several other microorganisms live within the biofilm adhering to teeth (Preza et al., 2008). They produce acids from fermentable sugars in dental plaque, and acid demineralizes enamel, cementum, and dentin. The acidic demineralization is more likely on the root surfaces of teeth as the loss of gingival attachment exposes the less resistant cementum and dentin. And, so, the likelihood of caries increases with advancing age and gingival recession when the frequency of sugar consumption is high and the effectiveness of toothbrushing is low.

Carious lesions expand and are seen as cavities when the organic matrix of a tooth collapses without adequate mineral support. Typically, inactive or quiescent lesions have smooth or rounded rather than sharp or ragged edges, probably because rough edges are smoothed by normal wear and tear when the lesion stops expanding (Fejerskov et al., 2008). Early carious lesions typically are not cavitated but have a yellowish-brown color (Figure 9.2, *arrow a*), but with time they becomes dark brown cavities as lesions expand under the enamel (Figure 9.2, *arrow b*).

A demineralized matrix allows the cariogenic bacteria to penetrate further into the dentin and underneath the enamel. If the lesion in the dentin is large and expanding slowly, the periphery will look rough and lightly yellow while the center is hard and a darker yellowish brown as the dentinal tubules are sclerosed with new mineral deposits.

In its more rampant state, caries attacks the coronal and root surfaces of most teeth, and if the lesions expand slowly the cavities will look black and ominous (Figure 9.3).

The color of the lesion reflects the mixture of organic and inorganic tooth structure infiltrated by food, medications, and other chemicals. Therefore, color is not a very reliable or sensitive indicator of pathological activity. The raggedness or smoothness of the lesion's periphery along with the feel or texture of the surfaces are better indicators of carious activity. Unfortunately, probing or curetting an incipient lesion will damage the matrix irreparably and eliminate the possibility of remineralizing the tooth to its natural contour, although it does not eliminate the possibility of

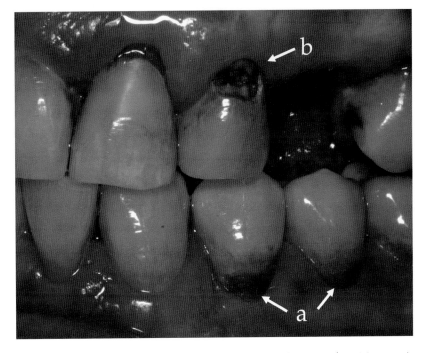

Figure 9.2 Early demineralized carious lesions on teeth #35 and #34 (*arrow a*); and cavitated lesion on tooth #24 (*arrow b*).

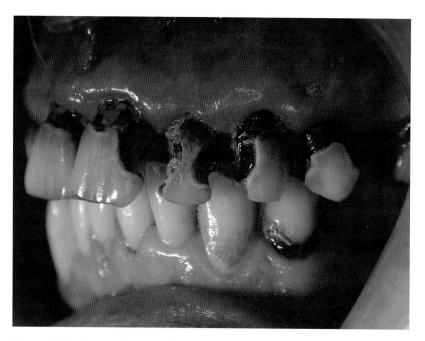

Figure 9.3 Rampant but slowly progressing caries.

remineralizing the damaged matrix to inactivate the carious process (Beighton et al., 1991, 1993). It is preferable, therefore, to judge carious activity by assessing the physical appearance and cavitation of the lesion's surface and periphery against the presence or absence of the behavioral risk factors, such as frequency of sugar consumption, medications, and oral hygiene.

DISTRIBUTION OF CARIES IN OLD AGE

Caries is a prevalent infection among elderly people as they grow frail. Recent data from the United States suggest that the average attack rate annually in older Americans over the last decade or so was about one new carious surface per person per year, which is similar to or higher than the attack rate reported on children (Griffin et al., 2005). The practical relevance of this attack rate to the incidence of the infection in the population is unclear because "late elder caries," like "early childhood caries," tends to occur rampantly within highly susceptible segments of the population, and much less aggressively or prevalently in the rest of the population (Wyatt and MacEntee, 1997). In any event, the infection can be very destructive in a short period of time for those who are susceptible to it (Frenkel et al., 2000; Wyatt, 2002a, b; Saub and Evans, 2001; Chalmers et al., 2002;

Carter et al., 2004). Therefore, it is necessary to take action to prevent the disease when the risk is high.

A major challenge to improving oral health in older populations is the lack of coordination between oral health, public health, and healthcare systems, and in particular, the overriding focus in dental practice on treatment rather than prevention of dental diseases. For many people, globally, dental treatment is simply unavailable or unaffordable (Institute of Medicine, 2009).

XEROSTOMIA AND SALIVARY GLAND HYPOFUNCTION

Dry mouth and dysfunctional salivary glands are usually the result of medications or radiation therapy that disturbs the flow or buffering capacity of saliva, and as a consequence they increase substantially the risk of caries (Chew et al., 2008; Turner and Ship, 2007). A remarkably large number of medications for a wide variety of chronic disorders interfere with salivary glands (Ikebe et al., 2005). Antidepressant and antipsychotic drugs prescribed for depression accompanying Alzheimer's disease, for example, lead almost inevitably to caries when compounded by the usual disinterest in personal hygiene and the cariogenic diets of people with severe dementia and depression (Anttila et al., 1999; Friedlander and Norman, 2002). Fortunately, for many of the disorders, there are alternative medications with much less impact on saliva (see Chapter 4).

PREVENTING CARIES

Preventing or reversing incipient and noncavitated carious lesion is achieved most effectively by a combination of altering the mineral structure of teeth, reducing the quantity and virulence of bacterial plaque on the teeth, and reducing the frequency of sugar consumption in the diet. These changes can be achieved by combinations of the following therapeutic strategies: (1) fluoride-containing toothpaste and mouthrinses; (2) oral hygiene; (3) sugar ingestions; (4) antimicrobial agents; and (5) pharmacological replacements. Fluoride applications alone might not be sufficient to prevent caries when salivary glands are dysfunctional, and it might be necessary to create a concentrated gradient of calcium and phosphate ions in saliva that will facilitate the diffusion of ions into the organic matrices of the teeth (Singh and Papas, 2009). The presence of statherin and the proline rich proteins in saliva promote a supersaturated concentration of calcium and phosphate ions and subsurface remineralization.

Fluoride

A concentration of fluoride ions in dental plaque and saliva simultaneously inhibits demineralization and enhances remineralization by promoting fluoroapatite. Fluoride, in one form or another, is the most effective chemical agent for remineralizing teeth and strengthening dental surfaces against demineralization (Ingram and Edgar, 1994). It is readily available in mouthrinses, toothpastes, gels, and varnishes, without evidence that any one form is therapeutically superior (Ravald and Birkhed, 1992).

Concentrations of fluoride, either as sodium fluoride or monofluorophosphate, in toothpastes sold in the United States range from 1,000 to 1,500 ppm (concentration of fluoride in toothpaste are presented usually in parts per million [ppm] because most toothpaste manufacturers report only the percentage of the fluoride compound in the tube of paste) (Centers for Disease Control and Prevention, 2009), whereas in Europe the concentrations are lower (~450 ppm) due to concerns about dental fluorosis in children (Dental Health Foundation—Ireland, 2010). Fluoride concentrations of 1,000 ppm or higher will prevent demineralization of dental surfaces and enable remineralization of incipient carious lesions if part of a daily health-promoting regimen (Jensen and Kohout, 1988). In addition, therapeutic concentrations of 5,000 ppm will double this protection and remineralization of the tooth structure within cavitated lesions (Stephen et al., 1988; Baysan et al., 2001). Similar dose-related protection and remineralization of coronal and root surfaces is possible with a daily mouthrinse of about 250 ppm (0.05%) to 500 ppm (0.2%) sodium fluoride (Ripa et al., 1987; Wyatt and MacEntee, 2004).

A mouthrinse of 920 ppm (0.2%) neutral sodium fluoride used daily will reduce the incidence of new caries and reverse demineralization of new lesions (Wyatt and MacEntee, 2004). Two daily applications of a 5,000 ppm fluoride toothpaste will also prevent caries, while a varnish containing 22,600 ppm (5%) of sodium fluoride applied once a month by a dentist or dental hygienist is similarly effective (Weintraub, 2003; Ekstrand et al., 2008). Alternatively, an acidic (pH ~3) gel containing 0.4% stannous fluoride will reduce the incidence of caries by disturbing the dental biofilm and helping fluoride ions penetrate the surface of the tooth. This strategy has been used effectively for root surfaces of overdenture abutments (Derkson and MacEntee, 1982; Willumsen et al., 2007). Daily use of a highly concentrated fluoride toothpaste or mouthrinse supplemented by a fluoridated varnish applied to the teeth at 3- to 6-month intervals by a dental professional is probably needed by elders at high risk of developing caries (Zero et al., 2010).

Oral hygiene

The physical and cognitive limitations of frailty render oral hygiene difficult to control (de Baat et al., 1993; Kay and Locker, 1996). Electric toothbrushes are helpful (Papas et al., 2007), but teeth with large restorations and exposed root surfaces are difficult to clean no matter what type of brush is used.

Reducing sugar ingestions

Frequent ingestions of refined carbohydrates greatly increase the risk of caries (Papas et al., 1995a, b). People who consume more than eight intakes of sugar throughout the day, for example, double the risk (Steele et al., 2001). It can be difficult to find the source of the sugar in the diet, especially among people who are cognitively impaired. However, we do know that more than half of the medications consumed by older people contain sugar to improve the taste of the medication, so this alone is a major source of occult sugar (Maguire and Baqir, 2000). On the other hand, a primary objective of long-term care is to maintain the weight of frail patients (Keller, 1993; Tierney, 1996); consequently, caregivers are reluctant to discourage any potential source of calories, even if they come as sugar in drinks or candies.

Xylitol is a sugar substitute that interferes with the metabolism of mutans streptococcus, and when combined with chlorhexidine in chewing gum that stimulates salivary flow, it disturbs the dental biofilm and the quantity of microbial plaque on teeth (Simons et al., 2001). However, we do not know that xylitol, with or without chlorhexidine, will prevent or help manage caries in elders.

Chlorhexidine

Chlorhexidine is a broad-spectrum antibiotic that binds to mucosa and to microorganisms, including mutans streptococci and other gram-positive microorganisms. It is used primarily in dentistry to control gingivitis by disturbing the cell membranes and killing microorganisms (Persson et al., 1991). Systemic side effects are rare, but users often experience discoloration of teeth and dentures, and taste alteration.

The practical value of chlorhexidine as an anticaries medication is controversial. There is limited evidence that at 0.12% concentration it reduces the numbers of mutans streptococci and lactobacilli (Persson et al., 1991; van Rijkom et al., 1996) and that it compliments the benefits of fluoride (Brailsford et al., 2002; Bizhang et al., 2007). A substantial reduction in root caries was obtained with a 10% chlorhexidine varnish (Banting et al., 2000). However, evidence is inconclusive from other studies of chlorhexidine as a mouthrinse or varnish for preventing root caries and tooth loss (Twetman, 2004; Wyatt et al., 2006; van Strijp et al., 2008).

RESTORING DENTAL CAVITIES

Debriding and recontouring a shallow carious lesion to produce an easily cleansable surface that can be remineralized with saliva and fluoride is preferable to restoring the dental surface with an amalgam, composite, or glass ionomer filling (Billings et al., 1985; Beighton et al., 1991, 1993; Anusavice, 1995). Alternatively, the "atraumatic restorative treatment" (ART) technique offers a relatively conservative approach to debriding and restoring deeper lesions. Originally advocated with considerable success for primary teeth (Frencken et al., 1996, 2007), it has been used successfully to debride carious lesions and restore the teeth of elders (Lo et al., 2006) and of patients with radiation-induced caries (Hu et al., 2005). The preferred restorative material for the ART is a high-viscosity fluoride-releasing glass ionomer because the adhesion of the filling to the tooth excludes carbohydrates from any residual bacteria in the lesion (Weerheijm et al., 1993; Weerheijm and Groen, 1999), while the fluoride strengthens the tooth against further remineralization (Cenci et al., 2008). In any event, the ease and speed with which the ART can be performed make it very suitable for patients who are restless or physically restricted. However, the adhesion of the filling to the tooth is compromised if the dentin is contaminated by saliva, gingival fluid, or blood.

A CLINICAL SCENARIO

Clinical scenario

The Director of Nursing in a local residential care facility requests a consultation with a dentist for Mrs. Switzer, who is 86 years old with a fractured maxillary left lateral incisor. Mrs. Switzer was admitted to the facility 3 weeks previously with moderate Alzheimer's disease, type II diabetes, and severe hypertension.

Mrs. Switzer attended her dentist 1 month before entering the facility but did not follow the dentist's recommendations for periodontal debridement, intracoronal dental restorations, and a fixed partial denture. Previous to this, Mrs. Switzer had not seen a dentist for 2 years, although she claims to have visited her dentist frequently over the years before then. Consequently, she is referred to the hospital's dentist for further assessment and treatment of the fractured tooth.

The dentist examined Mrs. Switzer to confirm that the maxillary lateral incisor has an asymptomatic, but complete, coronal fracture due to root caries (Figure 9.4).

He notes also that there is copious plaque and food debris around the teeth and mouth. On questioning, Mrs. Switzer reveals that she drinks tea sweetened with sugar constantly "for energy" and to be sociable in the facility, and she takes multiple medications for blood pressure, depression, and occasional memory loss.

The dentist requests the radiographs taken before she entered the facility to determine the extent of the carious lesions (Figure 9.5).

A diagnosis was made of extensive root caries involving all previously restored teeth. A treatment plan of extraction of the fractured maxillary left lateral incisor and replacement using an acrylic removable partial denture was made. The carious lesions were scheduled for restoration using resin-modified glass ionomer material. The patient's daughter was warned that excavation of caries on the roots might result in tooth fracture. If this occurs, then denture teeth can be added to the acrylic removable partial denture in the maxilla or an additional prosthesis will be needed for the mandible. Personalized diet and daily mouthcare counseling was discussed with the patient, daughter, and nursing staff. Daily use of 0.2% neutral sodium fluoride was prescribed for prevention of root caries.

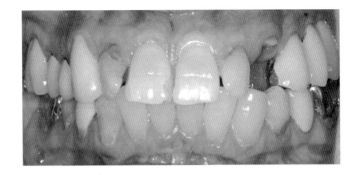

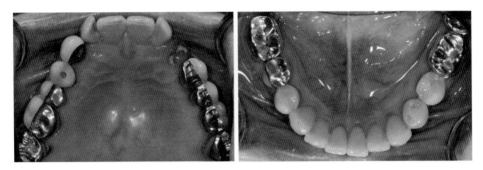

Figure 9.4 Mrs. Switzer's dentition.

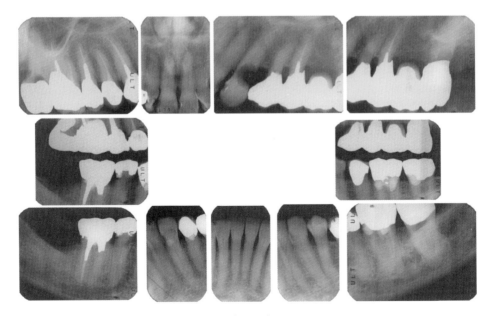

Figure 9.5 Mrs. Switzer's radiographs.

CONCLUSIONS

Caries is a challenging infection to manage, particularly when foods, drinks, and medications are cariogenic, saliva is abnormal, and oral hygiene is inadequate. Such are the conditions that confront many frail elders. In short, caries is an unpredictable disease that can produce defects in teeth at an alarming rate to weaken them beyond repair. Decisions to remineralize, restore, or extract teeth depend largely on the extent of the structural damage. Dental surfaces can be strengthened and remineralized with fluoride to withstand the assault of acidogenic bacteria, and antimicrobial agents, such as a chlorhexidine, might help reduce the number of cariogenic bacteria, although it is not clear yet how much impact antibacterial agents have on the incidence of caries (Wyatt et al., 2006). Management and restoration of carious lesions range from debridement of the lesions to restoration of cavities with dental materials, whereas long-term strategies to control the infection need careful surveillance of the diet supplemented by continuous application of fluorides.

REFERENCES

Anttila SS, Knuuttila ML, and Sakki TK. 1999. Depressive symptoms favour abundant growth of salivary lactobacilli. *Psychosom Med* 61:508–12.

Anusavice KJ. 1995. Treatment regimens in preventive and restorative dentistry. *J Am Dent Assoc* 126:727–743.

Banting DW, Papas A, Clark DC, Proskin HM, Schultz M, and Perry R. 2000. The effectiveness of 10% chlorhexidine varnish treatment on dental caries incidence in adults with dry mouth. *Gerodontology* 17:67–76.

Baysan A, Lynch E, Ellwood R, Davies R, Petersson L, and Borsboom P. 2001. Reversal of primary root caries using dentifrice containing 5000 and 1100 ppm fluoride. *Caries Res* 35:41–46.

Beighton D, Hellyer PH, Lynch EJ, and Heath MR. 1991. Salivary levels of mutans streptococci, lactobacilli, yeasts, and root caries prevalence in non-institutionalized elderly dental patients. *Community Dent Oral Epidemiology* 19:302–7.

Beighton D, Lynch E, and Heath MR. 1993. A microbiological study of primary root caries lesions with different treatment needs. *J Dent Res* 72:623–9.

Billings RJ, Brown LR, and Kaster AG. 1985. Contemporary treatment strategies for root-surface dental caries. *Gerodontics* 1:20–7.

Bizhang M, Chun YH, Heisrath D, Purucker P, Singh P, Kersten T, and Zimmer S. 2007. Microbiota of exposed root-surfaces after fluoride, chlorhexidine, and periodontal maintenance therapy: A 3-year evaluation. *J Periodontol* 78:1580–9.

Brailsford S, Fiske J, Gilbert S, Clark D, and Beighton D. 2002. The effects of the combination of chlorhexidine/thimol- and fluoride-containing varnishes on the severity of root caries lesions in frail institutionalized elderly people. *J Dent* 30:319–24.

Broadbent JM, Thomson WM, and Poulton R. 2006. Progression of dental caries and tooth loss between the third and fourth decades of life: a birth cohort study. *Caries Res* 40:459–65.

Carter G, Lee M, McKelvey V, Sourial A, Halliwell R, and Livingston M. 2004. Oral health status and oral treatment needs of dependent elderly people in Christchurch. *N Z Med J* 21:117.

Cenci MS, Tenuta LMA, Pereira-Cenci T, Del Bel Cury AA, ten Cate JM, and Cury JA. 2008. Effect of microleakage and fluoride on enamel-dentine demineralization around restorations. *Caries Res* 42:369–79.

Centers for Disease Control and Prevention. 2009. *Other Fluoride Products. Division of Oral Health, National Center for Chronic Disease Prevention and Health Promotion.* Available at www.cdc.gov/FLUORIDATION/other.htm (accessed January 5, 2010).

Chalmers JM, Hodge C, and Fuss JM, Spencer AJ, and Carter KD. 2002. The prevalence and experience of oral disease in Adelaide nursing home residents. *Aust Dent J* 47:123–30.

Chestnut I, Binnie V, and Taylor M. 2000. Reasons for tooth extraction in Scotland. *J Dent* 28:295–7.

Chew ML, Mulsant BH, Pollock BG, Lehman ME, Greenspan A, Mahmoud RA, Kirshner MA, Sorisio DA, Bies RR, and Gharabawi G. 2008. Anticholinergic activity of 107 medications commonly used by older adults. *J Am Geriatr Soc* 56:1333–41.

de Baat C, Kalk W, and Schuil GR. 1993. The effectiveness of oral hygiene programs for elderly people: A review. *Gerodontology* 10:109–13.

Dental Health Foundation—Ireland. 2010. *Oral Health Care Products, Fluoride Toothpastes.* Available at www.dentalhealth.ie/dentalhealth/index.tmpl?secid=20020821120259&subid=20020822145733 (accessed January 5, 2010).

Derkson G and MacEntee MI. 1982. Effect of a 0.4% stannous fluoride gel on the gingival health of overdenture abutments. *J Prosthet Dent* 48:23–6.

Ekstrand K, Martignon S, and Holm-Pedersen P. 2008. Development and evaluation of two root caries controlling programmes for home-based frail people older than 75 years. *Gerodontology* 25:67–75.

Fejerskov O and Nyvad B. 1986. Pathology and treatment of dental caries in the aging individual. In: Holm-Pederson P and Löe H (eds.), *Geriatric Dentistry*. Copenhagen: Munksgaard, pp. 238–62.

Fejerskov O, Nyvad B, and Kidd EAM. 2008. Clinical appearances of caries lesions. In: Fejerskov O and Kidd EAM (eds.), *Dental Caries: The Disease and Its Clinical Management*. Oxford: Blackwell Munksgaard Ltd., pp. 7–18.

Friedlander AH and Norman DC. 2002. Late-life depression: Psychopathology, medical interventions, and dental implications. *Oral Surg Oral Med Oral Pathol Oral Radiol Endod* 94:404–12.

Frencken JE, Pilot T, Songpaisan Y, and Phantumvanit P. 1996. Atraumatic restorative treatment (ART): Rationale, technique, and development. *J Public Health Dent* 56:135–40.

Frencken JE, van't Hof MA, Taifour D, and Al-Zaher I. 2007. Effectiveness of ART and traditional amalgam approach in restoring single-surface cavities in posterior teeth of permanent dentitions in school children after 6.3 years. *Community Dent Oral Epidemiol* 35:207–14.

Frenkel H, Harvey I, and Newcombe RG. 2000. Oral health care among nursing home residents in Avon. *Gerodontology* 17:33–38.

Fure S. 2003. Ten-year incidence of tooth loss and dental caries in elderly Swedish individuals. *Caries Res* 37:462–9.

Gift HC, Reisine ST, and Larach DC. 1992. The social impact of dental problems and visits. *Am J Public Health* 82(12):1663–8.

Griffin SO, Griffin PM, Swann JL, and Zlobin N. 2005. New coronal caries in older adults: Implications for prevention. *J Dent Res* 84:715–20.

Hu JY, Chen XC, Li YQ, Smales RJ, and Yip KH. 2005. Radiation-induced root surface caries restored with glass-ionomer cement placed in conventional and ART cavity preparations: Results at two years. *Aust Dent J* 50:186–90.

Ikebe K, Morii K, Kashiwagi J, and Nokubi T. 2005. Ettinger RL. Impact of dry mouth on oral symptoms and function in removable denture wearers in Japan. *Oral Surg Oral Med Oral Pathol Oral Radiol Endod* 99:704–10.

Ingram GS and Edgar WM. 1994. Interactions of fluoride and non-fluoride agents with the caries process. *Adv Dent Res* 8:158–65.

Institute of Medicine. 2009. *The U.S. Oral Health Workforce in the Coming Decade: Workshop Summary.* Washington, DC: The National Academies Press. Available at www.nap.edu/catalog.php?record_id=12669 (accessed February 1, 2010).

Jensen M and Kohout F. 1988. The effect of a fluoridated dentifrice on root and coronal caries in an older adult population. *J Am Dent Assoc* 117:829–832.

Kay EJ and Locker D. 1996. Is dental health education effective? A systematic review of current evidence. *Community Dent Oral Epidemiology* 24:231–5.

Keller HH. 1993. Malnutrition in institutionalized elderly: How and why? *J Am Geriatr Soc* 41:1212–8.

Lo EC, Luo Y, Tan HP, Dyson JE, and Corbet EF. 2006. ART and conventional root restorations in elders after 12 months. *J Dent Res* 85:929–32.

MacEntee MI. 1994. How severe is the threat of caries to old teeth. *J Prosthet Dent* 71:473–7.

Maguire A and Baqir W. 2000. Prevalence of long-term use of medicines with prolonged oral clearance in the elderly: A survey in northeast England. *Br Dent J* 189:267–72.

Miller J. 1978. Waste of dental pain. *Int Dent J* 28:66–71.

Papas AS, Joshi A, Palmer CA, Giunta J, and Dwyer JT. 1995a. Relationship of diet to root caries. *Am J Clin Nutr* 61(Suppl.):423S–9S.

Papas AS, Joshi A, Belanger A, Kent R, and DePaola, P. 1995b. Dietary models for root caries. *Am J Clin Nutr* 61(Suppl.):417S–22S.

Papas AS, Singh M, Harrington D, Ortblad K, de Jager M, and Nunn M. 2007. Reduction in caries rate among patients with xerostomia using a power toothbrush. *Spec Care Dentist* 27:46–51.

Persson RE, Truelove EL, Lereshe L, LeResche S, and Robinovitch MR. 1991. Therapeutic effects of daily or weekly chlorhexidine rinses on oral health of a geriatric population. *Oral Surg Oral Med Oral Pathol* 72:184–91.

Preza D, Olsen I, Aas JA, Willumsen T, Grinde B, and Paster BJ. 2008. Bacterial profiles of root caries in elderly patients. *J Clin Microbiol* 46:2015–21.

Ravald N and Birkhed D. 1992. Prediction of root caries in periodontally treated patients maintained with different fluoride programs. *Caries Res* 26:450–8.

Ripa L, Leske G, Forte F, and Varma A. 1987. Effect of a 0.05% NaF rinse on coronal and root caries in adults. *Gerodontology* 6:131–6.

Saub R and Evans R. 2001. Dental needs of elderly hostel residents in inner Melbourne. *Aust Dent J* 46:198–202.

Schüpbach P, Guggenheim B, and Lutz, F. 1990. Histopathology of root-surface caries. *J Dent Res* 69:1195–204.

Simons D, Brailsford S, Kidd E, and Beighton D. 2001. The effect of chlorhexidine/xylitol chewing gum on the plaque and gingival indices of elderly occupants in residential homes. *J Clin Periodontol* 28:101–105.

Singh ML and Papas AS. 2009. Long term clinical observation of dental caries in salivary hypofunction patients using supersaturated calcium phosphate remineralizing rinse. *J Clin Dent* 20:87–92.

Steele JG, Sheiham A, Marcenes W, Fay N, and Walls AW. 2001. Clinical and behavioural risk indicators for root caries in older people. *Gerodontology* 18:95–10.

Stephen KW, Creanor SL, Russell JI, Burchell CK, Huntington E, and Downie CF. 1988. A 3 year oral health dose-response study of sodium monofluoro-phosphate dentifrices with and without zinc citrate: Anti-caries results. *Community Dent Oral Epidemiol* 16:321–5.

Taylor GW, Loesche WJ, and Terpenning MS. 2000. Impact of oral diseases on systemic health in the elderly: Diabetes mellitus and aspiration pneumonia. *J Public Health Dent* 60:313–20.

Tierney AJ. 1996. Undernutrition and elderly hospital patients: A review. *J Adv Nurs* 23:228–36.

Turner MD and Ship JA. 2007. Dry mouth and its effects on the oral health of elderly people. *J Am Dent Assoc* 138(Suppl.):15S–20S.

Twetman S. 2004. Antimicrobials in future caries control? A review with special reference to chlorhexidine treatment. *Caries Res* 38:223–9.

van Rijkom HM, Truin GJ, and van't Hof MA. 1996. A meta-analysis of clinical studies on caries-inhibiting effect of chlorhexidine treatment. *J Dent Res* 75:790–5.

van Strijp AJ, Gerardu VA, Buijs MJ, van Loveren C, and ten Cate JM. 2008. Chlorhexidine efficacy in preventing lesion formation in enamel and dentine: an in situ study. *Caries Res* 42:460–5.

Weintraub J. 2003. Fluoride varnish for caries prevention: Community-based protocol. *Spec Care Dentist* 23:180–6.

Weerheijm KL and Groen HJ. 1999. The residual caries dilemma. *Community Dent Oral Epidemiol* 27:436–41.

Weerheijm KL, De Soet JJ, Van Amerongen WE, and De Graff J. 1993. The effect of glass ionomer cement on carious dentin: An in vivo study. *Caries Res* 27:417–23.

Willumsen T, Solemdal K, Wenaasen M, and Ogaard B. 2007. Stannous fluoride in dentifrice: An effective anti-plaque agent in the elderly? *Gerodontology* 24:239–43.

Wyatt CCL. 2002a. Elderly Canadians residing in long term care hospitals: Part I—Medical and dental status. *J Can Dent Assoc* 68:353–8.

Wyatt CCL. 2002b. Elderly Canadians residing in long term care hospitals: Part II—Dental caries status. *J Can Dent Assoc* 68:359–63.

Wyatt CCL and MacEntee MI. 1997. Dental caries in chronically disabled elders. *Spec Care Dentist* 17:196–202.

Wyatt CCL and MacEntee MI. 2004. Caries management for institutionalized elders using fluoride and chlorhexidine mouthrinses. *Community Dent Oral Epidemiol* 32:322–8.

Wyatt CCL, Maupome G, Hujoel PP, MacEntee MI, Persson GR, Persson RE, and Kiyak HA. 2006. Chlorhexidine and preservation of sound tooth structure in older adults: A placebo-controlled trial. *Caries Res* 41:93–101.

Zero DT, Fontana M, Martínez-Mier EA, Ferreira-Zandona A, Ando M, Gonzalez-Cabezas C, and Bayne S. 2010. The biology, prevention, diagnosis and treatment of dental caries. *J Am Dent Assoc* 140(Suppl. 1):25S–34S.

Contexts of body image and social interactions among frail elders

Leeann Donnelly, Laura Hurd Clarke, Alison Phinney, and Michael I. MacEntee

INTRODUCTION

Social relations are necessary for health and well-being (Berkman, 1995; Seeman et al., 1996; Bennett, 2005), and reduced social engagement is a threat to health that equates to smoking tobacco, high blood pressure, and reduced physical activity (House et al., 1988). Frail elders, probably more than most other groups, are at increased risk of becoming socially isolated as their physical and cognitive capacities decline, their accommodations change, and connections with family and friends severed (Havens and Hall, 2001). The chronic diseases of old age have a significantly negative impact on social interactions; however, the impact of oral health on social involvement has received very little attention from clinicians and researchers alike. We know that the social interactions of children, adolescents, and middle-aged adults are influenced by the appearance and health of their teeth, but it has been assumed widely that natural teeth are lost with advancing age, so that teeth are no longer a matter of much concern when old age leads to frailty and general disability. Consequently, the interrelationships between oral health and the social experiences of elders as they grow frail have all but been ignored.

Old age imposes multiple challenges on the mouth and on oral healthcare. Medications may reduce salivary flow, which increases the occurrences of caries, mucositis, and candidiasis (Turner and Ship, 2007). Physical and cognitive impairments interfere with personal hygiene, which heightens the risk of candidiasis, gingivitis, halitosis, periodontal disease, and to a lesser extent, caries, while impaired mobility limits access to oral

Oral Healthcare and the Frail Elder: A Clinical Perspective.
Edited by Michael I. MacEntee © 2011 Blackwell Publishing Ltd.

healthcare. Collectively, these challenges have a very significant physical impact, causing pain and discomfort, upsetting nutrition, and exacerbating other diseases. But just as importantly, these challenges to oral health can disrupt body image, reduce social interactions, and diminish quality of life. This chapter will describe what we know about associations between conditions of the mouth and social interactions among elderly people as they grow frail. In addition, we will introduce the concept of body image as a possible influence on social interaction in old age, and consider how it too is influenced by the oral healthcare administered to frail elders.

SOCIAL ISOLATION, EMOTIONAL ISOLATION, AND DEPRESSION

Social isolation, typically defined as a physical separation from others, becomes more common as people grow older because of the social and physical realities of retirement, declining health, impaired mobility, and the death of friends and relatives (de Jong Gierveld and Havens, 2004). Barriers to social interaction are potentially very damaging because of the strong links between health and social engagement. Lack of social contact predisposes to depression, neglectful health practices, and increased susceptibility to physical and cognitive disabilities (House et al., 1988; Cacioppo and Hawkley, 2003). Likewise, there are many health-related conditions, for instance, hearing impairment, incontinence, and pain, that impede social interactions (Weinstein and Ventry, 1982; Fultz and Herzog, 2001; Sofaer-Bennett et al., 2007). It is not clear, therefore, whether social isolation causes disease or if disease causes social isolation (House et al., 1988). Either way, social activities help prevent disability, which, in turn, enables further activity. Similarly, exercise, hygiene, and a good diet influence personal appearance, and an attractive appearance fosters social contacts (Umberson, 1987).

Emotional isolation or loneliness in contrast to social isolation is a feeling of social inadequacy and involuntary exile (de Jong Gierveld et al., 1987). They are feelings occurring in both an emotional and a social context (Weiss, 1973). Death of a spouse or a close friend produces strong emotions of isolation, grief, and loneliness, and they occur, to a lesser extent, for many people on retirement or separation from familiar surroundings (Tomaka et al., 2006). Elders can feel very isolated as they grow frailer with deteriorating health, and especially if they live alone or in residential care away from familiar friends and family (Jongenelis et al., 2004; Jylha, 2004; Routasalo et al., 2006).

Loneliness and depression frequently go hand in hand, and together they double the likelihood of early death (Stek et al., 2005). Consequently, the ill health attributed to a lack of social relationships is probably due more directly to loneliness and depression than to social isolation alone (Pinquart and Sorensen, 2001; Wenger and Burholt, 2004; Tomaka et al., 2006). However, this is not clear since the relationship between social isolation, loneliness, and depression is a complicated interaction. Depression is often precipitated by loneliness, but social isolation and loneliness do not always accompany each other as evidenced by some elders who are socially isolated and not lonely, whereas others feel lonely even in the midst of a crowd (Wenger and Burholt, 2004). Apparently, it is the quality rather than the quantity of social contacts that matter, and social contacts among close friends and confidants are frequently more protective of health than contacts with relatives who frequently impose more emotional stress than comfort (Giles et al., 2005; Routasalo et al., 2006).

ORAL HEALTH AND SOCIAL INTERACTIONS

Oral health and disease influence social interactions within all age groups (Linn, 1966; Vallittu et al., 1996; Newton et al., 2003). Malformed or misaligned teeth (Helm et al., 1985; Kiyak, 2000; Coffield et al., 2005), cleft lips and palates (Noar, 1992), and teeth damaged by caries (Filstrup et al., 2003) can increase self-consciousness, disturb body image and personal relationships, and generally disrupt social interactions. Halitosis or bad breath, whether from dental and gingival diseases or from more distant gastrointestinal or pulmonary disorders, is particularly disturbing to social interactions both for people with the disorder and others confronted by it (MacEntee et al., 1997; McKeown, 2003; van den Broek et al., 2008). Anaerobic bacteria can degrade organic residue in the mouth to produce volatile sulfur compounds that smell very unpleasant (Tonzetich, 1977). However, there are people who believe that they have halitosis even in the absence of an organic cause (Murata et al., 2002; Yaegaki and Coil, 2000), and they too feel embarrassed, lack self-confidence, and restrict their social relationships.

There is little doubt that oral disease and impairment can have a very serious effect on how people of all ages interact.

Clinical scenario 1

Mrs. Claude is 85 years old and has been living in a residential care facility for 5 years. Her family arranged for a dental hygienist to clean her teeth every few months because she seemed unable to do this for herself, although she seemed cognitively alert and physically robust. The nurse attending to her needs explained to the dental hygienist that Mrs. Claude had not spoken to anyone for at least 2 years, and that she suspected a stroke and "the isolation of old age," although there was no other evidence of cerebrovascular problems. The nurse commented on the smell of Mrs. Claude's breath but thought little more about it because, as she explained, "most old people have smelly breath." Apparently, Mrs. Claude had withdrew from most social encounters several months previously and communicated solely by nodding in response to questions.

The dental hygienist found that Mrs. Claude was very cooperative and appreciative of the treatment rendered but only through smiles and hand gestures—no words. There were deep layers of plaque and calculus on Mrs. Claude's teeth (Figure 10.1).

After the calculus was removed, she was encouraged to use a toothbrush every day despite the gingival bleeding. The nurse was instructed also on how to help Mrs. Claude's hygiene; however, very little had improved when the dental hygienist returned 1 month later. The plaque layers had returned, the gingiva continued to bleed when brushed, and Mrs. Claude seemed distressed. The nurse explained that she tried to get Mrs. Claude to use the toothbrush but they both were reluctant to brush thoroughly because of the bleeding. The nurse explained further that she suspected a bleeding disorder and that a physician had ordered blood tests and results were expected the next day. The dental hygienist on telephoning the next day was advised that Mrs. Claude's blood was normal. Consequently, she returned for another consultation with Mrs. Claude and her nurse, from which they agreed that a different approach to dental hygiene was needed. The nurse in Mrs. Claude's presence received additional instructions on gingivitis and dental plaque, and they were reassured that the bleeding would cease when the gingiva were no longer irritated by the plaque, but that this would require several days or weeks of thorough plaque removal from the teeth.

The dental hygienist returned 1 week later to find Mrs. Claude in the midst of a conversation with several other residents. The nurse explained enthusiastically that Mrs. Claude diligently cleaned her own teeth three times daily since the previous consultation (Figure 10.2). When Mrs. Claude saw the dental hygienist, she exclaimed, "My breath doesn't smell anymore."

Further discussions with staff and family revealed that over the course of her life, Mrs. Claude was fastidious about her personal grooming, and derived much pride and pleasure from her appearance, including her teeth. The neglect and deterioration of her oral health as she grew frail and moved to institutional life disturbed her so much that she refused to speak for fear of exposing the condition of her mouth. Subsequently, renewed attention to oral hygiene gave her the self-confidence she needed to speak openly with a confident smile and normal breath.

The impact of oral health and hygiene on social interactions among frail elders has received very little attention, considering the potential morbidity of social isolation and loneliness (Fiske et al., 1998; Gregory et al., 2005; Mollaoglu and Alpar, 2005; MacEntee, 2006). Elderly people are embarrassed by teeth that they see as ugly, breath that smells, dentures that move visibly when eating, and by the amount of time needed to finish a meal when teeth or dentures are not chewing comfortably or efficiently (MacEntee et al., 1997). Improvement in oral comfort and function can have a very positive, and as illustrated in our clinical scenario, overt influence on self-image and social interaction.

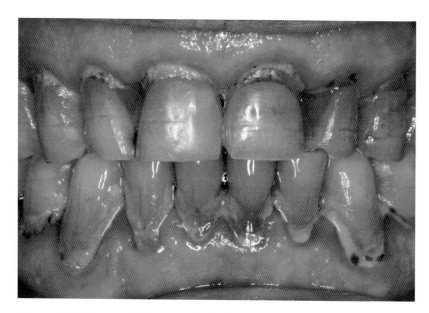

Figure 10.1 Layers of plaque and calculus causing gingivitis, periodontitis, and halitosis. (Photograph courtesy of Dr. B. Lamberts.)

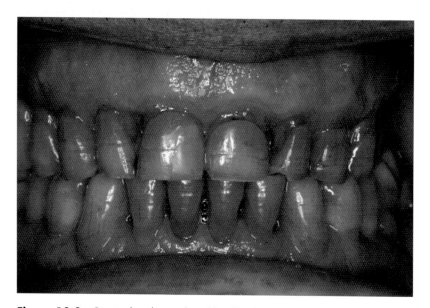

Figure 10.2 Gingival and periodontal health after removing plaque and calculus. (Photograph courtesy of Dr. B. Lamberts.)

It appears that the extent to which elders are bothered by their oral health and the degree to which impairments and disease disturbs their quality of life is not entirely associated with the physical or clinical status of the teeth as interpreted by dental professionals. Rather, the significant issues appear to revolve around the elder's perceptions and expectations (Lee et al., 2007). People in all stages of life construct their own priorities and expectations, and there is no reason to believe that elders differ as they grow frail. However, the consequences of thwarted priorities and unmet expectations in old age are likely to be especially threatening to self-image, confidence, and social interaction. Fortunately, frailty and social relations are influenced by an array of circumstances both past and present, but much remains to be known about how best to monitor and adjust the circumstances so that a self-imposed isolation does not become a morbid or even fatal loneliness.

BODY IMAGE AND ORAL HEALTH

The impact of oral impairment and disease in old age can be considered usefully in the context of body image. Defined initially in 1935 by Schilder, body image is "the picture of our body which we form in our mind" (Cash and Pruzinsky, 1990). It relates not only to how we view and project the appearance of our body, but also to how others perceive and react to us. Although interest tends to dwell on the shape (and weight) of younger women (Tiggemann and Kurring, 2004), there is awareness now of the interest that older women and men also have in projecting positive images of themselves (Hayslip et al., 1997; Farquhar and Wasylkiw, 2007). Concerns about personal appearances are influenced strongly by cultural standards of masculine and feminine attractiveness, with overemphasis today on youthful characteristics, such as physical fitness, slimness, smooth skin, and white teeth. As well as fueling the cosmetic and fitness industries, the current emphasis on youthfulness and appearance can lead to poor body image and decreased well-being among all ages. People young and old almost invariably find themselves lacking when compared with current ideals of male and female beauty. The unending drive to achieve the ideal body-beautiful produces, in the extreme, an expensive assortment of cosmetic creams and gels, excessive physical exercise, eating disorders, cosmetic surgery, and drug abuse (Hurd Clarke and Griffin, 2007). Similarly, the social emphasis on youthful appearances leads to the disparagement of aging and aged bodies, with associated and profound negative effects to the self-esteem of elders (Hayslip et al., 1997; Bedford and Johnson, 2006; Hurd Clarke and Griffin, 2007).

Information about the influence of oral health on body image relates mostly to young adults who have become, in recent years, increasingly attracted to teeth that are both straight and white. However, facial attractiveness is not the sole prerogative of youth. Older women and men also value "nice teeth" and a "nice smile" (MacGregor, 1990; Hurd Clarke, 2002). Appearance-related concerns about broken, missing, or crooked teeth can negatively affect how individuals view their bodies and can result in a reluctance to smile (Patel et al., 2007, 2008). Moreover, there is widespread belief that attractive people are more intelligent, successful, desirable, happy, socially integrated, kind, and sincere, and that "what is beautiful is good" (Dion et al., 1972). Smiling people, it is presumed, are more attractive, more sincere, sociable, and competent than people who do not or cannot smile, which leads to the conclusion that "what is smiling is beautiful and good" (Reis et al., 1990). Western society's ideal of good oral health is perpetuated everywhere by images of young, healthy, smiling people with straight, white teeth. Sadly, images that equate "good oral health" with youthful attractiveness are impossible for most elders to meet, and especially when physically disabled and poor. Worse still, the inability to meet these ideals can result in feelings of embarrassment, diminished self-confidence, shame, and failure (McKinley and Hyde, 1996). These feelings influence not only an individual's body image but also how they cope and behave in social situations. People with a normal appearance can go about their daily lives with relative anonymity, while those without are forced often to endure unwanted attention that blatantly disregards the common rules of social behavior (MacGregor, 1990; Houston and Bull, 1994; Rumsey et al., 2002). Disfigurement from head and neck cancer, for example, can lead to stigma and social exclusion (Clarke, 1999). It is no surprise, therefore, that elders with visible deformities of the mouth and decay of the teeth will feel stigmatized and if possible avoid social situations in an effort to minimize their psychosocial distress (Newell, 1999; Rumsey et al., 2002, 2004).

COGNITIVE BEHAVIORAL THERAPY AND SUPPORT

Dentistry is well equipped to manage, and even resolve, most oral disfigurements. Dental hygiene and periodontal treatments offer solutions for most instances of halitosis, while prosthodontics provides sophisticated solutions for unsightly broken or missing teeth. However, there are situations where frailty severely limits access to dentistry, or where a patient's expectations and circumstances overwhelm the abilities of even the most skilful dental professionals, and in this context, it is helpful to draw on other management techniques.

Cognitive behavioral therapy for those with disfigurements helps reduce fear, dispel negative beliefs, and provide strategies for coping positively in social situations (Newell and Marks, 2000). Stroke victims who experience facial disfigurement from paralysis, for example, can benefit from understanding that the stares they attract are simply rude curiosities rather than expressions of disgust or horror. Negative beliefs about how others judge our appearance can alter our body image and diminish self-esteem, resulting in miscommunication or avoidance of social situations. Cognitive behavioral therapy not only provides a realistic explanation for a stranger's behavior but also encourages open discussion about the disfigurement so that more positive interactions occur. Ultimately, repeated exposure to social situations with positive outcomes from appropriate responses to stares and questions can help maintain body image and self-esteem.

Cognitive behavioral therapy has been especially helpful for people with low self-esteem from relatively minor disfigurements such as missing or unsightly teeth. This therapy might prove beneficial for frail elders who believe they are unable to meet unrealistic ideals of good oral health.

Generally, people respond more favorably to emotional support that encourages self-efficacy than to offers of direct assistance with personal care. Compliance with a daily mouthcare regimen, for example, is more likely when dental hygiene supplies (toothbrushes, etc.) are available than when a nurse or care-aide is assigned to clean a patient's teeth (Connell et al., 2002). A supportive approach to the assistance of daily activities strengthens independence and self-efficacy even in the face of increasing frailty (Mendes de Leon et al., 1996). This support is demonstrated in the clinical scenario, where a supportive interaction between Mrs. Claude and her caregivers has a very positive effect on Mrs. Claude's well-being.

CONCLUSIONS

Social interactions are important to the health and well-being of frail elders who are physically and emotionally vulnerable. The comfort and support of family, friends, and professional caregivers are acknowledged parts of long-term care, but it is the constant social interactions with peers that provide the daily comfort and support necessary for good health and contentment. Oral infections, such as caries, gingivitis, and mucositis, are all potentially very disfiguring, and even more disturbing when accompanied by severe halitosis. Consequently, oral diseases can seriously alter personal perceptions of body image and restrict social interactions. Dental professionals as active participants on multidisciplinary healthcare teams can alert their colleagues to the disabling potential of these disturbances, and offer dental treatment as well as practical advice on therapeutic strategies to protect the lives of frail and vulnerable elders.

REFERENCES

Bedford JL and Johnson S. 2006. Societal influences on body image dissatisfaction in younger and older women. *J Women Aging* 18:41–5.
Bennett K. 2005. Social engagement as a longitudinal predictor of objective and subjective health. *Eur J Ageing* 2:48–55.

Berkman LF. 1995. The role of social relations in health promotion. *Psychosom Med* 57:245–54.

Cacioppo J and Hawkley L. 2003. Social isolation and health with an emphasis on underlying mechanisms. *Perspect Biol Med* 46(Suppl. 3):S39–52.

Cash TF and Pruzinsky T (eds.). 1990. *Body Images: Development, Deviance and Change*. New York: Guilford.

Clarke A. 1999. Psychological aspects of facial disfigurement. *Psychol Health Med* 4:127–42.

Coffield KD, Phillips C, Brady M, Roberts MW, Strauss RP, and Wright JT. 2005.The psychosocial impact of developmental dental defects in people with hereditary amelogenesis imperfect. *J Am Dent Assoc* 136:620–30.

Connell BR, McConnell ES, and Francis EG. 2002. Tailoring the environment of oral health care to the needs and abilities of nursing home residents with dementia. *Alzheimer's Care Q* 3:19–25.

de Jong Gierveld J and Havens B. 2004. Cross-national comparisons of social isolation and loneliness: Introduction and overview. *Can J Aging* 23:109–13.

de Jong Gierveld J, Kamphuis JE, and Dykstra P. 1987. Old and lonely. *Compr Gerontol B* 1:13–7.

Dion KK, Berscheid E, and Walster E. 1972. "What is beautiful is good". *J Pers Soc Psychol* 24:285–90.

Farquhar JC and Wasylkiw L. 2007. Media image of men: trends and consequences of body conceptualization. *Psychology of Men and Masculinity* 8:145–60.

Filstrup S, Briskie D, da Fonseca M, Lawrence L, and Inglehart M. 2003. Early childhood caries and quality of life—Child and parent perspectives. *Pediatr Dent* 25:431–40.

Fiske J, Davis DM, Frances C, and Gelbier S. 1998. The emotional effects of tooth loss in edentulous people. *Br Dent J* 184:90–3.

Fultz NH and Herzog AR. 2001. Self-reported social and emotional impact of urinary incontinence. *J Am Geriatr Soc* 49:892–9.

Giles LC, Glonek GF, Luszcz MA, and Andrews GR. 2005. Effect of social networks on 10 year survival in very old Australians: The Australian longitudinal study of aging. *J Epidemiol Community Health* 59:574–9.

Gregory J, Gibson B, and Robinson PG. 2005. Variation and change in the meaning of oral health related quality of life: A "grounded" system approach. *Soc Sci Med* 60:1859–68.

Havens B and Hall M. 2001. Social isolation, loneliness and the health of older adults in Manitoba, Canada. *Indian J Gerontol* 15:126–44.

Hayslip B, Cooper CC, Dougherty LM, and Cook DB. 1997. Body image in adulthood: A projective approach. *J Pers Assess* 68:628–49.

Helm S, Kreiborg S, and Solow B. 1985. Psychosocial implication of malocclusion: A 15 year follow-up study in 30-year old Danes. *Am J Orthod* 87:110–8.

House JS, Landis KR, and Umberson D. 1988. Social relationships and health. *Science* 241:540–5.

Houston V and Bull R. 1994. Do people avoid sitting next to someone who is facially disfigured? *Eur J Soc Psychol* 24:279–84.

Hurd Clarke L. 2002. Older women's perceptions of ideal body weights: The tensions between health and appearance motivations for weight loss. *Ageing Soc* 22:751–73.

Hurd Clarke L and Griffin M. 2007. The body natural and the body unnatural: Beauty work and aging. *J Aging Stud* 21:87–201.

Jongenelis K, Pot A, Eisses A, Beekman A, Kluiter H, and Ribbe M. 2004. Prevalence and risk indicators of depression in elderly nursing home patients: The AGED study. *J Affect Disord* 83:135–42.

Jylha M. 2004. Old age and loneliness: Cross-sectional and longitudinal analyses in the Tampere Longitudinal Study on Aging. *Can J Aging* 23:157–68.

Kiyak HA. 2000. Cultural and psychological influences on treatment demand. *Semin Orthod* 6:242–8.

Lee I, Sheih T, Yang Y, Tsai C, and Wang J. 2007. Individuals' perception or oral health and its impact on the health-related quality of life. *J Oral Rehabil* 34:79–87.

Linn E. 1966. Social meanings of dental appearance. *J Health Hum Behav* 7:295–8.

MacEntee MI. 2006. Missing links in oral healthcare for frail elders. *J Can Dent Assoc* 72:421–5.

MacEntee MI, Hole R, and Stolar E. 1997. The significance of the mouth in old age. *Soc Sci Med* 4:1449–58.

MacGregor FC. 1990. Facial disfigurement: Problems and management of social interaction and implications for mental health. *Aesthetic Plast Surg* 14:249–57.

McKeown L. 2003. Social relations and breath odour. *Int J Dent Hyg* 1:213–7.

McKinley NM and Hyde JS. 1996. The objectified body consciousness scale: Development and validation. *Psychol Women Q* 20:181–215.

Mendes de Leon CF, Seeman TE, Baker DI, Richardson ED, and Tinetti ME. 1996. Self-efficacy, physical decline and change in functioning in community-living elders: A prospective study. *J Gerontol B Psychol Sci Soc Sci* 51:S183–90.

Mollaoglu N and Alpar R. 2005. The effect of dental profile on daily functions of the elderly. *Clin Oral Investig* 9:137–40.

Murata T, Yamaga T, Iida T, Miyazaki H, and Yaegaki K. 2002. Classification and examination of halitosis. *Int Dent J* 52:181–6.

Newell RJ. 1999. Altered body image: A fear-avoidance model for psychosocial difficulties following disfigurement. *J Adv Nurs* 30:1230–8.

Newell RJ and Marks J. 2000. Phobic nature of social difficulty in facially disfigured people. *Br J Psychiatry* 176:177–81.

Newton J, Prabhu N, and Robinson P. 2003. The impact of dental appearance on the appraisal of personal characteristics. *Int J Prosthodont* 16:429–34.

Noar JH. 1992. A questionnaire survey of attitudes and concerns of three professional groups involved in the cleft palate team. *Cleft Palate Craniofac J* 29:92–5.

Patel R, Tootla R, and Inglehart M. 2007. Does oral health affect self perceptions, parental ratings and video-based assessments of children's smiles?
Community Dent Oral Epidemiol 35:44–52.

Patel R, Richards P, and Inglehart M. 2008. Periodontal health, quality of life
and smiling patterns—An exploration. *J Periodontol* 79:224–31.

Pinquart M and Sorensen S. 2001. Influences on loneliness in older adults: A
meta-analysis. *Basic Appl Soc Psych* 23:245–66.

Reis H, McDougal IW, Monestere C, Bernstein S, Clark K, and Seidl E.
1990. What is smiling is beautiful and good. *Eur J Soc Psychol* 20:259–
67.

Routasalo R, Savikko N, Tilvis, Strandbuerg T, and Pitkala K. 2006. Social
contacts and their relationship to loneliness among aged people—A
population-based study. *Gerontology* 52:181–7.

Rumsey N, Clarke A, and Musa M. 2002. Altered body image: The psychosocial
needs of patients. *Br J Community Nurs* 7:563–6.

Rumsey N, Clarke A, White P, Wyn-Williams M, and Garlick W. 2004. Altered
body image: Appearance related concerns of people with visible disfigurement. *J Adv Nurs* 48:23–7.

Seeman TE, Bruce ML, and McAvay GJ. 1996. Social network characteristics
and on-set of ADL disability: MacArthur studies of successful aging.
J Gerontol B Psychol Soc Sci Soc 51:S191–200.

Sofaer-Bennett B, Moore AP, Walker J, Lamberty J, Thorp TA, and O'Dwyer J.
2007. The social consequences for older people of neuropathic pain: A qualitative study. *Pain Med* 7:530–3.

Stek ML, Vinkers DJ, Gussekloo J, Beekman AT, van der Mast R, and
Westendorp R. 2005. Is depression in old age fatal only when people feel
lonely? *Am J Psychiatry* 162:178–80.

Tiggemann M and Kurring JK. 2004. The role of body objectification in disor-
dered eating and depressed mood. *Br J Clin Psychol* 4:299–311.

Tomaka J, Thompson S, and Palacios R. 2006. The relation of social isolation,
loneliness, and social support to disease outcomes among the elderly.
J Aging Health 18:359–84.

Tonzetich J. 1977. Production and origin of oral malodour: A review of the
mechanisms and methods of analysis. *J Periodontol* 48:13–20.

Turner MD and Ship JA. 2007. Dry mouth and its effects on the oral health of
elderly people. *J Am Dent Assoc* 138(Suppl. 1):15S–20S.

Umberson D. 1987. Family status and health behaviors: Social control as a
dimension of social integration. *J Health Soc Behav* 28:306–19.

Vallittu P, Vallittu A, and Lassila V. 1996. Dental aesthetics—A survey of attitudes in different groups of patients. *J Dent* 25:335–8.

van den Broek A, Feenstra L, and de Baat C. 2008. A review of the current
literature on management of halitosis. *Oral Dis* 14:30–9.

Weinstein BE and Ventry IM. 1982. Hearing impairment and social isolation in
the elderly. *J Speech Hear Res* 25:593–9.

Weiss R. 1973. *Loneliness: The Experience of Emotional and Social Isolation.*
Cambridge, MA: MIT Press.

Wenger GC and Burholt V. 2004. Changes in levels of social isolation and loneliness among older people in a rural area: a twenty-year longitudinal study. *Can J Aging* 23:115–27.

Yaegaki K and Coil J. 2000. Genuine halitosis, pseudo-halitosis, and halitophobia: Classification, diagnosis, and treatment. *Compend Contin Dent Educ* 21:880–6.

Communications and education for palliative care

Ronald L. Ettinger, Shiva Khatami, and Michael I. MacEntee

INTRODUCTION

New styles of communications and education have been identified as essential components of healthcare generally, but nowhere are they needed so obviously as in the context of managing the healthcare needs of frail elders. Appropriate communication networks are likely to include various health professionals, managers, educators, researchers, and policy makers, especially considering the political dimensions globally of so much of healthcare today (Best, 2010). This chapter will consider the impact of education and communications on the current and potential role of oral healthcare in palliative care.

PALLIATIVE CARE

Palliative care is any form of healthcare or treatment of disease that focuses on reducing the severity of symptoms, rather than curing, halting, or delaying progress of the disease (Merriam Webster's Collegiate Dictionary, 1993; World Health Organization, 1997). The aim is to prevent or reduce pain and discomfort and to improve quality of life, while affirming life and helping a patient and family to live in dignity with diseases and disabilities.

Oral Healthcare and the Frail Elder: A Clinical Perspective.
Edited by Michael I. MacEntee © 2011 Blackwell Publishing Ltd.

Hospice care

The *hospitium* or hospitality in ancient Greece and Rome established a close relationship of caring between the host and a visiting stranger. It evolved through medieval times in the context of the hospice as a philosophy of care and a place of shelter or respite for weary and ill travelers. Its current use stems from the specialized care for dying patients which Dame Cicely Saunders introduced in 1967 at St. Christopher's Hospice in a suburb of London (Dahlin, 2004). It has developed since then into a program of caring for the physical, spiritual, psychological, and social needs of incurably ill patients and their families. Hospice care includes palliative care. Although not all palliative care is hospice care, they both share similar goals to provide symptom relief and pain management (Wiseman, 2000).

The aim of palliative care in hospice care is to

- help families and patients accept dying as a normal process;
- provide care that neither hastens nor postpones death;
- integrate the psychological and spiritual aspects of care;
- support patients to live as actively as possible and with dignity until death;
- allow families to cope with illness and bereavement;
- provide multidisciplinary healthcare teams to care for patients and their families; and
- help patients and their families select appropriate treatments, and understand and manage clinical side effects.

Metaphysics and spirituality

Medical and nursing schools have recognized for many years the role of communications between mind and matter, and the positive contributions of spirituality to palliative and end-of-life care (Puchalski and Larson, 1998; Pettus, 2002). Spirituality, in contrast to external physical sensations, is a medium of communications between the inner "self" and the surrounding environment, where contemplative introspection occurs in the form of meditation or prayer. Advocates of spiritual communications are reacting typically to the dominance of scientific technology and cure-oriented healthcare (Puchalski, 2001). More broadly, they present spirituality as "the way individuals seek and express meaning and purpose" to life (Puchalski et al., 2009). However, practically, it is a very important form of communication for some patients, especially near the end-of-life where it can help immensely with decisions about healthcare and quality of life (McCord et al., 2004; Balboni et al., 2007). It shores up relationships, and allows patients and clinicians to communicate together collaboratively on treatment and care. Religion as a formal organization of spiritual beliefs, texts, rituals, and other formalities helps many people to conceptualize and express their spirituality in a particular way, whereas others gain similar comfort from a more personal introspection (Sulmasy, 2009).

Serious illness triggers questions about values and relationships. Dentists can help patients with serious illness by listening sympathetically and sensitively, and by alleviating pain and discomfort. This "empathetic witnessing" is beginning to infiltrate dental curricula generally, although not without a struggle, as a counter to the more traditional instrumental approach to dentistry (Khatami et al., 2008).

ORAL HEALTH IN PALLIATIVE CARE

It is unusual for dentists to attend to dying patients. Nonetheless, they offer an invaluable service to palliative care when the mouth is disturbed directly by the diseases or indirectly by treatments. Consequently, the focus of dentistry in palliative care is on quality of life (Larue et al., 1994). Patients want to eat and talk comfortably, to feel clean and at ease with their appearance, and of course to be free of pain (MacEntee, 2006; Brondani et al., 2007). Even patients who are fed through a gastrointestinal feeding tube value the role of anterior teeth in speech, normal appearance, and personal dignity.

Unfortunately, dental services are not part of the health benefits in many countries (Lapeer, 1990; Leake, 2000); consequently, dentists and other dental professionals play a very minor, if any, role on the interdisciplinary care teams that constitute the backbone of communications in most long-term care facilities.

Communications between members of an interdisciplinary healthcare team can take various forms (British Medical Association 2004; Rider et al., 2006). Verbal communications dictate mediation, negotiation, and advocacy. However, nonverbal communications are very pertinent to the success of clinical practice within interdisciplinary teams, especially in multicultural societies. Effective teams acknowledge the diversity of working cultures and professional languages that permeate most interdisciplinary teams in Western society today. There is also a skill to communicating with healthcare managers and administrators, and maneuvering effectively through the organizational hierarchy of a nursing facility. Dental professionals as lone practitioners are usually unfamiliar with these communication tactics, and so they often feel unwelcome or even threatened by the stance of administrators and other team members (Thorne et al., 2001). On a broader perspective, they need to communicate also with professional and governmental bodies, such as dental associations and health ministries, to promote policy change.

Clinical competencies for palliative care

Wiseman (2006) has identified several competencies that are especially relevant to palliative care where dentists need to

- prevent and manage oral mucositis and stomatitis, xerostomia, and candidiasis;
- manage nausea and vomiting;
- cope with the influence of depression and adverse effects of psychotropic drugs on oral care;
- help dieticians with nutrition, hydration, and taste disorders; and
- prevent and manage oral diseases.

Xerostomia, caries, gingivitis, mucosal ulceration, denture-induced trauma, along with disturbances of taste and swallowing are common findings in frail patients as they near death (Jobbins et al., 1992; Wyche and Kerschbaum, 1994; Chiodo et al., 1998; Paunovich et al., 2000). Unfortunately, hospice administrators, physicians, and nurses are very prone to underestimate the prevalence of oral concerns among their frail patients (Andersson et al., 2007). Indeed, medical care teams in general usually overlook the significance of teeth as an integral part of social communications and body image, and only a very small proportion of nursing administrators place any significance on the daily oral hygiene or mouth problems of their patients (Ettinger, 2000; Cohen-Mansfield and Lipson, 2002; MacEntee, 2005).

Clinical scenario

Mr. Franklin is aged 77 years, divorced, and lives in a long-term care center in a small town. His daughter has power of attorney over his affairs, and he has a "living will" with a "Do-Not-Resuscitate" and a "No-Tube-Feeding" directive.

He complains that his denture, which he usually wears day and night, is loose, his mouth is sore and dry, and he cannot eat comfortably. He was very annoyed also that he had difficulty eating the cookies that were a frequent treat during the day but especially before bed and when he could not sleep. He had been advised to reduce his sugar consumption, but he found this difficult.

He has several major health problems: congestive heart failure, diabetes mellitus type II, osteoarthritis, severe hearing loss, hypothyroidism, peroneal muscle atrophy, right total hip replacement, venous insufficiency, diabetic neuropathy, spinal stenosis, and muscular dystrophy. However, he can stand with help but needs a wheelchair to move around.

Mr. Franklin, along with his daughter, visited Dr. Aloysius, his dentist. His daughter told Dr. Aloysius that her father "was failing" and had about 3–6 months to live due to his deteriorating heart and kidneys. Mr. Franklin's blood pressure at mid-morning of the appointment was 195/98. Neither he nor his daughter could remember whether or not he took his medications that morning, nor did they know his blood sugar levels.

The nurse at the long-term care facility relayed the information to Dr. Aloysius that Mr. Franklin took the following medications daily: levothyroxine—125 mcg qd; acetaminophen—325 mg × 2 qid; aspirin (enteric coated) 325 mg qd; hydrocodone/APAP 5/500 1 tab 4–6 h; furosemide—80 mg qd; gabapentin—300 mg bid; glipizide—5 mg AM; glipizide—10 mg PM; metformin—500 mg bid; novolin—100 u/mL 15 units subcu AM; spirolactone—50 mg qd.

The nurse reported also that his blood pressure was usually high and unstable, and that he had not taken all of his medications that morning.

Mr. Franklin's mouth on examination revealed that he was cleaning his mouth effectively, and he had several crowns and an upper acrylic partial denture (Figure 11.1).

The periodontium of all of the teeth looked secure (Figure 11.2); however, there were carious lesions and a few cavities in several mandibular teeth.

The right lateral border of his tongue had leukoplakia, which he was aware of without change for many years, and had been examined by a dermatologist about a year ago. No lymph nodes were palpable one either side of his jaw;

The cast retainers of the maxillary partial denture had fractured (Figure 11.1).

Impact of medical problems

Hypertension and congestive heart failure

Dr. Aloysius monitored Mr. Franklin's blood pressure at all subsequent treatment appointments, and limited epinephrine in the local anaesthetic to 0.036 mg (approximately two carpules of lidocaine with 1/100,000 epinephrine). The appointments were scheduled for mid-morning, with considerable attention to prevent a cardiovascular event by keeping stress to a minimum.

Diabetes

Mr. Franklin was advised to have his breakfast and to take his medications before each appointment. The length of the treatment appointments, including traveling time from the facility to the dentist, was carefully limited to 90 min or less. His diabetes probably produced the atrophy of his peroneal muscles and the neuropathy of his feet, so Dr. Aloysius and his staff were careful not to accidently traumatize his feet because he cannot feel them.

Osteoarthritis and spinal stenosis

Mr. Franklin was taking hydrocodone and gabapentin to relieve pressure and pain for these related pathoses. The dental staff provided him with extra support in the dental chair to ease the pressure on his spine, and they instructed him on how to obtain a toothbrush with a thick handle to allow a more comfortable grip with arthritic fingers.

Oral pathoses and denture problems

The caries was managed by an atraumatic restorative technique to (1) strengthen the teeth with a daily 0.2% fluoride mouthrinse and occasional application of a fluoride varnish to help remineralize carious lesions and reduce the risk of caries; (2) debride the carious cavities to reduce the number of cariogenic bacteria in the saliva; and (3) place a fluoridated glass ionomer filling in the cavities to seal them from further infection.

The retainer on the partial denture was replaced with a wrought-wire retainer, and the denture was relined. He was advised, with his daughter present, that the retention of the denture is compromised by the inadequate salivary flow and dry mouth, which could be relieved a little by spraying water into his mouth from a small atomizer bottle. He could use a denture adhesive occasionally if needed for special occasions.

Dr. Aloysius gave him advice with his daughter present on the carcinogenicity of sugar when consumed frequently, and on the significance of using the fluoride rinse every day.

Dr. Aloysius sent a report to Mr. Franklin's physician and to the director of nursing at his facility advising them that several of Mr. Franklin's medications were disturbing the buffering capacity of his saliva and seriously elevating his risk for caries and diabetes.

A regular regimen of appointments was arranged subsequently at approximately 3-month intervals to monitor the risk of caries and the status of the leukoplakia.

Evaluation of treatment

This treatment improved the quality of his life by restoring the carious teeth, improving the stability of his maxillary denture, which gave him improved function as he had five chewing pairs of teeth on the left side and two on the right side. The treatment of the dry mouth made him more comfortable. The patient died comfortably in his sleep about 5 months after the first appointment with Dr. Aloysius.

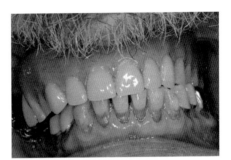

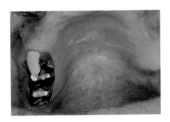
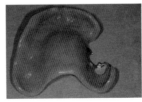
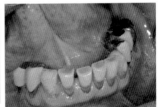

Figure 11.1 Mr. Franklin's mouth, teeth, and denture.

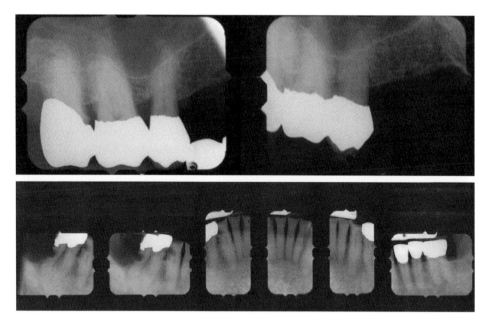

Figure 11.2 Radiographs of Mr. Franklin's teeth.

EDUCATION FOR PALLIATIVE CARE

About half of the physicians in Australia and in six European countries received formal training in palliative care (Löfmark et al., 2006). Hence, it is not surprising that education for dentists in hospice care requires substantial improvement. The absence of formal exposure to terminally ill patients is a serious omission in most dental curricula, which helps explain why so many dentists and dental hygienists are reluctant to treat frail elders (Weiss et al., 1993; Bryant et al., 1995; Strayer, 1995). The objectives of dental treatment in palliative care can be quite different from the objectives for more able elders, a difference that can conflict strikingly with the usual ritual of diagnosis and instrumental treatment of oral diseases and impairments (Khatami, 2010). Indeed, the conflict poses serious ethical and moral dilemmas for most dental professionals, and it demands sensitive strategies to cope with uncertain outcomes (Bryant et al., 1995; McNally, 2003). The need to communicate with patients, relatives, and other healthcare providers assumes greater significance than usual in dental practice to reach a shared understanding of the problems and treatment objectives. Rarely do dental students address these matters (MacEntee, 2010).

Educating dental professionals today

Recognizing palliative medicine as a unique specialty of the medical profession is under consideration in several countries where fellowship training programs are available in palliative medicine (Billings, 2000; LeGrand et al., 2003; Dickinson, 2007). In the United States, at present, there are about 50 such programs, along with plans to lobby the American Board of Medical Specialties for accreditation of the fellowship program leading to specialty status (Scharfenberger et al., 2008). Currently, there are no postgraduate training programs in palliative care for dentists in North America. General dental practice residents working in hospitals encounter patients who are terminally ill, but most hospice programs operate without a defined protocol for mouthcare or input from dental professionals (Paunovich et al., 2000). There are encouraging developments in some countries, with rare rays of hope for wider acceptance of dentistry as active and full members of interdisciplinary healthcare teams (Wiseman, 2006; Schimmel et al., 2008, Shah, 2010).

The heterogeneity of elderly populations and the diversity of their oral healthcare needs complicate the development of educational objectives in the broader context of dental geriatrics (Ettinger, 2010). Curricular overload and limited financial resources are ongoing barriers to geriatrics in most dental schools (Mohammad et al., 2003, Preshaw and Mohammad, 2005). Competency outlines for dentistry in general (Chambers and Gerrow, 1994, Plasschaert et al., 2005) and for dental geriatrics in particular (Kress and Vidmar, 1985) have helped establish educational objectives, although the diversity of curricular models compounded by the conflicting perspectives of discipline-based educators continually thwart all reasonable efforts to integrate dental geriatrics within the constructs of dental education (Khatami, 2010; MacEntee, 2010).

The undergraduate curriculum in many dental faculties addresses palliative and geriatric care together with one or two lectures supplemented by one or two clinical rotations through a long-term care facility. Typically, dental students observe frail elders without providing clinical care, while most of their clinical experience of "old patients" occurs with independent elders who attend clinics for restorative treatment in dental schools. Clinical rotations through long-term care, at best, offer most of the students a few opportunities to observe experienced dentists and dental hygienists interacting with patients who are frail and usually bedridden. Nonetheless, these brief encounters can have a positive impact on students' perspectives about the role and responsibilities they will have as dentists providing care for this vulnerable population (MacEntee, 2005).

The Iowa example

Dental students at the University of Iowa receive one lecture as part of a course on dental geriatrics. The lecture explains that palliative and end-of-life care should be humanistic, interdisciplinary, and interactive with family members. Students are introduced to the "rational dental care" model (Ettinger, 2000, 2006), with the following questions for assessing frail patients:

- What is the rate of decline and impending death?
- What are the medical comorbidities, and how do they influence life expectancy?
- What is the patient's quality of life, and how does oral healthcare improve it?
- What is the patient's cognitive function, and what level of assistance do they need with daily oral care?
- What dental products do they need? What is a realistic frequency for interceptive care?
- Will there be a need for physical or pharmacological restraint?
- How will the person's emotional and spiritual health and beliefs influence oral care?
- What is the patient's social support from family, carers, or others in providing access to dental services?
- What is the patient's ability to pay for oral healthcare products and professional services?

Students are alerted also to the significance of dysphagia in dehydration, malnutrition, weight loss, and aspiration pneumonia (Langmore et al., 1998; Yoneyama et al., 2002; Terpenning, 2005; Easterling and Robbins, 2008; Ishikawa et al., 2008). Explanations are offered on the role of dietitians in adjusting diets to ease swallowing, and of other specialists in assessing and managing speech and hearing problems. Overall, this is a small educational offering that opens the way for some students to expand their clinical services as dentists. However, it needs much more development in hospice and palliative care.

Future prospects for dental education

Dental education has a long history of struggle to balance biomedical science with psychosocial and human sensitivities (Hendricson and Cohen, 2001; MacEntee, 2007). The Institute of Medicine in the United States drew attention to this struggle and recommended expanding community service learning for dental students (Field, 1995). Slowly but increasingly, dental educators are adopting alternative approaches to curriculum design. Problem-based and competency-based curricula are popular examples that promote a comprehensive care model of dental practice where discipline-based knowledge is integrated with clinical competencies. Dental educators have also begun to address the challenges posed by access to oral healthcare for vulnerable and disadvantaged populations by offering opportunities for dental and dental hygiene students to work within the interdisciplinary and diverse contexts of community-based clinics (Bailit et al., 2005; Brondani et al., 2008; Khatami, 2010). Of course, the impact on dental practice of these new opportunities remains to be seen as the current generation of new dentists establish and fulfill their professional priorities.

SUMMARY

Several issues need to be addressed if dental professionals are to communicate effectively within the context of healthcare for frail elders. First, dental professionals should expand their active participation on interdisciplinary healthcare teams within palliative care clinics. Second, administrators and nursing staff should assume responsibility for the regular oral healthcare of their patients. Third, all dentists should be clinically competent to provide appropriate dental services in palliative care. Lastly, clinical education should prepare dental professionals for the pragmatic challenges of palliative care.

ACKNOWLEDGMENT

We are very grateful for the input and advice given to us by Dr. Helen Best as the chapter evolved.

REFERENCES

Andersson K, Furhoff AK, Nordenram G, and Wardh I. 2007. "Oral health is not my department." Perceptions of elderly patients' oral health by general medical practitioners in primary health care centres: A qualitative interview study. *Scand J Caring Sci* 21:126–33.

Bailit HL, Formicola AJ, Herbert KD, Stavisky JS, and Zamora G. 2005. The origins and design of the dental pipeline program. *J Dent Educ* 69:232–8.

Balboni TA, Vanderwerker LC, Block SD, Paulk ME, Lathan CS, Peteet JR, and Prigerson HG. 2007. Religiousness and spiritual support among advanced cancer patients and associations with end-of-life treatment preferences and quality of life. *J Clin Oncol* 25:555–60.

Best H. 2010. Education systems and the continuum of care for the older adult. *J Dent Educ* 74:7–12.

Billings JA. 2000. Palliative medicine fellowship programmes in the United States: Year 2000 survey. *J Palliat Med* 3:391–6.

British Medical Association. 2004. *Communication Skills Education for Doctors: An Update.* Available at www.bma.org.uk/images/communication_tcm41-20207.pdf (accessed January 12, 2010).

Brondani MA, Bryant SR, and MacEntee MI. 2007. Elders assessment of an evolving model of oral health. *Gerodontology* 24:189–95.

Brondani MA, Clark C, Rossoff L, and Aleksejuniene J. 2008. An evolving community-based dental course on professionalism and community service. *J Dent Educ* 72:1160–8.

Bryant SR, MacEntee MI, and Browne A. 1995. Ethical issues encountered by dentists in the care of institutionalized elders. *Spec Care Dentist* 15:79–82.

Chambers DW and Gerrow JD. 1994. Manual for developing and formatting competency statements. *J Dent Educ* 58:361–6.

Chiodo GT, Tolle SW, and Madden T. 1998. The dentist's role in end-of-life care. *Gen Dent* 46:560–5.

Cohen-Mansfield J and Lipson S. 2002. The underdetection of pain of dental etiology in persons with dementia. *Am J Alzheimers Dis Other Demen* 17:249–53.

Dahlin C. 2004. Oral complications at the end-of-life. *Am J Nurs* 104:40–7.

Dickinson GE. 2007. End-of-life and palliative care issues in medical and nursing schools in the United States. *Death Stud* 31:713–26.

Easterling OS and Robbins E. 2008. Dementia and dysphagia. *Geriatr Nurs* 29:275–85.

Ettinger RL. 2000. Dental management of patients with Alzheimer's disease and other dementias. *Gerodontology* 17:8–16.

Ettinger RL. 2006. Rational DENTAL CARE: Part 1. Has the concept changed in 20 years? *J Can Dent Assoc* 72:441–5.

Ettinger RL. 2010. Meeting oral health needs to promote the well-being of the geriatric population: Educational research issues. *J Dent Educ* 74:29–35.

Field MJ. 1995. *Dental Education at the Crossroads: Challenges and Change.* Washington, DC: National Academy Press, pp. 1–19.

Hendricson WD and Cohen PA. 2001. Oral healthcare in the 21st century: Implications for dental and medical education. *Acad Med* 76:1181–206.

Ishikawa A, Yoneyama T, Hirota K, Miyake Y, and Miyatake K. 2008. Professional oral healthcare reduces the number of oropharyngeal bacteria. *J Dent Res* 87:594–8.

Jobbins J, Bagg J, Finlay IG, Addy M, and Newcombe RG. 1992. Oral and dental disease in terminally ill cancer patients. *Br Med J* 304:1612.

Khatami S. 2010. *Clinical Reasoning in Dentistry: Across Levels of Expertise and Problems.* PhD thesis. Vancouver: University of British Columbia.

Khatami S, MacEntee, MI, and Loftus S. 2008. Clinical reasoning in dentistry. In: Higgs J, Jones M, Loftus S, and Christensen N (eds.), *Clinical Reasoning in the Health Professions*, 3rd edn. Oxford: Butterworth-Heinemann, pp. 257–64.

Kress GD Jr. and Vidmar GC. 1985. Critical skills assessment for the treatment of geriatric patients. *Spec Care Dentist* 5:127–9.

Langmore SE, Terpenning MS, Schork A, Chen Y, Murray JT, Lopatin D, and Loesche WJ. 1998. Predictors of aspiration pneumonia: How important is dysphagia. *Dysphagia* 13:69–81.

Lapeer GL. 1990. The dentist as a member of the palliative care team. *J Can Dent Assoc* 56:205–7.

Larue F, Brasseur L, Musseault P, Demeulerester R, Boniess L, and Bez G. 1994. Pain and symptoms during HIV disease. A French National Study. *J Palliat Care* 10:95.

Leake JL. 2000. The history of dental programs for older adults. *J Can Dent Assoc* 66:316–9.

LeGrand SB, Walsh D, Nelson KA, and Davis MP. 2003. A syllabus for fellowship education in palliative medicine. *Am J Hospice Palliat Care* 20:279–89.

Löfmark R, Mortier F, Nilstun T, Bosshard G, Cartwright C, Van Der Heide A, Norup M, Simonato L, and Onwuteaka-Philipsen B. 2006. Palliative care training: A survey of physicians in Australia and Europe. *J Palliat Care* 22:105–10.

MacEntee MI. 2005. Caring for elderly long-term care patients: Oral health-related concerns and issues. *Dent Clin North Am* 49:429–43.

MacEntee MI. 2006. An existential model of oral health from evolving views on health, function and disability. *Community Dent Health* 23:5–14.

MacEntee MI. 2007. Where science fails prosthodontics. *Int J Prosthodont* 20:377–81.

MacEntee MI. 2010. The educational challenge of dental geriatrics. *J Dent Educ* 74:13–9.

McCord G, Gilchrist VJ, Grossman SD, King BD, McCormick KE, Oprandi AM, Schrop SL, Selius BA, Smucker DO, Weldy DL, Amorn M, Carter MA, Deak AJ, Hefzy H, and Srivastava M. 2004. Discussing spirituality with patients: A rational and ethical approach. *Ann Fam Med* 2:356–61.

McNally M. 2003. Rights access and justice in oral health care: Justice toward underserved patient populations—the elderly. *J Am Coll Dent* 70:56–60.

Merriam-Webster's Collegiate Dictionary. 1993. 10th edn. Springfield, MA: Merriam-Webster Inc., p. 560.

Mohammad AR, Preshaw PM, and Ettinger RL. 2003. Current status of predoctoral geriatric education in U.S. dental schools. *J Dent Educ* 67:509–14.

Paunovich ED, Aubertin MA, Saunders MJ, and Prange M. 2000. The role of dentistry in palliative care of the head and neck cancer patient. *Tex Dent J* 117:36–45.

Pettus MC. 2002. Implementing a medicine-spirituality curriculum in a community-based internal medicine residency program. *Acad Med* 77:745.

Plasschaert AJ, Holbrook WP, Delap E, Martinez C, and Walmsley AD. 2005. Profile and competences for the European dentist. *Eur J Dent Educ* 9:98–107.

Preshaw PM and Mohammad AR. 2005. Geriatric dentistry education in European dental schools. *Eur J Dent Educ* 9:73–7.

Puchalski C. 2001. The role of spirituality in health care. *Proc (Bayl Univ Med Cent)* 14:352–7.

Puchalski C and Larson DB. 1998. Developing curricular in spirituality and medicine. *Acad Med* 73:970–4.

Puchalski C, Ferrell B, Virani R, Otis-Green S, Baird P, Bull J, Chochinov H, Handzo G, Nelson-Becker H, Prince-Paul M, Pugliese K, and Sulmasy D. 2009. Improving the quality of spiritual care as a dimension of palliative care: The report of the consensus conference. *J Palliat Med* 12:885–904.

Rider EA, Hinrichs MM, and Lown BA. 2006. A model for communication skills assessment across the undergraduate curriculum. *Med Teach* 28:e127–34.

Scharfenberger J, Furman CD, Rotella J, and Pfeifer M. 2008. Meeting American Council of Graduate Medical Education guidelines for a palliative medicine fellowship through diverse community partnerships. *J Palliat Med* 11:428–30.

Schimmel M, Schoeni P, Zulian GB, and Müller F. 2008. Utilization of dental services in a university hospital palliative and long-term care unit in Geneva. *Gerodontology* 25:107–12.

Shah N. 2010. Teaching, learning and assessment in geriatric dentistry: researching models of practice. *J Dent Educ* 74:20–8.

Strayer MS. 1995. Perceived barriers to oral health care among the homebound. *Spec Care Dentist* 15:113–8.

Sulmasy DP. 2009. Spirituality, religion and clinical care. *Chest* 135:1634–42.

Terpenning M. 2005. Geriatric oral health and pneumonia risk. *Clin Infect Dis* 40:1807–10.

Thorne S, Kazanjian A, and MacEntee MI. 2001. Oral health in long-term care: The implications of organizational culture. *J Aging Stud* 15:271–83.

Weiss RT, Morrison BJ, MacEntee MI, and Waxler-Morrison NE. 1993. The influence of social, economic and professional considerations on services offered by dentists to long-term-care residents. *J Public Health Dent* 53:70–5.

Wiseman MA. 2000. Palliative care dentistry. *Gerodontology* 17:49–51.

Wiseman M. 2006. The treatment of oral problems in the palliative patient. *J Can Dent Assoc* 72:453–8.

World Health Organization. 1997. *WHO Definition of Palliative Care*. Available at www.who.int/cancer/palliative/definition/en (accessed June 3, 2010).

Wyche CJ and Kerschbaum WE. 1994. Michigan hospice oral healthcare needs survey. *J Dent Hyg* 68:35–41.

Yoneyama T, Yoshida M, Ohrui T, Mukaiyama H, Okamoto H, Hoshiba K, Ihara S, Yanagisawa S, Ariumi S, Morita T, Mizuno Y, Ohsawa T, Akagawa Y, Hashimoto K, and Sasaki H. 2002. Oral care reduces pneumonia in older patients in nursing homes. *J Am Geriatr Soc* 50:430–3.

12

Prevention of oral diseases for a dependent population

Heather Frenkel, Debora C. Matthews, and Ina Nitschke

Heather Frenkel, Debora C. Matthews, and Ina Nitschke

INTRODUCTION

Frail elders, whether they reside in a long-term care facility or at home, have difficulty accessing timely and appropriate oral healthcare. (The terms "long-term care facility," "residential care facility," and "nursing home" are used to indicate collective residences where elders receive varying levels of assistance with daily activities and nursing care.) They face multiple challenges—limited physical and cognitive abilities, unclear values and priorities of caregivers, unstable politics and policies where they reside, sparse financial support, and doubtful jurisdictional control of care facilities (MacEntee, 2006). In the absence of insurance or personal resources, a large portion of the frail population will be unable to afford dental services, even if available. Publicly funded programs, such as Medicare in the United States, often do not provide adequate coverage for dentistry, and scarce finances are often spent transporting residents for emergency treatments when preventive care would be a more efficient use of funds. Clearly, there must be a response to the increasing oral health concerns of frail elders with special needs.

Even without physical, psychological, and financial limitations, many elders cannot access dentists or dental hygienists, either outside or within their residence. Therefore, the task of preventing disease usually falls to the nursing staff. However, dentistry and oral healthcare get scant attention in the education of most nurses and personal care-workers or care-aides. Current expectations are that "best available evidence" is based on randomized controlled trials to test all preventive and treatment strategies

Oral Healthcare and the Frail Elder: A Clinical Perspective.
Edited by Michael I. MacEntee © 2011 Blackwell Publishing Ltd.

(Sanson-Fisher et al., 2007). However, expectations are not always met when evidence relates to real life-events that are impossible to control fully or to observe without bias.

In this chapter, we consider the factors affecting maintenance of oral health in frail elders at home and in residential care, and the success of programs designed to prevent oral diseases. We conclude with recommendations for future policy and service development.

BARRIERS TO MAINTAINING ORAL HEALTH FOR FRAIL ELDERS

Frailty and dependence

Frail elders in residential care in North America typically have three chronic diseases, take numerous medications daily, and feel more unhealthy when compared with elders who are living independently (Shay and Ship, 1995). Some of them are fatalistic about losing their teeth, while others are offended when their oral hygiene is criticized (Schou and Eadie, 1991). Nonetheless, when elders grow frail almost invariably they have unhealthy mouths and teeth, probably because of visual impairment, loss of manual dexterity, cognitive impairment, or depression (Chalmers et al., 2008). The impact of this neglect can have a very deleterious effect on general health, particularly relating to vascular and coronary heart diseases, diabetes, and pneumonia (Russell et al., 1999; Scannapieco et al., 2003; Khader et al., 2004; Department of Health, 2005; Jablonski et al., 2005; Osterberg et al., 2008). It is also likely that the psychological impact of dental disability precipitates depression, negative self-image, and difficulties communicating and eating, which leads to apathy and social withdrawal (Department of Health, 2005).

Cognitive impairment intensifies preexisting oral problems, and individuals with dementia typically have poor oral hygiene, poor diets, and higher levels of oral diseases (Chalmers et al., 2008). Mouth problems arise when the dementia precipitates verbal or physical aggression, and the elders refuse oral hygiene and other care, and they are exacerbated further when the elders are unable to explain their discomforts and wish for dental care (Shimazaki et al., 2004).

When severely disabled, there is a tendency for some residents to accept care passively. However, many carers lack knowledge, training, and basic skills for identifying oral problems or brushing a patient's teeth (Frenkel, 1999; Fitzpatrick, 2000; Department of Health, 2005). It is not surprising, therefore, that assistance with oral hygiene is not readily available, nor that residents have dirty mouths as they grow frail and dependent (Figure 12.1).

Residents are frequently aware that their carers dislike or feel insecure with mouthcare, which increases their sense of vulnerability, heightens their concern about being a nuisance, and inhibits their requests for help (Frenkel, 1999). Consequently, even when their oral health is moderately

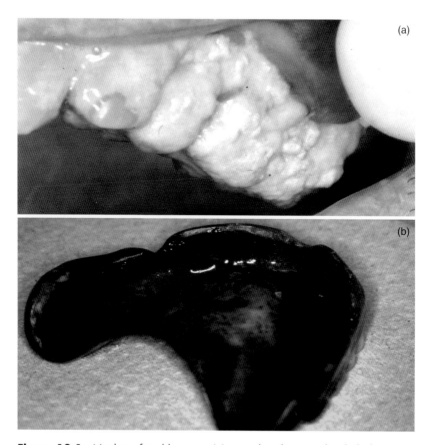

Figure 12.1   Neglect of oral hygiene: (a) natural teeth covered with thick, mature plaque; (b) a denture thickly coated with disclosed, mature plaque.

good on admission, it can deteriorate rapidly if they are dependent on others for the routine of daily oral hygiene and access to dental treatment (Jablonski et al., 2005).

About three-quarters of the elders in residential care are cognitively impaired and require help with three or more basic activities, such as bathing, dressing, toileting, or feeding (Jablonski et al., 2005). It is no surprise, therefore, that they need assistance to visit a dentist, and that they encounter physical barriers, such as difficult access to the dental chair or to the toilet when at a treatment center and despite the legislation supporting disabled people in many countries.

Finances

For retired people on low or restricted incomes, financing dental care is a significant problem. The culture of older generations often leads them to avoid physicians and dentists, except as a last resort (MacEntee et al., 1999).

Some elders in residential care cannot decide whether or not to have dental treatment, and occasionally, their relatives offer little encouragement because treatment seems unnecessary and expensive. Furthermore, in most countries, dentistry is not included as a benefit of medical insurance (Shay and Ship, 1995), and state-funded dental benefits, especially those with fee exemptions for people with low income, provide very limited care that is poorly understood by potential recipients (Jablonski et al., 2005).

There are many different social insurance systems and different payment methods for dentistry. For example, in Switzerland, dentistry is not insured, and everybody pays a fee for service unless they have a very low retirement income, which the state supplements with limited financial support for health services. In Germany, the Legal Social Insurance, which covers 95% of the population, pays for dental extractions, apicectomies, endodontics, composite and amalgam restorations, radiological examinations, and partial reimbursement of prosthodontic fees. Government Web sites usually contain information about the current regulations in force in individual jurisdictions.

Knowledge, attitudes, and training of dentists and carers

Professional limitations of dentists

There are dentists who manage the decline and death of their patients very effectively, even though death and dying are not normally part of their usual experiences (Nitschke et al., 2005). But there are many others who have difficulty coping with frail patients, especially if they have to leave the familiarity of a well-equipped dental clinic to attend elders who are frail and bedridden at home or in a long-term care facility (MacEntee et al., 1991; Bryant et al., 1995). Residential care administrators complain occasionally that dentists lack kindness, compassion, patience, and professional skills to treat residents with dementia and behavioral problems (Chalmers et al., 2001). Indeed, dentists receive very limited education in managing patients, whether young or old, who are physically or cognitively disabled (Chalmers et al., 2001; Department of Health, 2005; Nitschke et al., 2005). Furthermore, dentists generally are uninterested in residential care and its administrative complexities, and hesitate to work in unfavorable conditions for financial returns that are less than they receive in their more controlled and familiar clinics (MacEntee et al., 1999; Simons, 2003; Chalmers et al., 2001; Nitschke et al., 2005).

Nursing staff

Responsibility for daily mouthcare as an integral part of healthcare generally lies with nursing staff and care-aides or care-workers. Yet, there are barriers to fulfilling this responsibility, including lack of knowledge and training, general anxiety about causing harm to a resident's mouth, unco-operative residents, lack of time, staff shortages, and lack of appropriate supplies such as toothbrushes and toothpaste (Eadie and Schou, 1992; Weeks and Fiske, 1994; Chalmers et al., 1996; Wårdh et al., 1997; Frenkel, 1999; MacEntee et al., 1999). Furthermore, some nurses are misinformed about oral health, or they are unable to translate their knowledge into best practice (Hoad-Reddick and Heath, 1995). It is not uncommon for nurses and care-aides to use mouthwashes and swabs rather than toothbrushes and toothpaste when cleaning a patients teeth, and more often than not their knowledge about gingivitis and caries is poor (Weeks and Fiske, 1994; Adams, 1996). It is easier to remove and clean dentures than to brush natural teeth, although many nurses are uneasy about removing dentures from a patient's mouth (Vigild, 1990; Frenkel et al., 2001; Grimoud et al., 2005; Nicol et al., 2005; Peltola et al., 2007), possibly because they feel that this is a threat to the resident's privacy and dignity (Charteris and Kinsella, 2001). More likely, they are fearful of being bitten, or they avoid teeth because of their own traumatic experiences with dentistry (Frenkel, 1999). Residents who resist care by clamping lips together or by pushing away the carer's hands are particularly unsettling for many carers. Usually, this reaction is precipitated by confronting a resident without warning, whereas a nonthreatening explanation of the intent or purpose of the care will go a long way to getting the resident's cooperation and consent (Paley et al., 2004; Coleman and Watson, 2006). In general, mouthcare for elders who are demented can be a demanding and confusing task, which probably explains why most carers overlook oral hygiene as an essential part of daily hygiene (MacEntee et al., 1999).

Without doubt, there are many nursing facilities where the administra-tors and staff acknowledge the importance of a healthy mouth and the ideal of daily mouthcare for all (MacEntee et al., 1999). Consequently, appropriate training and clinical experience for nurses and care-aides should help enhance their knowledge and clinical skills for mouthcare, much as it helps overcome ignorance and prejudices around incontinence (MacDonald and Butler, 2007). Unfortunately, nursing practice of mouth-care falls well short of the ideal elsewhere, and nurses with their adminis-trators tend to seek help from dentists and dental hygienists rather than involve themselves in the daily preventive care of their residents (Eadie and Schou, 1992; MacEntee et al., 1999). There are facilities where special training in mouthcare is dismissed as unnecessary because it is "just common sense" (Weeks and Fiske, 1994; Frenkel, 1999). There are also carers who rate the oral health of their residents as fair or poor, yet when asked they seem satisfied with the "fair or poor" oral care they provide (Wårdh et al., 1997; Pyle et al., 2005).

Nursing journals offer good advice on oral healthcare (e.g., Fitzpatrick, 2000), but nursing textbooks in general are woefully neglectful of dentistry and basic oral care (Furr et al., 2004). Student nurses in the United Kingdom and the United States, for example, receive on average about 1 h of oral health-related education, almost half of them receive no instruction at all, while less than 10% receive postqualification tuition in oral healthcare (Hoad-Reddick and Heath, 1995; Adams, 1996). The tuition offered is delivered usually by nurses who advocate little more than swabbing the inside of the mouth and teeth with lemon and glycerine or dilute hydrogen peroxide (Moore, 1995). It is very likely that the neglect of mouthcare for elderly patients reflects a general uneasiness about geriatric care and lack of good practical education in geriatrics among nurses, at least in North America (Baumbusch and Andrusyszyn, 2002; Koren et al., 2008). Nearly all nursing schools in the United States integrate gerontology in the course curricula, but less than half of them offer it as an elective, and only a quarter of them require students to take a course in gerontology (Grocki and Fox, 2004).

In the United Kingdom, "care of old people/geriatrics" is part of basic nurse training, but specialized gerontological qualifications can be obtained in work-related courses (e.g., Higher National Diploma, Higher National Certificate) or as a 3- to 4-year university-based bachelor's degree; and in Germany, there is a 3-year training program leading to a certificate of geriatric nursing.

The emotional adjustments identified within the maternal relationship model of caring helps explain why some carers distance themselves from frail residents in whom they see a disturbing image of their own future (Edwards, 2008). The apathy of frail residents can also be used as an excuse for not bothering to offer assistance (Wårdh et al., 2002), while more alert residents can be discouraging by resenting or refusing offers of help from younger carers. The personal autonomy and independence of the residents is used also by carers as an excuse for not helping with mouthcare, but this is reasonable only if it supports the wishes of the resident. Indeed, occupational therapists should be consulted, if possible, when healthcare and personal autonomy are under review (Bellomo et al., 2005).

Care-aides

Long-term care-aides (also called care assistants) in most Western countries receive even less instruction about mouthcare than nurses, yet they work usually with minimal supervision and render most of the personal care for the residents (Chalmers et al., 1996; MacEntee et al., 1999). They are often recruited from immigrant populations whose culture and language can differ from the elders in their care. Moreover, they are a very mobile profession who may remain as carers only for short periods (Weeks and Fiske, 1994; Chalmers et al., 1996; Frenkel, 1999; Jablonski et al., 2005). Consequently, the mouthcare they provide can be very unpredictable and unstable.

Organizational barriers

Oral health policy, guidelines, and protocols

Administrators and managers of residential care facilities are concerned about the cost of dentistry, and they complain about the lack of information on the professional services available, along with apparent lack of interest among dentists and dental hygienists, and the need to transport residents out of the facility for dental treatment (MacEntee et al., 1999; Paley et al., 2004). Policy decisions about mouthcare rendered to frail elders are made usually by physicians and nurses, despite their limited expertise in oral healthcare. Rarely are dentists or dental hygienists part of policy deliberations, either at a local or national level (Fiske et al., 1996; Nitschke, 2001; Department of Health, 2005). Moreover, when oral healthcare guidelines are in place, all too frequently they are overlooked in some jurisdictions (Adams, 1996; Frenkel, 1999; MacEntee et al., 1999), in as much the same way as other "peripheral" services, such as management of pressure sores (Buss et al., 2004), are overlooked.

Organizational structure in nursing homes

Administrators of nursing facilities can feel insecure about monitoring oral health, and seek help from dental professionals as much as possible (MacEntee et al., 1999). However, others do not welcome dental professionals because of the expectations they might bring, or more practically and ethically, because they would abrogate the nurses' responsibility for daily oral healthcare. Dentists and dental hygienists in contrast have suggested that their participation in interdisciplinary care conferences would be useful to everyone in the nursing facility.

Providing accessible dental services

People are more easily upset physically and emotionally as they grow frail, so routine dentistry should be readily accessible to them without moving to remote dental clinics (MacEntee et al., 1999; Paley et al., 2004). Meals and medications are easily missed when they have to travel afar to a dentist, which is doubly difficult if they are incontinent. Disturbances of dementia are exacerbated by strange people and places. Domiciliary care, therefore, allows continuity of regular treatment even when individuals have significant problems with mobility and health. Nonetheless, there are occasions when it is necessary to transport a frail resident for special care at another clinic or private dental practice.

On-site dentistry with mobile equipment

A dental professional with good mobile dental equipment can serve patients at home or in a facility (Figure 12.2).

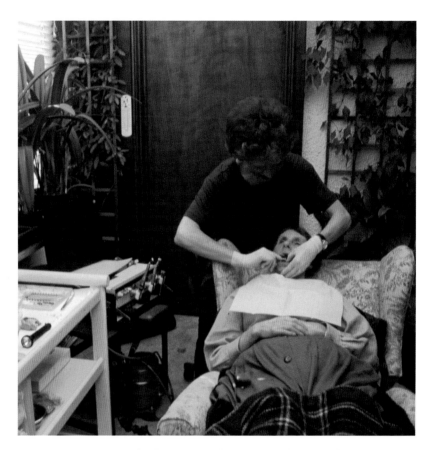

Figure 12.2 A portable dental unit with compressor being used by a dentist to treat a patient with multiple sclerosis at home in her own reclining chair.

Access to residents who are bedridden is more difficult and ergonomically demanding, but it certainly is possible (Figure 12.3).

A typical portable or mobile dental unit will include a reclining chair with headrest, an intense light, high- and low-speed handpieces, air and water syringes with air compressor, and a self-contained high-vacuum suction with vacuum pump, while some come also with a radiographic unit (Figure 12.4).

Typically, the facility provides a private space with electricity and water, and if possible a staff member or volunteer will be available to transport residents to and from the mobile clinic. The type and quantity of treatment possible with portable equipment is influenced more by the frailty and health status of the patients than on the equipment or location. In general, dentists who become familiar with this context of clinical care find it comfortable and productive (Bee, 2004), although not everyone agrees about the productivity of domiciliary care (Chalmers et al., 2001).

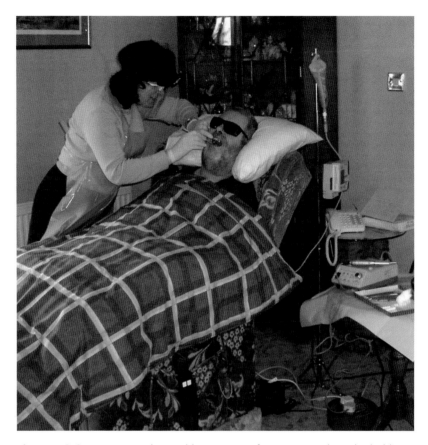

Figure 12.3   Dentistry with portable equipment for a patient who is bedridden.

Challenges in delivering successful oral care to frail elders

Oral health assessments

A regular system of oral assessment for all frail elders is essential for a successful oral health service. It serves as a screening process to identify existing problems and suggest interventions and treatments. When the assessment is performed by nondental healthcare workers, the assessment tool or clinical guide should be simple and brief, yet focused on significant observations relevant to physical status and quality of life. The assessment can be a simple structured interview to identify an elder's general mouth problems (Hoad-Reddick, 1991; Fiske et al., 1996), or it can involve carers recording observations of the elder's mouth and teeth against a checklist, such as the validated Oral Health Assessment Tool (Chalmers et al., 2005). However, all suspected problems should be referred to a dentist for further investigation.

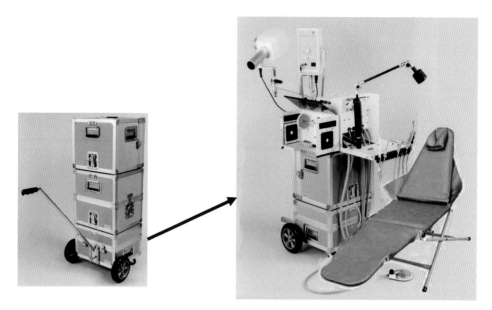

Figure 12.4   Portable dental unit (Mobile Dental Systems PortOP III Portable Dental Unit, MDSysCo, LLC, Austin, TX). (Reprinted with permission.)

The Resident Assessment Instrument (RAI) is used widely on admission to nursing facilities in North America and Europe, and the Minimum Data Set (MDS) is the basic data collection instrument within the RAI (Morris et al., 1990). The MDS has been revised several times, and currently (MDS 3.0) addresses 19 domains, including six oral/dental problems—broken or loose dentures; missing or fragmented teeth; abnormal mouth tissues; dental cavities and broken teeth; inflamed gums; mouth or facial pain and chewing difficulties (Minimum Data Set, 2010). Unfortunately, inconsistent application of the MDS is a widespread concern because, at best, only half of the dental problems are detected by nurses (Ettinger et al., 2000).

The "Clinical Oral Disorder in Elders (CODE) index" designed for use by dentists or dental hygienists focuses more deeply on oral health and disease but needs further clinical validation before it can be adopted widely as a useful oral health screening instrument and predictor of treatment needs (MacEntee and Wyatt, 1999).

Daily oral care and treatments

A plan for daily oral care and treatment should be developed based on the assessment of each resident. An effective daily care routine requires about 5 min (Sumi et al., 2002), although even this regular commitment seems more than many facilities can make, despite established guidelines or best practices (MacEntee et al., 1999; Frenkel et al., 2001). Unfortunately, it is not unusual for carers in some parts of the United States to spend less than 30s rather than the recommended 2min cleaning a resident's teeth, and even then, only a small proportion of residents get this care (Coleman and Watson, 2006). A higher commitment to mouthcare by nondental staff in a facility can be achieved when a "champion" is assigned particular responsibility for the task (MacEntee et al., 1999; Charteris and Kinsella, 2001; Frenkel, 2003; Wårdh et al., 2003), and it also helps to have the different disciplines in a facility agree that oral care for the residents requires a collective approach to manage (Edwards, 2008).

Educating care-staff of residential care facilities

The responsibility for maintaining and monitoring daily oral healthcare of dependent elders resides with the care-staff (Hoad-Reddick and Heath, 1995; Wårdh et al., 1997). Educating the staff to clean the mouth, teeth, and dentures of frail residents is a difficult and unpredictable task, especially when the carers are not fluent in the dominant language of the residents (Cowan et al., 2004). Some educational training programs are well received by participating staff and seem to raise awareness of oral health for a while (Woodall, 1997; Frenkel et al., 2002). However, evidence of practical and sustained improvements in oral healthcare is inconclusive (MacEntee et al., 2007).

There are reports of sustained benefits to mucosal and gingival health among nursing home residents for periods of 6months to 2years following educational programs for care-staff (Vigild, 1990; Charteris and Kinsella, 2001; Frenkel et al., 2001; Grimoud et al., 2005; Nicol et al., 2005; Peltola et al., 2007). Yet, educational programs in this setting do not always succeed (Simons et al., 2000; Wårdh et al., 2003; MacEntee et al., 2007), and there is widespread belief that this education needs repetition and regular reinforcement to sustain the benefits (Vigild, 1990; Nicol et al., 2005).

Use of varied and individualized educational techniques

Organizational policy tends to come from the top of the administrative scheme. Consequently, an innovative oral healthcare policy needs promotional support from above to succeed. Support involves participation of nursing directors and other managers in educational programs to emphasize to other staff their commitment to oral care (Frenkel et al., 2001, 2002; Frenkel, 2003). The format of the educational program depends on the general environment and culture of each facility. Small groups of learners foster interactions and personal commitments, while mixed formal presentations entice wider interest and enthusiasm. Most nursing home directors prefer to have their staff trained on-site if possible. However, there are distinct advantages to locating educational programs for staff away from the facility where there are no disruptions (Woodall, 1997; Frenkel, 2003; Edwards, 2008). Above all, clinical personnel generally prefer personal demonstrations and practical applications of knowledge rather than theory or facts alone. Informational booklets provide "takeaway" sources of reference, and attendance certificates provide records of achievement, reminders of responsibility, and boosts to self-esteem.

There are several oral healthcare-related programs available. The German Association for Gerodontology, for example, has a two-stage educational program suitable in German, French, and Italian for nurses, physicians, patients, and relatives. It consists of a 45-min presentation by a dentist, followed by an extensive computer-aided informational package for private study. Each chapter concludes with a simple test, and when completed successfully, the participant can print a certificate of accomplishment. Finally, participants are encouraged to perform practical exercises in small groups of colleagues and resident patients. A similar informational program (www.elders.dentistry.ubc.ca/education/products/materials.asp) is available in Canada from the University of British Columbia.

Evidence-based preventive strategies

Ideally, preventive strategies will ensure the stability of a frail oral environment as illustrated by the following two clinical scenarios highlighting evidence-based techniques that can be incorporated into daily personal care routines.

Clinical scenario 1

Mrs. Schmidt is an 89-year-old widow. She has type 2 diabetes, for which she takes a sulfonurea drug. She also takes bezafibrate—a cholesterol-lowering medication; atenolol—a beta-blocker; and nonsteroidal anti-inflammatory drugs (NSAIDs) regularly because her hands are severely affected by rheumatoid arthritis. Her mouth feels dry, so she sucks lemon candies to stimulate her saliva. She has difficulty eating and, occasionally, pain when chewing. A visual examination of her mouth and teeth reveals that she has several broken teeth with obvious large carious cavities and a thick layer of plaque and food debris. Her mucosa looks dry and her gingiva look slightly swollen and they bleed on probing.

Mrs. Schmidt's dry mouth is most likely a consequence of one or more of her medications, probably atenolol, whereas the caries are due to the acidogenic potential of the lemon candies and bacteria in the absence of saliva. She could switch to an alternative beta-blocker—perhaps acebutolol—that does not disturb salivation (see Chapter 4).

In addition, she would be well advised as a diabetic to use sugar-free candies with frequent sips of water to compensate for the dry mouth. Some people like to use a mouthrinse to keep the mouth moist, but the alcohol content of most over-the-counter rinses can exacerbate the feeling of mucosal dryness. Chewing sugar-free gum might stimulate salivation; however, chewing gum is not popular among elders with missing, broken, and sensitive teeth.

The bleeding gingiva should heal quite quickly with effective oral hygiene if the diabetes is controlled. Mrs. Schmidt might find it easier and more effective to use a toothbrush with a large handle, which is easier to grasp with her arthritic hand. Alternatively, she might be better able to manage an electric toothbrush. But if neither instrument is suitable, she will need physical help each day to remove the plaque from her teeth, preferably before she goes to bed at night.

A capful (~5 mL) of a neutrally based 0.2% sodium fluoride mouthrinse used daily for about 1 min will help resist the acidogenic demineralization of her teeth (Wyatt and MacEntee, 2004). She can use also a 5,000 ppm fluoridated toothpaste daily. If she cannot use the rinse or the highly fluoridated toothpaste, a dentist can maintain the protection against caries with a fluoride varnish applied every few months to all exposed dental surfaces.

Finally, in most situations, a dentist will be required immediately to debride the carious cavities and restore or extract the broken teeth (Frencken et al., 1996).

Clinical scenario 2

Mr. Belliveau is 74 years old with dementia. He looks physically healthy, but for the last year he has been taking donepezil, an anticholinesterase inhibitor, for Alzheimer's disease. He wears complete upper and lower dentures. He has had several sets of dentures over many years since his first set were made for him as a youth. He had a new set made 2 years ago that were comfortable until his dementia deteriorated, when he began to complain about pain on eating and loose dentures.

Over the last few months, he has been eating only soft foods, and keeps pushing the lower denture to one side of his jaw or removing it. He has lost one set of dentures during the previous year because he would remove and forget where he placed them. His wife reports that he prefers more often than not to leave them out of his mouth, especially the lower denture, which she finds very disturbing because he is losing weight and she believes that he looks even more demented and old without teeth. She reports also that she is very distressed by his dementia, which appears to have worsened over the last month. However, she wants her husband to look normal and to eat a wider range of healthy foods.

On examination, both dentures are obviously loose and unstable when Mr. Belliveau smiles and talks. He has clinical signs of angular cheilitis bilaterally, along with drooling stains on his clothing. The dentures occlude reasonably effectively, but they are covered in plaque and material alba. His wife explains with reassurance about his independence that he cleans the dentures frequently but alone by rinsing them under the tap. In fact, she said, "he always seems to be cleaning them when they're not lost!"

His mouth seems abnormally dry, and his palatal mucosa is mildly inflamed. On the left mylohyoid ridge, there is a small ulcer beneath the denture, which is obviously painful when he brings his teeth together.

The dry mucosa undoubtedly disturbs retention of the upper denture, and is likely to upset the overall comfort of both dentures. The hyposalivation might be caused by the donepezil, which is an anticholinesterase inhibitor with salivary gland hypofunction as a side effect. Perhaps Mr. Belliveau's physician should consider an alternative inhibitor, such as galantamine, that does not disturb salivary glands.

Hygiene is obviously inadequate and the risk of oral fungal infections is high, which probably explains the palatal edema and the angular cheilitis. Mr. Belliveau's unsupervised denture hygiene is ineffective, and his wife will need instruction on how to brush the dentures with soap and water. The dentures can be soaked daily for a short while in water with a "denture-soaking tablet," or in a 0.5%–1.0% solution of sodium hypochlorite for 10 min (Buergers et al., 2008). However, cleaning them daily with soap and water is most important, and they should be stored in a dry container when not worn to reduce the growth of candida fungi (Stafford et al., 1986).

Removable dentures should be labeled with the patient's name preferably when the dentures are made, and the name can be embedded within the denture base and covered with clearly transparent acrylic resin (Figure 12.5a).

Alternatively, but less permanently, the name can be written directly on the surface of "pink" acrylic resin, usually on the lingual surface of a lower denture or the distobuccal surface of the upper denture, with indelible ink (MacEntee and Campbell, 1979; Takahashi et al., 2008). A light abrading of the surface with sandpaper will help retain the ink, which is covered with a layer of clear autopolymerizing methyl methacrylate (Figure 12.5b–d).

There is a range of preventive strategies for individualized care plans involving risk reductions for caries, denture stomatitis, and candidiasis (Table 12.1).

Consent and accommodating residents' preferences

Many elderly residents of long-term care facilities are too frail to express their need for help (Department of Health, 2005). Some believe that the nurses and care-aides are too busy, while others are simply apathetic, or they are disturbingly fearful that their demands will precipitate subtle discriminations from the staff. Yet, nearly everyone who is frail will accept help if offered empathetically and with respect for their autonomy (Frenkel, 1999; Fitzpatrick, 2000). However, there are residents who resist help because they are capable of cleaning their own teeth if they have a toothbrush, toothpaste, washbasin, and towel. The principles of personal autonomy allow assistance only with the consent of the recipient following a clear explanation of the service or care offered (Etchells et al., 1996).

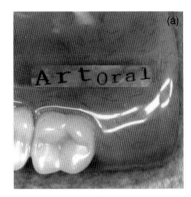

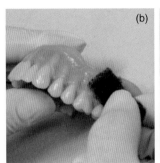 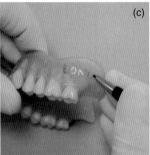 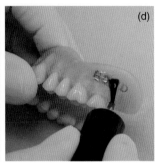

Figure 12.5 Identification labels embedded in denture base (a) or written with indelible ink on the surface of the denture (b–d).

Essentially, people, no matter how frail, are entitled to decline offers of help.

Carers usually need instruction on how to explain the essentials of good oral hygiene and how to render assistance from an ergonomically comfortable working position (Figure 12.6), although if a patient is in a wheelchair or lying in bed, it is not always possible to clean the mouth from a comfortably unstrained position (Figure 12.3).

Residents with cognitive impairment pose the most difficult challenges. They cannot express their needs and wishes clearly, and they can misinterpret the intentions and actions of the carer. Consent must be obtained from a legal guardian before rendering any care other than removal of immediate threats to life.

A quiet ambience and an empathetic approach with gentle verbal and physical reassurances in the presence of a familiar carer or friend can help calm anxious and disoriented elders (Chalmers et al., 2008). Physical resistance such as shouting, punching, and kicking indicate acute anxiety and confusion, and can be managed by postponing the interaction and, perhaps, spending more time establishing rapport and a less threatening relationship between the demented elder and the carer. Other strategies include

Table 12.1 Strategies to prevent dental, gingival, and periodontal diseases.

Strategy	Purpose
Manual and electric toothbrushing	Removes dental plaque and biofilm from surfaces of teeth, dentures, and mucosa
Cotton or sponge mouth swab	Helps • deliver fluoride and chlorhexidine; • moisten the mouth with water; • dislodge gross material alba and plaque from surfaces in the mouth
Fluoride: • daily applications of 0.2% sodium fluoride mouthrinse; • 5,000 ppm fluoride toothpaste; • twice annual application of 0.4% stannous fluoride gel or 5% sodium fluoride varnish	Resists demineralization of teeth and risk of caries
Alcohol-free antibacterial 0.12% or 0.2% chlorhexidine glucinate mouthrinse or spray twice daily at least 30 min after toothbrushing	Reduces gingivitis and periodontitis
Reduce frequency of sugars and other refined carbohydrates in medications, foods, and drinks	Resists dental demineralization and caries
Salivary stimulants, such as sugar-free candies or chewing gum	Stimulates salivary flow
Sip or spray water or suck ice chips	Compensates for salivary gland hypofunction and xerostomia to reduce discomfort of dry mouth
Denture care: • dentures should be removed at night and cleaned; • dentures should be allowed to dry when out of the mouth apart from a brief period soaking in a dilute bleach solution	Reduces fungal infections and stomatitis

communicating through simple and familiar phrases, and performing mouthcare when the elder is obviously more cooperative and restful. A plastic mouth prop, or an improvised prop with surgical tape wrapped around a tongue depressor, supports the lower jaw comfortably for a patient who has difficulty controlling the mandible and also reduces the risk of bites to the carer (Figure 12.7).

If treatment for a distressed and uncooperative patient cannot be postponed, it is possible sometimes for two or three carers working together

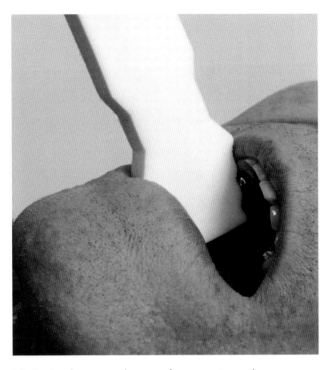

Figure 12.6 A plastic mouth prop for a patient who cannot control his mandible.

to talk calmingly to gently restrain arm and feet movements, and perform the necessary task efficiently and safely (Fiske et al., 2006). However, regulations on the use of physical and pharmacological restraints to treat uncooperative patients vary from jurisdiction to jurisdiction. A review of the literature in 2003 concluded "that restraint should only be used as a last resort, minimal level of restraint be used, for the minimal duration and that the restrained person should be closely monitored" (Evans et al., 2003). Furthermore, the legal status of physical restraint has been challenged in the United States where the courts in North Carolina, for example, have ruled that physical restraint on a handicapped patient infringes the patient's autonomy and violates the principle of social justice (Shuman and Bebeau, 1996).

CONCLUSIONS

- Frail elders often have high levels of oral disease, particularly if they have natural teeth, and the risk increases as they become frailer and consume more medications.

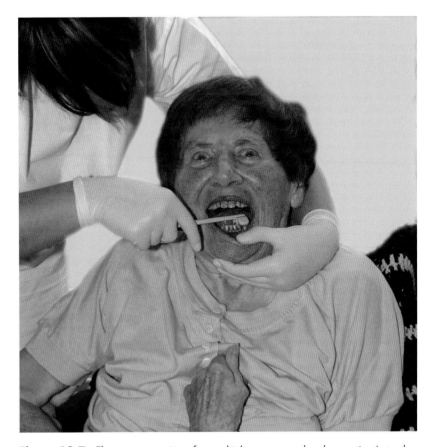

Figure 12.7 The correct position from which carers can brush a patient's teeth.

- Dental pain and oral problems are significantly underdiagnosed and undertreated in this population, and especially in people with dementia who cannot easily communicate their discomfort.
- Oral inflammation and infection in the mouths of frail elders increases morbidity, unnecessary suffering, and premature death.
- Promotion of oral health and healthcare is a low priority in many long-term care facilities.
- Nurses and other care staff are usually unacquainted with effective strategies for oral healthcare, and it is not easy to educate them in the cultural context of most facilities.
- Dental professionals feel challenged by the task of monitoring and providing acceptable oral care for the frail elders.
- The dental profession does not have effective and sustainable strategies to manage the oral health of frail elders.
- Improved services for frail elders require
  - planners, clinicians, and policy makers who understand the significance and underlying causes of oral neglect in people who are frail;

- integration of dental services with other healthcare services;
- systems for regular oral examinations, daily oral care, and ready access to dental treatments, including domiciliary care, suitable for frail elders;
- education of dental, nursing, and social care personnel to enable them to understand and meet the challenges of daily mouthcare and to recognize problems that need treatment.

REFERENCES

Adams R. 1996. Qualified nurses lack adequate knowledge related to oral health, resulting in inadequate oral care of patients on medical wards. *J Adv Nurs* 24:552–60.

Baumbusch JL and Andrusyszyn MA. 2002. Gerontological content in Canadian baccalaureate nursing programs: Cause for concern? *Can J Nurs Res* 34:119–29.

Bee JF. 2004. Portable dentistry: A part of general dentistry's service mix. *Gen Dent* 52:520–6.

Bellomo F, de Preux F, Chung JP, Julien N, Budtz-Jørgensen E, and Müller F. 2005. The advantages of occupational therapy in oral hygiene measures for institutionalised elderly adults. *Gerodontology* 22:24–31.

Bryant SR, MacEntee MI, and Browne A. 1995. Ethical issues encountered by dentists in the care of institutionalized elders. *Spec Care Dentist* 15:79–82.

Buergers R, Rosentritt M, Schneider-Brachert W, Behr M, Handel G, and Hahnel S. 2008. Efficacy of denture disinfection methods in controlling Candida albicans colonisation in vitro. *Acta Odontol Scand* 66:174–80.

Buss IC, Halfens RJG, Abu-Saad HH, and Kok G. 2004. Pressure ulcer prevention in nursing homes: Views and beliefs of enrolled nurses and other healthcare workers. *J Clin Nurs* 13: 668–76.

Chalmers JM, Levy SM, Buckwalter KC, Ettinger RL, and Kambhu PP. 1996. Factors influencing nurses' aides provision of oral care for nursing facility residents. *Spec Care Dentist* 16: 71–9.

Chalmers JM, Hodge C, Fuss JM, Spencer AJ, Carter KD, and Mathew R. 2001. Opinions of dentists and directors of nursing concerning dental care provision for Adelaide nursing homes. *Aust Dent J* 46:277–83.

Chalmers JM, King PL, Spencer AJ, Wright FAC, and Carter KD. 2005. The Oral Health Assessment Tool—Validity and reliability. *Aust Dent J* 50:191–9.

Chalmers JM, Carter KD, and Spencer AJ. 2008. Oral diseases and conditions in community-living older adults with and without dementia. *Spec Care Dentist* 23:7–17.

Charteris P and Kinsella T. 2001. The oral care link nurse: A facilitator and educator for maintaining oral health for patients at the Royal Hospital for Neuro-disability. *Spec Care Dentist* 21:68–71.

Coleman P and Watson NM. 2006. Oral care provided by certified nursing assistants in nursing homes. *J Am Geriatr Soc* 54:138–43.

Cowan DT, Roberts JD, Fitzpatrick JM, While AE, and Baldwin J. 2004. The approaches to learning of support workers employed in the care home sector: An evaluation study. *Nurse Educ Today* 24:98–104.

Department of Health. 2005. Meeting the challenges of oral health for older people: A strategic review. *Gerodontology* 22(Suppl. 1):9S–39S.

Eadie DR and Schou L. 1992. An exploratory study of barriers to promoting oral hygiene through carers of elderly people. *Community Dent Health* 9:343–8.

Edwards T. 2008. The reflections and dilemmas of a seasoned practitioner: Improving mouth care for dependent individuals. *National Oral Health Promotion Group Journal* (Autumn):22–3.

Etchells E, Sharpe G, Burgess MM, and Singer PA. 1996. Bioethics for clinicians: 2. Disclosure. *Can Med Assoc J* 155:387–91.

Ettinger RL, O'Toole C, Warren J, Levy S, and Hand JS. 2000. Nursing directors' perceptions of the dental components of the minimum data set (MDS) in nursing homes. *Spec Care Dentist* 20:23–7.

Evans D, Wood J, and Lambert L. 2003. Patient injury and physical restraint devices: A systematic review. *J Adv Nurs* 41:274–82.

Fiske J, Griffiths JE, Jamieson R, and Manger D. 1996. *Guidelines for Oral Care for Long Stay Patients and Residents*. British Society of Disability and Oral Health. Available at www.bsdh.org.uk/guidelines/longstay.pdf (accessed January 3, 2010).

Fiske J, Frenkel HF, Griffiths J, and Jones V. 2006. Guidelines for the development of local standards of oral healthcare for people with dementia. *Gerodontology* 23(Suppl. 1):30S.

Fitzpatrick J. 2000. Oral healthcare needs of dependent older people: Responsibilities of nurses and care-staff. *J Adv Nurs* 32:1325–32.

Frencken JE, Pilot T, Songpaisan Y, and Phantumvanit P. 1996. Atraumatic restorative treatment (ART): Rationale, technique, and development. *J Public Health Dent* 56:135–40.

Frenkel HF. 1999. Behind the screens: Care-staff observations on delivery of oral healthcare in nursing homes. *Gerodontology* 16:75–80.

Frenkel HF. 2003. Oral healthcare: Can training improve its quality? *Nurs Residential Care* 5:268–71.

Frenkel HF, Harvey I, and Newcombe R. 2001. Improving oral health in institutionalised elderly people by educating caregivers: A randomised controlled trial. *Community Dent Oral Epidemiol* 29:289–97.

Frenkel HF, Harvey I, and Needs KM. 2002. Oral healthcare education and its effect on caregivers' knowledge and attitudes: A randomised controlled trial. *Community Dent Oral Epidemiol* 30:91–100.

Furr LA, Binkley CJ, McCurren C, and Carrico R. 2004. Factors affecting quality of oral care in intensive care units. *J Adv Nurs* 48:454–62.

Grimoud AM, Lodter JP, Marty N, Andrieu S, Linas MD, Rumeau M, and Cazard JC. 2005. Improved oral hygiene and Candida species colonisation level in geriatric patients. *Oral Dis* 11:163–9.

Grocki JH and Fox GE Jr. 2004. Gerontology coursework in undergraduate nursing programs in the United States: A regional study. *J Gerontol Nurs* 30:46–51.

Hoad-Reddick G. 1991. A study to determine oral health needs of institutionalised elderly patients by non-dental healthcare workers. *Community Dent Oral Epidemiol* 19:233–6.

Hoad-Reddick G and Heath JR. 1995. Identification of elderly in particular need: Results of a survey undertaken in residential homes in the Manchester area. *J Dent* 23:273–9.

Jablonski RA, Munro CL, Grap MJ, and Elswick RK. 2005. The role of biobehavioral, environmental and social forces on oral health disparities in frail and functionally dependent nursing home elders. *Biol Res Nurs* 7:75–82.

Khader YS, Albashaireh ZS, and Alomari MA. 2004. Periodontal diseases and risk of coronary heart and cerebrovascular diseases: A meta-analysis. *J Periodontol* 75:1046–53.

Koren ME, Hertz J, Munroe D, Rossetti J, Robertson J, Plonczynski D, Berent G, and Ehrlich-Jones L. 2008. Assessing students' learning needs and attitudes: Considerations for gerontology curriculum planning. *Gerontol Geriatr Educ* 28:39–56.

MacDonald CD and Butler L. 2007. Silent no more: Elderly women's stories of living with urinary incontinence in long-term care. *J Gerontol Nurs* 33:14–20.

MacEntee MI. 2006. Missing links in oral healthcare for frail elderly people. *J Can Dent Assoc* 72:421–5.

MacEntee MI and Campbell T. 1979. Personal identification using dental prostheses. *J Prosthet Dent* 41:377–80.

MacEntee MI and Wyatt CCL. 1999. An index of Clinical Oral Disorder in Elders (CODE). *Gerodontology* 16:85–96.

MacEntee MI, Hill PM, Wong G, Mojon P, Berkowitz J, and Glick N. 1991. Predicting concerns for the mouth among institutionalized elders. *J Public Health Dent* 51:82–91.

MacEntee MI, Thorne S, and Kazanjian A. 1999. Conflicting priorities: Oral health in residential care. *Spec Care Dentist* 19:164–72.

MacEntee MI, Wyatt CCL, Beattie BL, Paterson B, Levy-Milne R, McCandless L, and Kazanjian A. 2007. Provision of mouth-care in residential care facilities: an educational trial. *Community Dent Oral Epidemiol* 35:25–34.

Minimum Data Set. 2010. *Minimum Data Set (MDS)—Version 3.0. Resident Assessment And Care Screening All Item Listing.* Available at www.ascp.com/resources/index/upload/MDS3.0.pdf (accessed May 27, 2010).

Moore J. 1995. Assessment of nurse-administered oral hygiene. *Nurs Times* 91:40–1.

Morris JN, Hawes C, Fries BE, Phillips CD, Mor V, Katz S, Murphy K, Drugovich ML, and Friedlob AS. 1990. Designing the national resident assessment instrument for nursing facilities. *Gerontologist* 30:293–307.

Nicol R, Sweeney MP, McHugh S, and Bagg J. 2005. Effectiveness of healthcare worker training on the oral health of elderly residents of nursing homes. *Community Dent Oral Epidemiol* 33:115–24.

Nitschke I. 2001. Geriatric oral health issues in Germany. *Int Dent J* 51:235–46.

Nitschke I, Ilgner A, and Müller F. 2005. Barriers to provision of dental care in residential facilities: The confrontation with ageing and death. *Gerodontology* 22:123–9.

Osterberg T, Carlsson GE, Sundh V, and Mellström D. 2008. Number of teeth— A predictor of mortality in 70-year-old subjects. *Community Dent Oral Epidemiol* 36:258–68.

Paley GA, Slack-Smith LM, and O'Grady MJ. 2004. Aged care-staff perspectives on oral care for residents: Western Australia. *Gerodontology* 21:146–54.

Peltola P, Vehkalahti MM, and Simoila R. 2007. Effects of 11-month interventions on oral cleanliness among the residential hospitalised elderly. *Gerodontology* 24:14–21.

Pyle MA, Jasinevicius TR, Sawyer DR, and Madsen J. 2005. Nursing home executive directors' perception of oral care in residential care facilities. *Spec Care Dentist* 25:111–7.

Russell SL, Boylan RJ, Kaslick RS, Scannapieco FA, and Katz RV. 1999. Respiratory pathogen colonisation of the dental plaque of institutionalized elders. *Spec Care Dentist* 19:128–34.

Sanson-Fisher RW, Bonevski B, Green LW, and D'Este C. 2007. Limitations of the randomized controlled trial in evaluating population-based health interventions. *Am J Prev Med* 33:155–61.

Scannapieco FA, Bush RB, and Paju S. 2003. Associations between periodontal disease and risk for nosocomial bacterial pneumonia and chronic obstructive pulmonary disease: A systematic review. *Ann Periodontol* 8:54–67.

Schou L and Eadie D. 1991. Qualitative study of oral health norms and behaviour among elderly people in Scotland. *Community Dent Health* 8:53–8.

Shay K and Ship JA. 1995. The importance of oral health in the older patient. *J Am Geriatr Soc* 43:1414–22.

Shimazaki Y, Soh I, Koga T, Miyazaki H, and Takehara T. 2004. Relationship between dental care and oral health in institutionalised elderly people in Japan. *J Oral Rehabil* 31:837–42.

Shuman SK and Bebeau MJ. 1996. Ethical and legal issues in special patient care. *Dent Clin North Am* 38:553–75.

Simons D. 2003. Who will provide dental care for housebound people with oral problems? *Br Dent J* 194:137–8.

Simons D, Baker P, Jones B, Kidd EAM, and Beighton D. 2000. An evaluation of an oral health training programme for carers of the elderly in residential homes. *Br Dent J* 188:206–10.

Stafford GD, Arendorf T, and Huggett R. 1986. The effect of overnight drying and water immersion on candidal colonization and properties of complete dentures. *J Dent* 14:52–6.

Sumi Y, Yasunori N, and Yukihiro M. 2002. Development of a systematic oral care program for frail elderly persons. *Spec Care Dentist* 22:151–5.

Takahashi F, Koji T, and Morita O. 2008. A new method for denture identification. *Dent Mater J* 27:278–83.

Vigild M. 1990. Evaluation of an oral health service for nursing home residents. *Acta Odontol Scand* 48:99–105.

Wårdh I, Andersson L, and Sörensen S. 1997. Staff attitudes to oral healthcare: A comparative study of registered nurses, nursing assistants and home care aides. *Gerodontology* 14:28–32.

Wårdh I, Berggren U, Andersson L, and Sörensen S. 2002. Assessments of oral healthcare in dependent older persons in nursing facilities. *Acta Odontol Scand* 60:330–6.

Wårdh I, Hallberg LR-M, Berggren U, Andersson L, and Sörensen S. 2003. Oral health education for nursing personnel; experiences among specially trained oral care aides: one-year follow-up interviews with oral care aides at a nursing facility. *Scand J Caring Sci* 17:250–6.

Weeks JC and Fiske J. 1994. Oral care of people with a disability: A qualitative exploration of the views of nursing staff. *Gerodontology* 11:13–7.

Woodall D. 1997. Some oral health education experiences. *Gerodontic Study Group Newsletter* June, p. 1.

Wyatt CCL and MacEntee MI. 2004. Caries management for institutionalized elders using fluoride and chlorhexidine mouthrinses. *Community Dent Oral Epidemiol* 32:322–8.

Prosthodontics, endodontics, and other restorative care for frail elders

George Zarb, Shane N. White, Nico H.J. Creugers, Frauke Müller, and Michael I. MacEntee

GUIDELINES TO CARE

"Come, grow old with me, the best is yet to be" opines the poet but not the experienced dentist to her or his frail patients. The physiological parameters of old age, which still include functional abilities and remedial potential, are frequently eclipsed by disease. All too suddenly, management strategies based on routine dental treatment formulae are passé and must be replaced by more eclectic and humanitarian care outside our traditional boundaries.

It is one thing to cope with the technical challenges encountered when treating elderly patients, but quite another to manage the oral healthcare of frail elders. The former's requirements for health maintenance are not dissimilar from those for other age groups. They are variations on the themes of traditional dental ingenuity, albeit with subtle differences in patient management irrespective of whether the clinical initiative involves retention of teeth or their replacement. The needs of all elderly patients vary greatly and should be considered within the context of general health and social circumstances, which change as our patients grow frailer. These flux and uncertainty require mature clinical aptitude and experience together with a high level of interpersonal skills in all aspects of healthcare. As a result, maintenance of oral health for frail elders demands an optimal convergence of realistic concerns and desires from the elders and their caregivers complemented by competent professional skills and judgments.

Frail elders, when managed appropriately, require stronger doses of compassion, common sense, and clinical pragmatism. Their expectations, and often those of their caregivers, of comfort and function are unlikely to warrant "herodontic" interventions or even major aesthetic concerns. Automatic reliance on the sort of "comprehensive treatment" repertoire that includes extensive fixed prostheses and complex implant restorations should be avoided in patients who are systemically brittle and obviously fragile. Frail elders are also unlikely to be managed suitably by dentists whose convictions regarding optimal professional care preclude simpler and less invasive management strategies. There is very little rigorous evidence to support a particular course of treatment for patients who are frail and dependent. Consequently, dentists must rely on personal and borrowed best practices from more robust patients with similar impairments and disabilities. However, the most prudent and sensible perceptions of care must focus on comfort and function without risking additional morbidity.

There are ethical and legal considerations that challenge a dentist's remit even further when managing the needs of this vulnerable population. Clinical judgments leading to dental treatment need to be made as correctly as possible and, preferably, in consultation with caregivers along with family and friends who have a close and affectionate relationship with the patient. The old maxim "treat the patient as you would if he or she was your own parent" is an admirable humanitarian substitute for the absence of a specific scientific measure for gauging a patient's adaptive potential. The concept of reconciling normative with realistic treatment needs for frail patients offers a prudent example for managing the oral healthcare needs of patients with, for example, Alzheimer's disease (Nordenram et al., 1997). It is based on a comparable escalating level of intervention that initially deals with immediate and necessary concerns, such as relief of pain and control of infection (Table 13.1).

Indeed, this conceptual approach acknowledges "no treatment" as an appropriate management strategy when there is no evidence of pain or risk, and particularly if the patient is uncooperative. Interceptive or corrective treatments, when needed, can be selected from a repertoire of modest protocols to correct and manage oral impairments and disabilities. And finally, there is a wide range of prosthodontic treatments available to meet most expectations of function and comfort.

Other than people with surgical maxillofacial defects, there is probably no other group demanding of so much wisdom, compassion, and clinical skill from dental professionals than the growing population of frail elders. And yet, our knowledge is far from adequate to offer them a defensible "best prosthodontic practice." Regrettably, there is a prevailing view that technological innovations offer quasi-panaceas that eclipse all other concerns. However, we believe that we have a compellingly professional obligation to balance technical skill with humanitarian priorities and common sense when attending to the needs of this particularly vulnerable population.

This chapter deals with the management of oral healthcare for frail elders under the following headings: dental restorations for individual

Table 13.1 Normative compared with realistic treatment needs for frail elders.

Patients in this category have stable systemic health and good cognitive function. They also demonstrate a capacity to make independent decisions.

Overall management objectives respond to pain, discomfort, and compromised function in the context of ensuring symptom relief and instituting preventive and corrective measures that maintain oral health, comfort, and aesthetics, as requested by the patient.

1   Immediate:
     Relief of pain and management of oral infections (extractions, endodontic treatment, relief of sore spots related to dentures, etc.)
2   None:
     Pain or disease is not present and oral function is satisfactory
3   Minor:
     Preventive measures to support and maintain oral health modifications
     Repairs/modifications/cleaning of prostheses
4   Major:
     Traditional clinical responses to sequelae of caries, periodontal, pulpal, or mucosal diseases by relieving discomfort and preventing bacterial dissemination
     Fabrication of new prostheses with consideration for implant support design

Critical concerns here are the patient's systemic health and cognitive capacities, as well as the availability and ability of caregivers to provide routine and frequent oral hygiene.

Overall management objectives are the same as those employed in normative needs. However, impaired cognition and/or inability to cooperate will determine the extent of intervention.

1   Immediate:
     Relief of pain and management of oral infections (extractions, relief of sore spots related to dentures, etc.). Interventions are minimal and seek to improve overall function and quality of life.
2   None:
     The patient is uncooperative, but treatment is unnecessary if the patient's oral environment is judged to be harmless or free of pain.
3   Modest:
     Only palliative care is rendered if the patient is uncooperative, and operative or prosthodontic treatment is likely to compromise the patient's overall well-being. Even the most minimal interventions might require general anesthesia, which raises a need for more general management decisions with broader medical implications.
4   Extensive:
     The patient wants treatment and is cooperative. The intervention seeks to maintain or improve oral health, and prosthodontic treatment might be feasible.

teeth, endodontic interventions to prolong the life of useful teeth, teeth replacement with fixed or removable prostheses, and recruiting oral implants to optimize prosthodontic prognoses.

DENTAL RESTORATIONS FOR INDIVIDUAL TEETH

Process and product in restorative and operative treatments

Teeth function for frail elders no differently than for other age groups. Whether sound or restored, they affect appearance, mastication, and other functions of the dentition as a whole. And while some teeth are more important than others (Käyser, 1994; Witter et al., 1999), dental restorations in general repair compromised teeth and protect them from further disease and trauma. Decisions to restore teeth for frail patients depend on a balance of input (effort, cost, and risk for unwanted side effects) and outcome (functional effectiveness, durability, comfort, etc.). However, the propensity or willingness of patients to cope with all the inevitable burdens of restorative treatment is often diminished (Mojon and MacEntee, 1994; Ettinger, 1996; MacEntee et al., 1997). For this reason, all operative interventions should be kept to a minimum wherever possible and adapted to the patient's general expectations and propensities.

In general, the important parameter or defining characteristic of operative dentistry for an able-bodied patient is the clinical product or treatment outcome. Typically, this should be long lasting and of high quality. However, frail patients require a different set of parameters that are physically and psychologically less demanding, relatively less durable, and repeatable at low cost if necessary (Table 13.2).

Direct or indirect restorations

Direct adhesive restorations are the first choice in the treatment of primary caries (Selwitz et al., 2007). However, a large proportion (50%–65%) of

Table 13.2 Context of restorative treatments for elders who are robust or frail.

	Elders	
Context	Robust	Frail
Overall objectives	Restore	Maintain
Treatment		
• Range	Unrestricted	Restricted
• Burden	Limited	Extensive
Adaptability of patient	Good	Moderate to poor
Expected longevity of results	>5 years	<5 years

restorations made for older patients are replacements, and as the restorations are enlarged, teeth are weakened (Brantley et al., 1995; Mjor et al., 2002; Forss and Widstrom, 2004). Indirect restorations are used to repair posterior teeth with large structural defects (Stavropoulou and Koidis, 2007), but anterior teeth that have been endodontically treated are more likely to be weakened further by metal ceramic or all ceramic crowns because of the amount of enamel and dentine removed to accommodate them (Sorensen and Martinoff, 1984). Nonetheless, there seems to be no significant difference overall in the clinical survival of direct and indirect restorations associated with endodontically treated teeth (Mannocci et al., 2002; Fokkinga et al., 2007, 2008). Indirect cast posts are probably more durable clinically than direct posts of composite resin (Jung et al., 2007), but the difference has little practical relevance to the dental needs of frail elders. Probably of greater relevance is the fact that directly bonded resin composites and amalgam restorations can be repaired effectively with minimal intervention to increase their longevity (Gordan et al., 2006; Moncada et al., 2009).

Cracks can occur in teeth with or without large restorations (Roh and Lee, 2006), and they can be treated with equal success by direct and indirect restorations if the tooth cusps are covered (Signore et al., 2007; Opdam et al., 2008). Finally, there is no compelling evidence favoring routine use of crowns to prevent fracture of teeth (Bader et al., 1996).

Abutment teeth

Abutment teeth for removable prostheses can carry heavy occlusal loads especially in denture-wearers who grind or brux their teeth. Consequently, if they are damaged and structurally weak, they can be crowned with indirect restorations to prevent further damage from stressful loads. However, the effectiveness of this preventive treatment, which seems reasonable, has been tested only for abutment teeth with precision attachments (Vermeulen et al., 1996). Overdenture abutment are subjected also to heavy loads in some patents, but here there is evidence that access to the root canal orifices can be closed effectively for at least 4 years with amalgam, composite, or glass ionomer restorations (Keltjens et al., 1999).

ENDODONTICS

Pulpal and periradicular disease is very common in adults; so is root canal treatment. In Denmark, Taiwan, and the United States, the annual incidence of endodontics lies somewhere between 1% and 7% of the adult population (Kirkevang et al., 2006; Tilashalski et al., 2006; Chen et al., 2007), while the prevalence is approximately 11% of all surviving teeth. Apparently, people accumulate periradicular disease and need root canal treatments as they age, and awareness of this need seems to be increasing

(Goodis et al., 2001; Vysniauskaite and Vehkalahti, 2006). Therefore, where endodontic treatment is readily accessible, it is likely that frail elders with natural teeth will have teeth with endodontic restorations.

Underdiagnosis and undertreatment of periradicular pathoses is common, especially in elderly populations (Petersson et al., 1989), although many of the periapical radiolucencies are healing rather than failing lesions. As a result, radiolucencies reflecting healing lesions accumulate as people grow old. Moreover, it is also likely that patients tolerate incompletely healed endodontic treatments without seeking additional intervention. Of course, an endodontic failure with extant pathosis should be addressed by orthograde endodontic retreatment or by extraction of the tooth.

Outcomes of endodontic treatment

Endodontic interventions are very successful with about 97% surviving comfortably for at least 6 years (Torabinejad et al., 2007; Iqbal and Kim, 2008). Failed root canal treatments are best addressed by cleaning and obturating the canals again rather than by surgical endodontics (Torabinejad et al., 2009). Success of on-surgical retreatment increases over time as patients heal, whereas surgical successes appear to decrease steadily over time. Endodontic surgery should be considered very selectively and only when retreatment fails or there is an immovable impediment, such as a post, in the canal of a strategically important tooth. The invasiveness of surgery in contrast to endodontic retreatment is an important consideration for frail patients, and there is little doubt that root canal treatment is inherently less traumatic than extraction of a tooth.

Endodontics as a foundation for prosthodontics

Pulpal and periradicular health should be confirmed before predicting the prognosis of an abutment tooth, and the prognosis of endodontic treatment is based collectively on a patient's history, the relative response of similar teeth to percussion, palpation, periodontal probing, electrical and thermal stimuli, and on radiographic observations. The absence of a pulpal response to cold, heat, or electrical stimuli does not necessarily mean that the pulp is necrotic. It can indicate also that there is thermal and electrical insulation by secondary or reparative dentin around the root canal—a common finding in old age. The correct interpretation of test results depends on clear communications to and from the patient, although communications can be challenging when patients are deaf, confused, or cognitively impaired.

Root canals calcify with age, which changes the technical difficulty rather than the prognosis of treatment (Goodis et al., 2001). The concept of the "stressed pulp" has been attributed to advancing age, but there is no convincing evidence that it exists in any way to justify "preventive endodontics" or "corrective endodontics." Endodontic treatment for a patient at any age and in any state of health is justified only if it addresses pulpal and periradicular pathoses diagnosed firmly on the patient's symptoms and clinical signs.

Medical and patient considerations for endodontics

The key to successful endodontics is removal of sufficient bacteria to allow normal healing, whereas instruments, materials, and techniques appear to be relatively unimportant. Few medical conditions are linked to this success (Quesnell et al., 2005). Healing, especially of periradicular lesions, is compromised in patients with diabetes (Fouad and Burleson, 2003), whereas bleeding disorders, radiation therapy, and high doses of bisphosphonates all favor root canal treatment over dental extractions or other surgical procedures. Indeed, root canal treatment is only precluded by severe and life-threatening illness or if a patient cannot understand and cooperate with the dentist's directions. And even when cooperation is absent, sedation or general anesthesia can enable the treatment.

Restoring endodontically treated teeth

The risk of vertical fracture in a posterior tooth can be reduced by covering the occlusal surface with a metallic or ceramic crown (Stavropoulou and Koidis, 2007), but anterior teeth with endodontic restorations can be weakened further by the preparation needed to accommodate crowns (Sorensen and Martinoff, 1984). Survival of an endodontically treated tooth depends on the integrity and structure of its crown and of its root (Nagasiri and Chitmongkolsuk, 2005; Fokkinga et al., 2007). A coronoradicular amalgam alloy or resin-composite restoration is a conservative, simple, useful, and inexpensive way to maintain a tooth with an endodontic restoration (Nayyar et al., 1980; Kane et al., 1990). Occasionally, it is necessary to place a post in the root canal to retain and stabilize the coronal restoration, despite the risk of an untreatable vertical root fracture. Currently, there is a lack of long-term evidence to favor fiber over metal posts (Cagidiaco et al., 2008). Fiber posts are relatively flexible, which might reduce the risk of root fracture, but their flexibility could also leave them prone to retentive or structural failure.

Artificial crowns on endodontic posts are rarely reliable abutments for removable dentures with distal extensions because the stress is likely to dislodge the post and crown. It is much less stressful to seal the root canal above the endodontic filling with an amalgam alloy or resin-composite restoration, and to contour the occlusal surface as a dome protruding approximately 3 mm above the gingiva so that it is easily cleaned when the denture is removed (Figure 13.1).

Managing discolored teeth

The appearance of discolored teeth after endodontics can be improved with bonded composite or porcelain veneers supplemented by internal

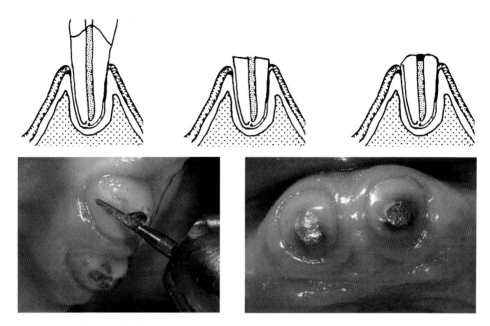

Figure 13.1   Overdenture abutments with amalgam restorations.

bleaching of dentine. A white or light opaque core of composite material placed deeply within the access cavity to the pulp chamber will improve the color of an abnormally dark tooth. Internal bleaching is safe with an aqueous slurry of sodium perborate without superoxyl or heat if a resin or glass ionomer cement base is placed above the level of the periodontal attachment.

TEETH REPLACEMENT

Prudent prosthodontics for any age group should be driven by reconciling a patient's needs and desires with a thorough knowledge of health, disease, and the likely outcomes of all treatments. The unavoidable risk of adverse ecological change dictates that treatment should be planned with concern for adverse biomechanical and aesthetic disturbances. The latter can take place in the context of possible time-dependent risks of further changes to the entire oral environment (Zarb et al., 1978). A history of caries and periodontal diseases increases further the challenge of repairing or replacing teeth and associated structures. Physical and cognitive disabilities reduce personal autonomy and the ability to handle and maintain oral prostheses, while compromising the ability and motivation for invasive and lengthy treatments. Muscle coordination and adaptation to dentures appears to decrease as dementia progresses (Taji et al., 2005). Limited finances—real or imagined—occasionally restrict treatment options even further. Nonetheless, preliminary or exploratory treatments can be useful for assessing a patient's resiliency and ability to cope with a proposed treatment, which, in turn, could lead to further accommodations as frailty and dependency increase (Riesen et al., 2002).

Healthy elders today in many countries see themselves as consumers of healthcare who expect to pay a professional fee for correct and ethical guidance along with the treatment itself. They often expect to participate in developing the treatment plan, and the outcome can be influenced substantially by their commitment to it. Hence, the dentist's responses to presumed treatment needs, such as "Let's save all of the remaining teeth and replace the missing ones," or "We'll remove the hopeless ones and just wait and see," are not always readily or uncritically received. On the other hand, explaining the time-dependent ecological implications of any form of provisional, partial, or extensive plan of treatment—and preferably for treatment that is as innocuous as possible—to frail patients and other caregivers demands a particularly prudent and resilient approach.

An axiom of modern dentistry is that caries and periodontal disease can be reduced, indeed even relatively easily managed, by means of correctly applied personal and professional initiatives. This conviction reflects current insights into the pathogenesis of both diseases supplemented by clinical ingenuity, which can almost guarantee the useful life of most teeth. The demineralizing effects of cariogenic bacteria can be minimized and frequently prevented altogether by the appropriate use of fluoride (Ettinger and Qian, 2004; Wyatt and MacEntee, 2004). Moreover, periodontal disease is now regarded as relatively easily managed with routine hygiene protocols administered by a dental hygienist, selective surgical pocket reductions, and a dentist's prescription pad (Loesche et al., 2005). Even advanced periodontitis can be managed successfully in older adults for over 5-year periods and even longer. However, the success of therapy demands extensive professional resources and personal abilities, neither of which comes easily to frail elders. Consequently, there is the temptation to extract teeth with pulpal or periodontal infections in the belief that endodontic treatment is extravagant, long-term periodontal maintenance unattainable, and prosthodontic treatment relatively simple.

The views presented up to this point in the chapter provide a background for the different management scenarios referred to in Table 13.1, and they can be conveniently summarized as a rational clinical protocol (Ettinger, 1996). However, "reluctant prosthodontics" might be a more apt way to describe our approach (Table 13.3).

Shortened dental arch

We probably need only a few pairs of opposing anterior teeth to chew adequately and comfortably, so the relative risks of wearing removable or fixed dental prostheses (FDPs) can be avoided altogether (Käyser, 1994; Witter et al., 1999). The concept of a "shortened dental arch" (SDA) in

Table 13.3 Prosthodontic options for frail elders.

Shortened dental arch
Removable prostheses
• Removable partial prosthesis
• Complete prosthesis
• Overdentures
Fixed partial prosthesis, including adhesive prostheses
Implant prostheses

Kennedy Classes 1 and 2 partial edentulism is remarkably stable and has particular benefits for patients who have difficulty cleaning microbial plaque from their teeth. However, there are patients, and even very frail patients, who are greatly bothered without molar teeth, either because their ability to chew feels inadequate or more typically because they dislike the appearance of an edentulous space posterior to the premolars.

Several factors influence the acceptance of an SDA with 8–10 anterior teeth in the opposing jaws. For example, the occlusal contacts and chewing movements might be functionally and aesthetically acceptable to patients with an Angle Class I jaw relationship but completely unacceptable for someone with an Angle Class II relationship. Consequently, dentists need a wider selection of prosthodontic options beyond simply prescribing the acceptance of an SDA for all patients with missing molars. A balance is required between the subjective demands of the patient and the clinical judgement as supplemented by the dentist's technical skills. In short, the SDA is a "minimalist" treatment strategy that aims to avoid the adverse ecological affect of a dental prosthesis (MacEntee, 1993), but it is not a helpful option for everyone.

Removable prostheses

Modifying dentures

Patients with removable partial or complete prostheses are usually willing to have minor or even major modifications to improve the prosthesis (Table 13.4).

Removing sore spots and relining dentures are among the most frequently performed maintenance measures in denture-wearers. The necessity for a reline can be attributed to rapid loss of body weight, indicating neurodegenerative decline or other morbidities. Loss of retention in a recent well-functioning maxillary complete denture (CD) over a relatively short period might be an especially valuable clinical indicator of more serious problems, and should be communicated to the patient's physician (Magri et al., 2003; Brubacher et al., 2004).

Shortening of teeth from attrition, abrasion, erosion, or a combination of two or more of these phenomena is encountered often in aging denti-

Table 13.4   Clinical methods of modifying dental prostheses to improve tolerance, comfort, and function for frail patients.

1. Reduce acrylic resin that is unnecessarily bulky or causing pressure sores.
2. Address patient perceptions regarding the bulk or weight of the prosthesis through selective steps that include modification or removal of excess material and metallic components (e.g., retainers or reciprocating arms)—especially if the materials or components interfere with movements of the tongue and other soft tissues.
3. Adjust the occlusion—on an articulator if adjustments are extensive—to provide comfortable bilateral contacts at or close to centric relation, and allow multidirectional contact movements without interference.
4. Add tooth-colored acrylic resin to increase and maintain a new vertical dimension of occlusion (VDO) and to optimize and stabilize occlusal contacts.
5. Replace severely damaged or worn prosthetic teeth.
6. Add soft lining material to improve retention and stability of the denture base and, if necessary, to restore a comfortable and aesthetically acceptable vertical dimension of occlusion.

Clinical scenario 1

Mrs. Zammit is 75 years old and frail but cognitively alert. She complained of aesthetic and functional problems with her upper teeth. Her face was "collapsing," she reported, as she could not wear her upper dentures comfortably. She was also worried by chronic grating sounds in both jaw joints.

On clinical examination, her vertical dimension of occlusion (VDO) had no posterior support and a deep anterior overbite (Figure 13.2), and there were signs on palpation of degenerative arthritis in both jaw joints.

She accepted prosthodontic treatment designed to increase the VDO with a removable prosthesis in both jaws. Subsequently, new dentures were made at a more comfortable VDO (Figure 13.3), and she was given advice on how to manage the osteoarthritic joints with rest and nonsteroidal anti-inflammatory drugs.

tions. The crowns of the teeth are abnormally short with sharp, broad incisal and occlusal edges, cervical wear, plus labial enamel changes. Long-term consumption of numerous medications can also induce xerostomia, which in turn counters the buffering effect of saliva and renders the teeth vulnerable to acidic erosion. Gastroesophageal reflux disorder (GERD) also produces erosion, noticeably around the edges of dental restorations so that tooth structure looks as if it has "retracted" from the restorations.

Pain in the jaw joints can occasionally respond favorably to increasing the vertical dimension of occlusion (VDO) (Zarb et al., 1994). This is achieved either with repeated applications of soft-liners over several weeks, and by improving posterior occlusal support in both removable partial and complete prostheses (see clinical scenario 1). However, this

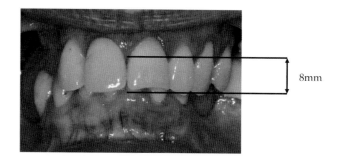

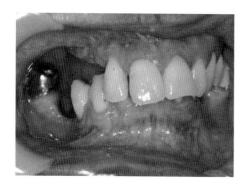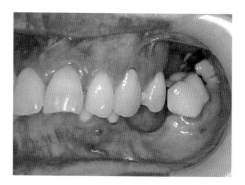

8mm

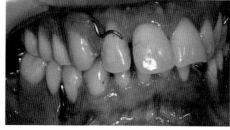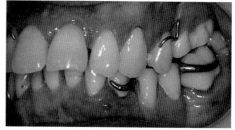

Figure 13.2 Mrs. Zammit's overbite without posterior dental support.

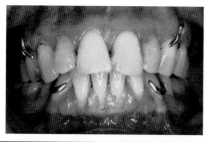

Figure 13.3 Mrs. Zammit's overbite with posterior prosthodontic support.

approach is neither always successful nor feasible. For example, patients who cannot tolerate wearing their dentures because of inadequate salivary flow or poor tissue tolerance may have to wear their dentures only intermittently, which is unlikely to improve their joint pain.

An abraded or eroded crown that is shortened does not necessarily imply that the VDO is excessively reduced or "collapsed." It is possible that the teeth have erupted to compensate for the loss of occlusal tooth structure. The concern here is not only to remove the cause through preventive measures (if these are indeed feasible) but also to address the restorative needs of individual teeth. An additional consideration could be an acrylic guard to protect soft tissues from sharp teeth, and to carry a fluoride gel into regular and intimate contact with enamel and dentin.

Partial dentures are intrusive and can cause a spectrum of adverse intraoral ecological changes (Zarb et al., 1978). Well-documented clinical and research experience underscores the simple fact that even the best "bikini" framework designs (as opposed to "Victorian bathing suit") can cause tissue damage if plaque control and regular servicing of the removable partial denture (RPD) are not scrupulously applied (Bergman et al., 1982; MacEntee, 1993). It is clear that the major determinant of adverse outcomes associated with long-term use of an RPD is poor oral hygiene, although the materials and design of the prosthesis can add to the problems. Avoidance of an RPD is often preferable for many able patients and an even more compelling *modus operandi* for frail elders.

Soft-liners

Soft lining materials (so-called tissue conditioners) are indispensable in removable prosthodontics. They play an essential role in the management of mucosal problems and loose dentures, at least for the short term. They permit easy and immediate changes to the fit of a denture base, and provide a helpful prognostic assessment of tolerance to a denture. The three different and progressive physical stages of most commercially available soft-liners account for their versatility and effectiveness. (1) The plastic stage permits movement of the denture base so that it is more compatible with the existing occlusion while flowing to cover the supporting residual ridges. This also allows displaced tissues to recover their original position. (2) The elastic stage helps attenuate adverse stresses on the ridge and prolongs the period of tissue recovery. Hence the arguably incorrect reference to "tissue conditioning," since what is really happening is a recovery of tissue form with a better-fitting denture. (3) Finally, the firm stage is influenced by the powder/liquid mix and functions as an interim reline of the denture pending a decision on the need for further treatment.

The strength of the underlying processed resin base occasionally needs reinforcement with additional hard resin before applying the soft-liner. Moreover, several denture cleansers can damage the soft porous material, which compromises hygiene even further. Typically, a soft toothbrush and soapy water used regularly will keep the material clean. The durability and hygiene of soft materials are prolonged by gentle polishing the surface with a soft pumice after 1–2 weeks, while antifungal creams can also be incorporated into the material to counter the abundant growth of *Candida* and other fungi, particularly for patients who are immunologically compromised (Geerts et al., 2008). In summary, frequent replacement of the soft-liner, supplemented by an effective effort to keep the mouth and the denture clean, will help fungi and stomatitis. However, neither the soft lining nor oral hygiene is always successful when the immune system is faulty.

Removable partial prostheses

Teeth in Kennedy Classes 1, 2, and 4 partially edentulous categories are best replaced with removable partial prostheses (RPPs) if chewing or appearance is disturbed by the inadequate distribution or condition of the remaining teeth. RPPs are made mostly of acrylic resin with or without cast cobalt–chromium components. The acrylic resin is strong, easily repaired, readily adjusted, and relatively inexpensive. Dental prostheses are stabilized usually by intimate contact with the underlying mucosa and adjacent teeth, and they are retained by the proximal surfaces of the adjacent teeth supplemented by cast alloy or wrought wire retainers engaging infrabulge undercuts on the abutment teeth.

Complete dentures

CDs are used widely by older people (Mojon et al., 2004). In Switzerland, for example, most (86%) of the population by age 85 years wear removable dentures, of which slightly more than one-third (37%) are complete prostheses (Zitzmann et al., 2008).

The technical aspects of making, relining, or copying a new CD are relatively straightforward and generally successful (Davenport and Heath, 1983). Soft-liners and the relative ease with which prosthetic teeth can add to old denture bases prolong their useful life even further. Residual alveolar ridges resorb continuously and are inherently unstable (Tallgren, 1972); hence, it is not surprising that older people have difficulty with CDs as they grow frail.

Denture adhesives

Denture adhesives can help patients who are struggling to control CDs (Grasso, 2004). They do not compensate for ill-fitting dentures, but they can compensate in part for neurological and morphological disturbances. Nonetheless, there are lingering concerns that denture adhesives contribute to mucosal inflammation by simply masking the source of the physical problems with ill-fitting dentures (Ai et al., 2005).

Denture hygiene

The health of the mucosa underlying CDs is compromised by poor denture hygiene, a maladapted base, unstable occlusion, and continuous denture-wearing (especially in the maxilla). Systemic diseases also contribute to mucosal vulnerability from pressure and facultative microorganisms. The combined effect of compromised immunity and poor oral hygiene often leads to angular cheilitis (Budtz-Jorgensen et al., 2000), which is best managed by meticulous denture hygiene and drying the dentures when out of the mouth overnight (Stafford et al., 1986).

Overdentures

Complete overdentures greatly benefit from the stability provided by underlying abutment teeth (Goodis et al., 1990). Abutment stimulation prevents resorption of alveolar bone, offers proprioceptive awareness of jaw activity, and improves masticatory efficiency (Fontijn-Tekamp et al., 2004). The catastrophic impact of multiple tooth loss from periodontal disease and excessive tooth mobility can be eased considerably by retaining a few teeth with a reasonably good periodontal attachment as abutments to support and stabilize a denture. If an abutment is lost, the consequences are usually relatively easy to manage by relining the denture over the site of the abutment socket. Moreover, the stability offered by an overdenture abutment, even for short periods, eases the transition from partial to complete tooth loss.

Clinical scenario 2

Ms. Murphy has been scheduled for extractions of most of her maxillary teeth due to severe periodontal disease (Figure 13.4a). She was very upset about the impending loss of her upper natural teeth, and because of her Parkinson's disease, she believed that she might not be able to control an upper CD. All of her maxillary teeth were disturbingly (≥Class II) mobile due to loss of periodontal bone. However, the periodontal pockets around teeth 13, 21, and 23 were ≤3 mm deep. Consequently, treatment was modified to retain the three teeth as abutments for a complete overdenture. The teeth were decoronated after endodontic treatment. Amalgam alloy restorations were placed to seal the access canals, and the "occlusal" surfaces domed before the other maxillary teeth were extracted (Figure 13.4b–d). The overdenture was modified immediately with autopolymerizing resin to rest stably on the abutments when Ms. Murphy was occluding firmly on the denture (Figure 13.4e, f).

    The abutments are managed with routine oral hygiene supplemented by daily application of a 0.4% stannous fluoride gel.

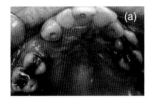
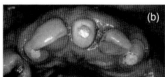
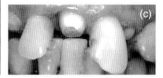

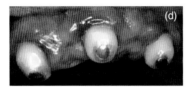
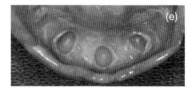

Figure 13.4 Ms. Murphy's teeth before (a), in transition (b, c), and as abutments for an overdenture (e).

Maintaining overdenture abutments

Patients with overdentures almost invariably have a long history of dental disease, but the risk of caries and periodontal disease is especially high in this population due to the pathogenic virulence of the protected biofilm underneath the dentures. Consequently, hygiene and daily applications of fluoride are very important. Indeed, caries risk can be reduced substantially by regular applications of fluoride, in a varnish, gel, or mouthrinse (Derkson and MacEntee, 1982; Ettinger and Qian, 2004), and the denture base is a convenient and effective medium for carrying the fluoridated gel to the abutment teeth. The dome-shaped and polished surface of each abutment helps to limit the accumulations of plaque and to facilitate the removal of the biofilm (MacEntee, 1978; Derkson and MacEntee, 1982). Problems with teeth under dentures are likely to increase with frailty, and it is not uncommon to find that caries recurs aggressively (Budtz-Jorgensen, 1995; Ettinger and Jakobsen, 1996; Brkovic-Popovic et al., 2008). However, the abutment teeth can be extracted and the denture can be modified quite easily to maintain or restore comfort and function.

Fixed dental prostheses

Conventional and resin-bonded FDPs typically require lengthy appointments, so it has limited applications for frail elders if there are concerns about fatigue. Success of the resin-bonded FDP depends heavily on enamel for adhesion, interocclusal space to accommodate the prosthesis, and normal rather than hyperactive or parafunctional jaw activity. Many dentists believe that fixed prostheses for older patients are too time-consuming and expensive considering the technical and biological risk of failure in mouths that are unstable.

Implant dentures

The documented effectiveness and versatility of implant-stabilized dentures have profoundly influenced the way in which prosthodontic treatment is planned and delivered (Zarb and Schmitt, 1990a,b; Zarb and Schmitt, 1996a,b; Attard et al., 2005). In fact, an almost complete dental and psychosocial rehabilitation appears to be possible after implant stabilization of a mandibular denture, which allows patients to live more comfortable social lives (Wismeijer et al., 1997). It is tempting to interpret the success of implant prosthodontics as confirmation of the treatment objective that the best prostheses are those which are securely retained and stable. Consequently, the spectrum of implant numbers and design possibilities offers enormous scope for addressing almost everyone's needs. While this is a very encouraging possibility, it remains a challenging procedure for a frail population, since implant treatment usually demands considerable time along with major surgical, fiscal, and behavioral commitments.

We have very limited information on the performance and fate of implant dentures in elders, although age alone does not seem to influence the osseointegration, health, survival, or function of the implants (Kondell et al., 1988; Meijer et al., 2001; Bryant and Zarb, 2003; Engfors et al., 2004). The decision made by people to accept or reject treatment involving implants is also influenced by many factors. Besides the usual physical and social barriers to care, such as illness, financial limitations, and cultural expectations, there are many deeply seated psychological apprehensions around fear of surgery and ability to cope with disability. It is best to place implants when a patient is still independent and systemically robust and resilient. It is clearly not only limited finances that prevent elders from oral implant treatment (Walton and MacEntee, 2005), but also a range of factors including anxiety about the progress of their frailty.

There are, nonetheless, distinct advantages offered by oral implants to all age groups whether robust or frail. The increased popularity of placing implants in edentulous mandibles has facilitated the technique's versatile implementation (e.g., one-stage surgical placement, easy site access, impressive imaging). While the challenge of providing stable prostheses has now been overcome, efforts to determine specific and optimal protocols continue with numerous attempts to create new overdenture orthodoxy. Clinical researchers argue whether comparable documented long-term clinical outcomes can be achieved using more or fewer implants, combined with diverse and ingenious retentive mechanisms (Figure 13.5).

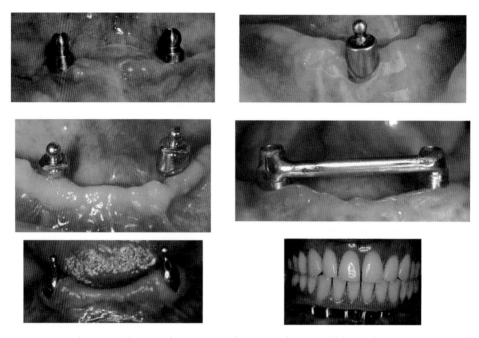

Figure 13.5 Endosseous implants in the mandible with various retentive mechanisms.

However, there is compelling evidence that the most important feature for patient-reported success is a stable prosthesis irrespective of implant numbers, retentive ingenuity, or time to loading (Zarb and Schmitt, 1996a,b; Attard and Zarb, 2004a,b; Attard et al., 2005; Attard et al., 2006; Liddelow and Henry, 2007; Walton et al., 2009).

Prolonged use of adhesives cannot be reconciled with predictable management of the consequences of aging and frailty as manifested in edentulous jaws. Implants offer a much better solution than adhesives to loose dentures, but frailty can inhibit surgery. This predicament highlights the need to consider implants in an edentulous mandible before frailty limits the feasibility of surgery (Lindquist et al., 1988; Naert et al., 1991; Jemt et al., 1996).

Microbial plaque around an implant is neither an automatic precursor of peri-implant bone loss nor a predictable cause of implant failure. This observation is a significant benefit to frail elders whose oral hygiene is neglected completely or very limited. Apparently, the soft-tissue response to microbes seems different around implants and less damaging than the response around teeth (Chvartszaid et al., 2008).

Motor control decreases as frailty increases, which can make it more difficult than usual to manage and control CDs. Moreover, this becomes a very significant threat to denture-wearers with dysphagia who struggle with the risk of aspiration pneumonia and who now run the risk of inhaling a broken denture (Arora et al., 2005; Chapman, 2006). Strategically placed oral implants can greatly reduce this risk by retaining the denture independently of weakened and uncoordinated muscles.

Oral implants usually improve the chewing efficiency very significantly, and offer the expanded possibility for selecting and consuming foods that are more nutritious and enjoyable than the soft foods typically consumed by complete denture-wearers (van Kampen et al., 2004; van der Bilt et al., 2006). Whether or not denture-wearers change their eating habits when they receive implants or an improved dentition is less certain (Moynihan et al., 2000). Nutritional intake depends on a variety of factors, such as appetite, cognitive state, general health, education, mobility, financial resources, and cultural and religious beliefs, as well as cooking skills. Consequently, chewing efficiency is only one of the many contributors to good nutrition (Sheiham et al., 2001).

Clearly, dental implants will continue to play an important role in the management of tooth loss; however, they are no panacea for the various problems and functional limitations that some denture-wearers experience (Owen, 2009), and as frailty increases, so do the difficulties of coping with dental prostheses.

CONCLUSION

The four common traditional life phases—childhood, adolescence, adulthood, and old age—are currently widely regarded as passé. They have now expanded to at least six, with the phases of odyssey (that unique time of pause and often travel-driven search for meaningful direction) and active retirement inserted on either side of the adulthood phase. The human life cycle remains a fluid one of course, and the profession of dentistry has evolved remarkably effectively to address oral health throughout all life's phases. It is therefore tempting to presume that correct and routine dental care will ensure relatively easily manageable oral health even through later stages of old age. However, socioeconomic realities complicated by disease and disability during any phase of life can quickly usurp optimistic expectations in scenarios that seek to reconcile patients' propensity for care with professional skills and accessibility.

Postponing the maintenance of oral healthcare and attendant needs for operative, endodontic, and prosthodontic interventions becomes increasingly risky even for the elderly patient who is robust. A point can be reached where professional skills, compassion, and pragmatism are exceedingly complex and often inadequate to the consequences of aging and dental neglect. Hence, the importance of addressing the oral health needs, and especially the prosthodontic needs, of elderly patients before frailty renders the feasibility of dental care a little better than palliative.

REFERENCES

Ai H, Lu HF, Liang HY, Wu J, Li RL, Liu GP, and Xi Y. 2005. Influences of bracket bonding on mutans streptococcus in plaque detected by real time fluorescence-quantitative polymerase chain reaction. *Chin Med J (Engl)* 118:2005–10.

Arora A, Arora M, and Roffe C. 2005. Mystery of the missing denture: An unusual cause of respiratory arrest in a nonagenarian. *Age Ageing* 34:519–20.

Attard NJ and Zarb GA. 2004a. Long-term treatment outcomes in edentulous patients with implant-fixed prostheses: The Toronto study. *Int J Prosthodont* 17:417–24.

Attard NJ and Zarb GA. 2004b. Long-term treatment outcomes in edentulous patients with implant overdentures: The Toronto study. *Int J Prosthodont* 17:425–33.

Attard NJ, Zarb GA, and Laporte A. 2005. Long-term treatment costs associated with implant-supported mandibular prostheses in edentulous patients. *Int J Prosthodont* 18:117–23.

Attard NJ, Laporte A, Locker D, and Zarb GA. 2006. A prospective study on immediate loading of implants with mandibular overdentures: Patient-mediated and economic outcomes. *Int J Prosthodont* 19:67–73.

Bader JD, Shugars DA, and Roberson TM. 1996. Using crowns to prevent tooth fracture. *Community Dent Oral Epidemiol* 24:47–51.

Bergman B, Hugoson A, and Olsson CO. 1982. Caries, periodontal and prosthetic findings in patients with removable partial dentures: A ten-year longitudinal study. *J Prosthet Dent* 48:506–14.

Brantley CF, Bader JD, Shugars DA, and Nesbit SP. 1995. Does the cycle of rerestoration lead to larger restorations? *J Am Dent Assoc* 126:1407–13.

Brkovic-Popovic S, Stanisic-Sinobad D, Postic SD, and Djukanovic D. 2008. Radiographic changes in alveolar bone height on overdenture abutments: A longitudinal study. *Gerodontology* 25:118–223.

Brubacher D, Monsch AU, and Stahelin HB. 2004. Weight change and cognitive performance. *Int J Obes Relat Metab Disord* 28:1163–7.

Bryant SR and Zarb GA. 2003. Crestal bone loss proximal to oral implants in older and younger adults. *J Prosthet Dent* 89:589–97.

Budtz-Jorgensen E. 1995. Prognosis of overdenture abutments in elderly patients with controlled oral hygiene. A 5 year study. *J Oral Rehabil* 22:3–8.

Budtz-Jorgensen E, Mojon P, Rentsch A, and Deslauriers N. 2000. Effects of an oral health program on the occurrence of oral candidosis in a long-term care facility. *Community Dent Oral Epidemiol* 28:141–9.

Cagidiaco MC, Goracci C, Garcia-Godoy F, and Ferrari M. 2008. Clinical studies of fiber posts: A literature review. *Int J Prosthodont* 21:328–36.

Chapman L. 2006. Another case of missing dentures. *Age Ageing* 35:205.

Chen SC, Chueh LH, Hsiao CK, Tsai MY, Ho SC, and Chiang CP. 2007. An epidemiologic study of tooth retention after nonsurgical endodontic treatment in a large population in Taiwan. *J Endod* 33:226–9.

Chvartszaid D, Koka S, and Zarb GA. 2008. Osseointegration failure. In: Zarb GA, et al. (eds.), *Osseointegration: On Continuing Synergies in Surgery, Prosthodontics and Biomaterials*. Chicago, IL: Quintessence, pp. 157–64.

Davenport JC and Heath JR. 1983. The copy denture technique. Variables relevant to general dental practice. *Br Dent J* 155:162–3.

Derkson GD and MacEntee MM. 1982. Effect of 0.4% stannous fluoride gel on the gingival health of overdenture abutments. *J Prosthet Dent* 48:23–6.

Engfors I, Ortorp A, and Jemt T. 2004. Fixed implant-supported prostheses in elderly patients: A 5-year retrospective study of 133 edentulous patients older than 79 years. *Clin Implant Dent Relat Res* 6:190–8.

Ettinger R. 1996. Geriatric considerations in prosthetic dentistry. In: Owall B, Käyser AF, Carlsson GE (eds.), *Prosthodontics: Principles and Management Strategies*. London: Mosby-Wolfe, pp. 9–19.

Ettinger RL and Jakobsen J. 1996. Periodontal considerations in an overdenture population. *Int J Prosthodont* 9:230–8.

Ettinger RL and Qian F. 2004. Postprocedural problems in an overdenture population: A longitudinal study. *J Endod* 30:310–4.

Fokkinga WA, Kreulen CM, Bronkhorst EM, and Creugers NH. 2007. Up to 17-year controlled clinical study on post-and-cores and covering crowns. *J Dent* 35:778–86.

Fokkinga WA, Kreulen CM, Bronkhorst EM, and Creugers NH. 2008. Composite resin core-crown reconstructions: An up to 17-year follow-up of a controlled clinical trial. *Int J Prosthodont* 21:109–15.

Fontijn-Tekamp FA, van der Bilt A, Abbink JH, and Bosman F. 2004. Swallowing threshold and masticatory performance in dentate adults. *Physiol Behav* 83:431–6.

Forss H and Widstrom E. 2004. Reasons for restorative therapy and the longevity of restorations in adults. *Acta Odontol Scand* 62:82–6.

Fouad AF and Burleson J. 2003. The effect of diabetes mellitus on endodontic treatment outcome: Data from an electronic patient record. *J Am Dent Assoc* 134:43–51; quiz 117–8.

Geerts GA, Stuhlinger ME, and Basson NJ. 2008. Effect of an antifungal denture liner on the saliva yeast count in patients with denture stomatitis: A pilot study. *J Oral Rehabil* 35(9):664–9.

Goodis HE, Rossall JC, and Kahn AJ. 1990. Endodontic considerations when fabricating overdentures. *Gerodontology* 9:25–8.

Goodis HE, Rossall JC, and Kahn AJ. 2001. Endodontic status in older U.S. adults. Report of a survey. *J Am Dent Assoc* 132:1525–30; quiz 95–6.

Gordan VV, Shen C, Riley J 3rd, and Mjor IA. 2006. Two-year clinical evaluation of repair versus replacement of composite restorations. *J Esthet Restor Dent* 18:144–53; discussion 54.

Grasso JE. 2004. Denture adhesives. *Dent Clin North Am* 48:721–33, vii.

Iqbal MK and Kim S. 2008. A review of factors influencing treatment planning decisions of single-tooth implants versus preserving natural teeth with non-surgical endodontic therapy. *J Endod* 34:519–29.

Jemt T, Chai J, Harnett J, Heath MR, Hutton JE, Johns RB, McKenna S, McNamara DC, van Steenberghe D, Taylor R, Watson RM, and Herrmann

I. 1996. A 5-year prospective multicenter follow-up report on overdentures supported by osseointegrated implants. *Int J Oral Maxillofac Implants* 11:291–8.

Jung RE, Kalkstein O, Sailer I, Roos M, and Hammerle CH. 2007. A comparison of composite post buildups and cast gold post-and-core buildups for the restoration of nonvital teeth after 5 to 10 years. *Int J Prosthodont* 20:63–9.

Kane JJ, Burgess JO, and Summitt JB. 1990. Fracture resistance of amalgam coronal-radicular restorations. *J Prosthet Dent* 63:607–13.

Käyser AF. 1994. Limited treatment goals—Shortened dental arches. *Periodontol 2000* 4:7–14.

Keltjens HM, Creugers TJ, van't Hof MA, and Creugers NH. 1999. A 4-year clinical study on amalgam, resin composite and resin-modified glass ionomer cement restorations in overdenture abutments. *J Dent* 27:551–5.

Kirkevang LL, Vaeth M, Horsted-Bindslev P, and Wenzel A. 2006. Longitudinal study of periapical and endodontic status in a Danish population. *Int Endod J* 39:100–7.

Kondell PA, Nordenram A, and Landt H. 1988. Titanium implants in the treatment of edentulousness: Influence of patient's age on prognosis. *Gerodontics* 4:280–4.

Liddelow GJ and Henry PJ. 2007. A prospective study of immediately loaded single implant-retained mandibular overdentures: Preliminary one-year results. *J Prosthet Dent* 97(Suppl. 6):S126–37.

Lindquist LW, Rockler B, and Carlsson GE. 1988. Bone resorption around fixtures in edentulous patients treated with mandibular fixed tissue-integrated prostheses. *J Prosthet Dent* 59:59–63.

Loesche WJ, Giordano JR, Soehren S, and Kaciroti N. 2005. The nonsurgical treatment of patients with periodontal disease: Results after 6.4 years. *Gen Dent* 53:298–306.

MacEntee MI. 1978. Practical considerations in the preparation of overdenture abutments. *Dent J* 44:462–4.

MacEntee MI. 1993. The biological sequelae of tooth replacement with removable partial dentures: A case for caution. *J Prosthet Dent* 70:132–4.

MacEntee MI, Hole R, and Stolar E. 1997. The significance of the mouth in old age. *Soc Sci Med* 45:1449–58.

Magri F, Borza A, del Vecchio S, Chytiris S, Cuzzoni G, Busconi L, Rebesco A, and Ferrari E. 2003. Nutritional assessment of demented patients: A descriptive study. *Aging Clin Exp Res* 15:148–53.

Mannocci F, Bertelli E, Sherriff M, Watson TF, and Ford TR. 2002. Three-year clinical comparison of survival of endodontically treated teeth restored with either full cast coverage or with direct composite restoration. *J Prosthet Dent* 88:297–301.

Meijer HJ, Batenburg RH, and Raghoebar GM. 2001. Influence of patient age on the success rate of dental implants supporting an overdenture in an edentulous mandible: A 3-year prospective study. *Int J Oral Maxillofac Implants* 16:522–6.

Mjor IA, Shen C, Eliasson ST, and Richter S. 2002. Placement and replacement of restorations in general dental practice in Iceland. *Oper Dent* 27:117–23.

Mojon P and MacEntee MI. 1994. Estimates of time and propensity for dental treatment among institutionalized elders. *Gerodontology* 11:99–107.

Mojon P, Thomason JM, and Walls AW. 2004. The impact of falling rates of edentulism. *Int J Prosthodont* 17:434–40.

Moncada G, Martin J, Fernandez E, Hempel MC, Mjor IA, and Gordan VV. 2009. Sealing, refurbishment and repair of Class I and Class II defective restorations: A three-year clinical trial. *J Am Dent Assoc* 140:425–32.

Moynihan PJ, Butler TJ, Thomason JM, and Jepson NJ. 2000. Nutrient intake in partially dentate patients: The effect of prosthetic rehabilitation. *J Dent* 28:557–63.

Naert I, Quirynen M, Theuniers G, and van Steenberghe D. 1991. Prosthetic aspects of osseointegrated fixtures supporting overdentures. A 4-year report. *J Prosthet Dent* 65:671–80.

Nagasiri R and Chitmongkolsuk S. 2005. Long-term survival of endodontically treated molars without crown coverage: A retrospective cohort study. *J Prosthet Dent* 93:164–70.

Nayyar A, Walton RE, and Leonard LA. 1980. An amalgam coronal-radicular dowel and core technique for endodontically treated posterior teeth. *J Prosthet Dent* 43:511–5.

Nordenram G, Ryd-Kjellen E, Ericsson K, and Winblad B. 1997. Dental management of Alzheimer patients. A predictive test of dental cooperation in individualized treatment planning. *Acta Odontol Scand* 55:148–54.

Opdam NJ, Roeters JJ, Loomans BA, and Bronkhorst EM. 2008. Seven-year clinical evaluation of painful cracked teeth restored with a direct composite restoration. *J Endod* 34:808–11.

Owen P. 2009. Standards of care—Good or evil? *Int J Prosthodont* 22:328–9.

Petersson K, Lewin B, Hakansson J, Olsson B, and Wennberg A. 1989. Endodontic status and suggested treatment in a population requiring substantial dental care. *Endod Dent Traumatol* 5:153–8.

Quesnell BT, Alves M, Hawkinson RW Jr., Johnson BR, Wenckus CS, and BeGole EA. 2005. The effect of human immunodeficiency virus on endodontic treatment outcome. *J Endod* 31:633–6.

Riesen M, Chung JP, Pazos E, and Budtz-Jorgensen E. 2002. Interventions bucco-dentaires chez les personnes âgées. *Med Hyg (Geneve)* 2414:2178–88.

Roh BD and Lee YE. 2006. Analysis of 154 cases of teeth with cracks. *Dent Traumatol* 22:118–23.

Selwitz RH, Ismail AI, and Pitts NB. 2007. Dental caries. *Lancet* 369:51–9.

Sheiham A, Steele JG, Marcenes W, Lowe C, Finch S, Bates CJ, Prentice A, and Walls AW. 2001. The relationship among dental status, nutrient intake, and nutritional status in older people. *J Dent Res* 80:408–13.

Signore A, Benedicenti S, Covani U, and Ravera G. 2007. A 4- to 6-year retrospective clinical study of cracked teeth restored with bonded indirect resin composite onlays. *Int J Prosthodont* 20:609–16.

Sorensen JA and Martinoff JT. 1984. Intracoronal reinforcement and coronal coverage: A study of endodontically treated teeth. *J Prosthet Dent* 51:780–4.

Stafford GD, Arendorf T, and Huggett R. 1986. The effect of overnight drying and water immersion on candidal colonization and properties of complete dentures. *J Dent* 14:52–6.

Stavropoulou AF and Koidis PT. 2007. A systematic review of single crowns on endodontically treated teeth. *J Dent* 35:761–7.

Taji T, Yoshida M, Hiasa K, Abe Y, Tsuga K, and Akagawa Y. 2005. Influence of mental status on removable prosthesis compliance in institutionalized elderly persons. *Int J Prosthodont* 18:146–9.

Tallgren A. 1972. The continuing reduction of residual alveolar ridges in complete denture wearers: A mixed longitudinal stydy covering 25 years. *J Prosthet Dent* 27:120–32.

Tilashalski KR, Gilbert GH, Boykin MJ, and Shelton BJ. 2006. Root canal treatment in a population-based adult sample: Differences in patient factors and types of teeth treated between endodontists and general dentists. *Community Dent Health* 23:21–5.

Torabinejad M, Anderson P, Bader J, Brown LJ, Chen LH, Goodacre CJ, Kattadiyil MT, Kutsenko D, Lozada J, Patel R, Petersen F, Puterman I, and White SN. 2007. Outcomes of root canal treatment and restoration, implant-supported single crowns, fixed partial dentures, and extraction without replacement: A systematic review. *J Prosthet Dent* 98:285–311.

Torabinejad M, Corr R, Handysides R, and Shabahang S. 2009. Outcomes of nonsurgical retreatment and endodontic surgery: A systematic review. *J Endod* 35:930–7.

van der Bilt A, van Kampen FM, and Cune MS. 2006. Masticatory function with mandibular implant-supported overdentures fitted with different attachment types. *Eur J Oral Sci* 114:191–6.

van Kampen FM, van der Bilt A, Cune MS, Fontijn-Tekamp FA, and Bosman F. 2004. Masticatory function with implant-supported overdentures. *J Dent Res* 83:708–11.

Vermeulen AH, Keltjens HM, van't Hof MA, and Kayser AF. 1996. Ten-year evaluation of removable partial dentures: Survival rates based on retreatment, not wearing and replacement. *J Prosthet Dent* 76:267–72.

Vysniauskaite S and Vehkalahti MM. 2006. First-time dental care and the most recent dental treatment in relation to utilisation of dental services among dentate elderly patients in Lithuania. *Gerodontology* 23:149–56.

Walton JN and MacEntee MI. 2005. Choosing or refusing oral implants: A prospective study of edentulous volunteers for a clinical trial. *Int J Prosthodont* 18:483–8.

Walton JN, Glick N, and MacEntee MI. 2009. A randomized clinical trial comparing patient satisfaction and prosthetic outcomes with mandibular overdentures retained by one or two implants. *Int J Prosthodont* 22:331–9.

Wismeijer D, Van Waas MA, Vermeeren JI, Mulder J, and Kalk W. 1997. Patient satisfaction with implant-supported mandibular overdentures. A comparison of three treatment strategies with ITI-dental implants. *Int J Oral Maxillofac Surg* 26:263–7.

Witter DJ, van Palenstein Helderman WH, Creugers NH, and Käyser AF. 1999. The shortened dental arch concept and its implications for oral health care. *Community Dent Oral Epidemiol* 27:249–58.

Wyatt CC and MacEntee MI. 2004. Caries management for institutionalized elders using fluoride and chlorhexidine mouthrinses. *Community Dent Oral Epidemiol* 32:322–8.

Zarb GA and Schmitt A. 1990a. The longitudinal clinical effectiveness of osseo-integrated dental implants: The Toronto study. Part II: The prosthetic results. *J Prosthet Dent* 64:53–61.

Zarb GA and Schmitt A. 1990b. The longitudinal clinical effectiveness of osseo-integrated dental implants: The Toronto study. Part III: Problems and complications encountered. *J Prosthet Dent* 64:185–94.

Zarb GA and Schmitt A. 1996a. The edentulous predicament. I: A prospective study of the effectiveness of implant-supported fixed prostheses. *J Am Dent Assoc* 127:59–65.

Zarb GA and Schmitt A. 1996b. The edentulous predicament. II: The longitudinal effectiveness of implant-supported overdentures. *J Am Dent Assoc* 127:66–72.

Zarb GA, Bergman B, Clayton JA, and MacKay HF. 1978. *Prosthodontic Treatment for Partially Edentulous Patients*. St. Louis, MO: Mosby.

Zarb GA, Carlsson GE, Mohl N, and Sessle B. 1994. *Temporomandibular Joint and Masticatory Muscle Disorders*, 2nd ed. Copenhagen: Munksgaard.

Zitzmann NU, Staehelin K, Walls AW, Menghini G, Weiger R, and Zemp Stutz E. 2008. Changes in oral health over a 10-yr period in Switzerland. *Eur J Oral Sci* 116:52–9.

Ethnocultural diversity

Stella Kwan, Rodrigo Mariño, H. Asuman Kiyak, Victor Minichiello, and Michael I. MacEntee

INTRODUCTION

This chapter, in three parts, explores the influence of culture on health beliefs, behaviors, and outcomes in frail elders who are part of an immigrant population. The first part presents the concept of culture and acculturation. It explores the models used to explain the health and social outcomes of immigrant groups, and it describes the demographics of immigrant groups with an emphasis on several multicultural countries. The second part examines the health, particularly oral health, of ethnocultural minority groups and explains how oral health can relate to cultural background. These include oral health status, beliefs, attitudes, and knowledge, as well as oral health-related practices, use of general healthcare services, and barriers to care. The last section identifies the gaps in our current knowledge about the systemic and oral health of older immigrants and discusses future challenges to health promotion and clinical practice.

POPULATION CHANGE AND DIVERSITY

Most Western countries are culturally diverse, composed of numerous ethnocultural groups (e.g., indigenous people, recent immigrants, established immigrants and their descendents) coexisting within a larger, predominant culture, and creating multicultural and multiracial societies. In any given year, hundreds of thousands of people migrate across national borders to a new environment. As a result, the size and diversity of ethnic

Oral Healthcare and the Frail Elder: A Clinical Perspective.
Edited by Michael I. MacEntee © 2011 Blackwell Publishing Ltd.

mix in various countries are increasing. Whether this movement is voluntary or involuntary, temporary or permanent, these people are "cultural strangers" in an unfamiliar environment.

Changes in the composition of the population create a new demand for appropriate content in multicultural policies affecting all aspects of society—political, social, economic, and academic (United Nations, 2004). Sociologists and anthropologists identify the quality and nature of social interactions, while psychologists study the impact of culture on perceptions and attitudes. Gerontologists and demographers have noted the impact immigration has had on the aging of populations. In some countries, such as Australia and Canada, immigration by older adults is one of the factors contributing to the graying of that society (Minichiello and Coulson, 2005). In contrast, immigration has protected the United States from becoming an "aging" country because of the influx of younger families, and higher birthrates among immigrants.

In response to both the opportunities and challenges of multicultural societies, government officials seek to establish policies and allocate resources, while educators and service providers attempt to deal with multilingual and multicultural needs. For health professionals and healthcare providers, this trend involves working with different cultures and across cultural borders to create more sensitive and appropriate healthcare. However, more than that, they need strategies to facilitate rapport with people who are culturally different from themselves. This has set an agenda of educating the workforce to be more responsive to ethnocultural differences.

Health needs of immigrants are exacerbated by a number of factors. Immigrant populations not only bring with them hopes and aspirations to their new country, but also a set of traditions, values, and beliefs from their native culture. Settlement experiences vary for each immigrant, depending on factors such as language and communication skills, migration circumstances, the support of family and friends, financial resources, and the geographical location of immigrant communities. For some immigrants, the settlement period prior to living independently can be relatively short, while for others, it can last several years or forever. Immigrants with cultural characteristics markedly different from the dominant society will experience greater difficulties relative to immigrant groups whose cultural values are closer to the dominant society. These and other barriers—real or perceived—such as language and communication; lack of familiarity with the nature and location of health services; fear of, and hostility toward, the mainstream society; premigration cultural beliefs; and knowledge of the dominant culture's customs, all have a potential impact on every aspect of life to create a unique set of health risks for immigrant groups. Moreover, in many situations, the risks cannot be reduced by established procedures in the host country, so it is not difficult to accept and expect that different approaches may be required for immigrants from different cultures.

The impact of increasing diversity on social and health services, and on the health of immigrants, is all but unknown, although certainly not inconsequential. Elderly immigrants pose special challenges for health workers because they have difficulty adapting to their new surroundings and often maintain unrealistic psychosocial expectations (Mariño et al., 2001; Soldov and Poon, 2001; Waxler-Morrison et al., 2005). There is little doubt, for example, that elderly members of ethnic minorities are prone to social isolation, which is linked to an increased risk of morbidity and mortality (Cacioppo and Hawkley, 2003). Furthermore, when considering the mediating factors and experiences of older immigrants, consideration should be given to the diverse reasons why older people emigrate. Mostly they move to join their children under a family reunion or family reunification visa, or to seek asylum as refugees (United Nations, 2004). However, no matter how or when they arrive, older immigrants are likely to have different experiences and needs than the indigenous residents of the host country.

WHAT IS CULTURE?

The past quarter century has witnessed worldwide changes that highlight the relevance of culture in healthcare. Terms such as "culture," "race," "language spoken," or "country of origin" have been used interchangeably and often without clarity. Race, for example, is a biological concept based on genetic features, while "culture" embraces the values, beliefs, ceremonies, and ways of life characteristic of a given group (Giddens, 2006). However, to assume that all black people, whether from Africa, the Caribbean, or the United States, have the same health values and beliefs is stereotyping that can negatively influence health outcomes. Perhaps more importantly, it is potentially offensive and politically inappropriate to operate on this assumption.

Ethnicity in this chapter is defined as "the shared sense of belonging, based on characteristics such as: common religion, language, ancestry, national or geographic origin and/or other cultural attribute" (Parrillo, 1994), and an ethnic group has one or all of these elements in common. For example, it is not unusual for second or subsequent generations to maintain the identity with their ethnic group. The terms "ethnic populations" or "ethnic groups" are often misused in reference to minority populations as if other groups do not have an ethnicity. It is also frequently confused with nationality or with immigrant status (Kedar et al., 1996). For example, there are 165 different ethnic groups within the single racial group of Chinese, so the term "Chinese" certainly does not designate homogeneity. This misuse of words and assumptions of homogeneity can lead to problems when using "race" or country of birth as variables for ethnicity, or even identifying all Chinese as one ethnic group, or the more common error of categorizing all Asians as one group. The U.S. census, for instance, identifies Asians as one ethnic group that includes people of Chinese, Vietnamese, Korean, Japanese, and other national backgrounds.

Culture is an essential element of the concept of ethnicity and is used often to refer to combinations of differences in country of origin, language, customs, and even socioeconomic class (Triandis and Brislin, 1984). It has been defined as the shared knowledge, behaviors, beliefs, customs, traditions, meanings, value orientations, and norms held by a group of people, who use it to see the world in a certain way, and it is transmitted to other members of the group through time as the basis for communication and mutual understanding (Leininger, 1993; Purnell and Paulanka, 1998).

Culture is a dynamic concept that constantly incorporates new values, beliefs, and attitudes relevant only in given situations. Therefore, it is neither homogeneous nor static, nor do all members of an ethnic group necessarily strive for the same cultural elements (Erez and Early, 1993). When the cultural environment changes, so too can people change or *acculturate* as they adapt to varying degrees from one culture to another (Redfield et al., 1936).

Behavioral or sociocultural acculturation relates to learning and adopting the observable aspects of the dominant culture, including social skills and the ability to "fit in" or negotiate aspects of the new sociocultural reality (Searle and Ward, 1990). It is affected by the level and length of contact with the host culture, cultural similarities, and dissimilarities, along with various personal characteristics. Psychological acculturation, in contrast, reflects the degree of personal satisfaction or agreement with defined norms of the host culture. It is a much more complicated phenomenon than behavioral acculturation, although it is less dependent on the length or level of exposure to the host culture.

Acculturation can be considered from two conceptual perspectives: a "bipolar unidimensional" model and a "two-dimensional" model, which incorporates and extends the bipolar model (Laroche et al., 1998). In the bipolar model, the acculturation process varies along a single continuum with the original culture at one end and the receiving or host society at the other on the assumption that strengthening one pole requires weakening the other (Laroche et al., 1998; Vega et al., 1998). This means that an individual becomes so integrated into the host society that newcomers and hosts are indistinguishable or assimilated. In contrast, the two-dimensional model presents the original and receiving cultures independently (Berry, 1998), whereby increased involvement in the host society does not necessarily entail rejection of the original culture. Within this model, it is possible to integrate, assimilate, separate, or marginalize in one way or another (Berry, 1998). In real life, however, the acceptance and rejection of the original and host cultures probably fluctuate dynamically between one another in a complex interplay of behaviors and beliefs (Figure 14.1). For example, an elderly immigrant might have assimilated into the host society but remain separated from the larger culture by language and food preferences.

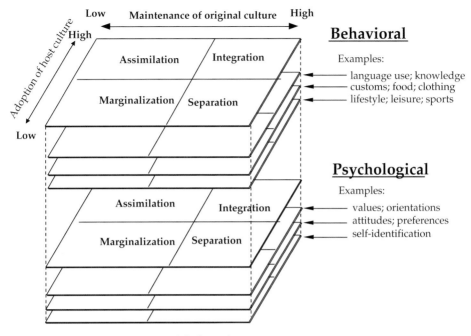

Figure 14.1 A model of acculturation.

DEMOGRAPHY OF IMMIGRANT GROUPS

Immigrants form a substantial proportion of the population in most countries within the Organization for Economic Cooperation and Development (OECD) and, particularly, in Australia, Canada, and New Zealand, where immigration policies support the workforce (Dummont and Lemaître, 2005). Nearly 20% of the residents, young and old, in Australia, Canada, New Zealand, Luxembourg, and Switzerland today were born elsewhere. Indeed, by 2026, it is projected that perhaps one in three of all elders in Australia will have been born overseas. Similarly, in the United States by 2050, more than one-third of the older population will identify themselves as immigrants or ethnic minorities (Latinos: 17%, African-Americans: 12%, Asians: 8%) born in the United States (Passel and Cohn, 2008).

Numbers will fluctuate of course reflecting the various waves of immigration from different countries (Victorian Ethnic Affairs Commission, 1995). In the United Kingdom, the 2001 census found that about 8% of the population identified with an ethnic minority—an increase of nearly 50% since the 1991 census (ONS, 2003; Dorling and Thomas, 2004; Simpson et al., 2006). Immigrants tend to concentrate in regions as a protective strategy of "group density," which seems to benefit health, probably by enhancing access to culturally competent healthcare and social services (Pickett and

Wilkinson, 2008). The family reunification component of Canada's immigration policy since 1994 accounts for about one-in-four immigrants, and has brought large numbers of Chinese and South Asian elders to the major cities (Ip, 2008).

GENERAL HEALTH OF ETHNOCULTURAL MINORITY GROUPS

Migrant populations in many countries are granted equal access to the healthcare system, along with the right to cultural recognition and freedom from discrimination. However, despite these supportive policies, healthcare systems do not always meet the dynamic needs of a culturally and linguistically diverse society, nor do they produce equivalent health outcomes for all ethnocultural groups (Migrant-friendly Hospitals, 2005).

The health status of immigrants is affected by ethnicity, gender, age, socioeconomic status, and migration (Julian, 2004). Recent immigrants to Australia, for example, are less healthy than other Australians if they are elderly and live alone in rented accommodation, with low income, limited social support, and inadequate English (Julian, 2004). Moreover, health disparity is compounded further by the genetic disposition of some groups to caries (Shuler, 2001). Although there is evidence that genetic disposition to disease is associated with ethnicity (Smith et al., 2000; Sproston and Mindell, 2006), it is not yet clear that it extends to the more common oral diseases.

Complementary and alternative medicines are used more often by some immigrant groups, particularly by Chinese elders, who typically combine it with Western medicine (Lai and Chappell, 2007).

Health screening of potential immigrants creates the "healthy immigrant effect" through selection of relatively healthy people—even among those who qualify under the family reunification policy operating in many countries (McDonald and Kennedy, 2004; United Nations, 2004; AIHW, 2006). Nonetheless, immigrants as they age tend more toward conditions such as diabetes, ischemic heart disease, and cerebrovascular disease, compared with the indigenous population (AIHW, 2006).

ACCULTURATION AND ORAL HEALTH

Typically, oral health is worse in older minority groups than among majority groups who live in Western societies (MacEntee et al., 1993; Mariño et al., 2001; Persson et al., 2004; Swoboda et al., 2006; Lai and Hui, 2007). Although immigrant elders have relatively fewer caries and tooth loss— probably because of traditional diets low in sugar and limited access to dentists (Newton et al., 1999)—their experiences of toothaches and other mouth problems are relatively numerous (Newton et al., 2003).

The level of acculturation is a good predictor of health-related outcomes (Liou and Contento, 2001; Mariño et al., 2001). Some cultural behavior is beneficial while others are detrimental to health and well-being (Marmot and Syme, 1976). Consequently, efforts to promote health in immigrant populations should combine traditional practices with Western concepts of care. Diets, for example, are likely to be more palatable and healthy if based on traditional foods and recipes. Likewise, health-related information is best presented in written and spoken formats that are familiar to the group and in cultural contexts that extend beyond simple translation of Western concepts and words (Guillemin et al., 1993; Mallard et al., 1997).

There is evidence that the majority of elders (not necessarily immigrants) in the United States have serious difficulties understanding and using written health materials in a prose format, finding and processing information based on numbers, or interpreting forms, lists, charts, and graphs (Rudd and Horowitz, 2005). Indeed, remarkably little attention has been paid to the oral health literacy of immigrants whether young or old, but it seems clear now that the process of acculturation should be considered carefully when framing appropriate health policies, developing health promotion and preventive and treatment programs, and planning health services for the elders in a multicultural society.

ORAL HEALTH-RELATED BELIEFS, KNOWLEDGE, AND ATTITUDES

Culturally specific beliefs in most instances are limited to people who live, congregate, and interact where a specific culture is concentrated. There are many cultural beliefs associated with susceptibility to and seriousness of dental disease. Body humor, *yin* and *yang*, and *qi*, for example, play a role in oral health as in general health for people from China. Losing teeth in old age is widely expected and accepted in Chinese culture, even to the point where it is considered bad luck *not* to lose teeth with advancing age (Kwan and Holmes, 1999). Older immigrants also worry about burdening their families; consequently, they tend to isolate themselves, use home remedies, and suffer silently. They often delay dental visits and seek professional help only when home remedies fail (Lucas, 1987; Lee et al., 1993; Schwarz and Lo, 1995; Chen, 2001). Traditional Chinese beliefs and values emphasize self-control, fate, and fatalism. Some believe that gingival bleeding results from disequilibrium between the yin and yang, which can be balanced by dietary and herbal remedies, such as cooling teas, to reduce the "hot air" from the stomach that inflames the gingiva. There are traditional concerns also about prolonged bleeding from tooth extractions and other bloodletting treatments that drain away vital energy (*qi*) and weaken the body (Kwan and Holmes, 1999). These concerns do not necessarily negate the value placed by immigrants on Western medicine and dentistry, but they can delay effective treatments from Western-educated physicians and dentists (Lam, 2001).

ORAL HEALTH-RELATED PRACTICES

The majority of immigrants adopt some oral hygiene habits from the host country, including toothbrushing with fluoridated toothpaste. However, some prefer traditional methods of dental hygiene with chewing sticks, tree bark, burnt breadcrumbs, and tea leaves (Summers et al., 1996; Mariño et al., 2002a, b). They also use traditional remedies for oral problems, including traditional healers to ward off evil spirits, prescribed herbal medicines and home remedies (Figure 14.2), or extract teeth or grind them with herbal medicines (Kwan and Holmes, 1999; Kwan and Bedi, 2000; Amruthesh, 2008).

Elders from South Asia who chew betel quid or "pan" have a higher risk of oral cancer, but they believe that it improves digestion, cures dysentery, expels worms, relieves pain, and reduces fever; and it relieves toothache and bad breath (Summers et al., 1994; Warnakulasuriya and Johnson, 1996). Therefore, a health promotion strategy mounted against this practice in a community of immigrants from South Asia should address the underlying beliefs before condemning it strongly.

USE OF DENTAL SERVICES

Immigrants from Asia are unlikely ever to visit a dentist in the host country, or to do so only when in pain (Erens et al., 2001; Newbold and Patel, 2006), and when compared with the "white" majority in the United Kingdom, at least they are less satisfied with available services (Erens et al., 2001; Sproston et al., 2001; Shah and Cook, 2008). This restricted use of Western dentistry has been observed also among elderly Greek and Italian immi-

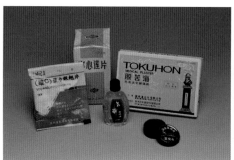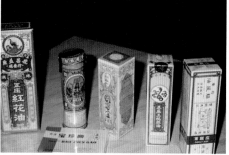

Figure 14.2 Traditional Chinese remedies for dental and gingival disorders.

grants in Melbourne despite the fact that they are entitled in Australia to public dental services at a reduced fee (Mariño et al., 2005). However, in Canada, elderly immigrants made more visits to a dentist than Canadian-born elders, which confirms again the weakness of assumptions about homogeneity in the beliefs and practices of immigrants (Newbold and Patel, 2006).

BARRIERS TO ORAL HEALTHCARE

The various meanings surrounding oral health are created within the sociocultural environments in which immigrants live, both before and after immigration. Access to dentistry is affected by financial, structural, informational, and attitudinal barriers. Recent immigrants, especially if they are frail, face daunting language barriers complicated by ignorance of the healthcare system and a general mistrust of "officials" such as dentists and physicians (Kwan and Williams, 1998; Pearson et al., 1999; Newton et al., 2001; Croucher and Sohanpal, 2006). Fear and anxiety from previous encounters with dentists, and from rumors of the high financial cost of dentistry, are additional disincentives to seek dental care, and of course, there is a constant concern among elderly parents about burdening their children. The language barrier and mistrust can lead to feelings of uncertainty about the care received and can restrict a patient's ability to challenge treatment plans (Kwan and Holmes, 1999).

There are, of course, elders in minority groups who value oral health and who seek preventive care, and they are likely to continue using dental services regularly, especially if they visited a dentist in the host country and are eligible for government-sponsored dental benefits (Kiyak, 1986, 1987; Holm-Pedersen et al., 2005). Therefore, part of the acculturation process should include opportunities if available to become familiar with the dental services in the host country, and especially in countries where dental care is offered as part of a government-sponsored health service. Yet, barriers to dental services can be daunting to all immigrants, and probably more so for frail elders. Elderly immigrants from Greece who had settled in Melbourne, for example, complained about the length of time it takes to get on a dentist's waiting list, the waiting time for treatment, and the cost of services (Table 14.1).

Immigrants from Italy or China, in contrast, were more disturbed by the cost of dentistry and by communication barriers, while others saw no barriers to accessing dental care. Some immigrants prefer to be treated by healthcare providers with the same background of culture and language. Others hold false beliefs or myths supporting strong negative attitudes toward dentistry and, in particular, toward public oral health services, but these are often reinforced and supported by peers from their cultural background (Williams et al., 1995; Kwan and Williams, 1998; Mariño et al., 2002a, b).

Clinical scenario 1

A group of elders from China are chatting at their luncheon club meeting. One woman complains about toothache and loose teeth that disturbs her ability to eat comfortably. She explains that she will not go to the dentist because she is worried that one of her teeth might be a "blood tooth," which could weaken her vital energy or "qi" or, worse, cause her to bleed to death if it was extracted.

Another woman interrupts this complaint and concern by exclaiming: "What do you expect when you get old? Your teeth will fall out. You can't keep your teeth because, if you do, they will eat away your children's fortune, bringing bad luck to the family." However, she explains further that she has difficulty eating her favorite dish—chicken feet—because her new dentures are hurting her gums. She thinks her dentist is "no good" because her dentures are so uncomfortable. Another friend asks: "Do you not realize that you can go back for adjustments to the dentures free of charge?" to whom she replies that she finds it embarrassing to go back to see her dentist and that she does not wish to bother the dentist or to become an "unpopular patient."

Now, everybody has something to say about their dentists and past dental experiences. Some believe that it is a good idea to consult with several dentists because in Hong Kong going "doctor/dentist shopping (hopping)" is common. It is apparent from the conversation that many of the lunchers have little faith in "Western" dentists who do not respect their culture and needs.

This sentiment was echoed by a man who stopped visiting dentists after his tooth was extracted many years ago. He said that "one minute [the dentist] was asking if I was OK, next minute he took my tooth out." He continued to explain that he was very distrustful of local dentists because he does not speak English. When the dentist spoke before the tooth was extracted all he understood was "gobbledegook and OK," which he thought was the dentist asking if he was alright, but when he nodded and said "OK!", the dentist extracted the tooth! Since then, he takes herbal tea, tonic soup, Tiger Balm, and White Flower® Embrocation (Pak Fah Yeow) when he has dental problems.

His friends at the luncheon all agreed that White Flower Embrocation cures everything from toothache, infection, flu and cold, tummy upset, indigestion, motion sickness, headache, muscle pain, and insect bites! They felt good also about this opportunity to exchange experiences and reinforce their cultural roots!

Table 14.1 Percentage distribution and rank of primary barriers to dental healthcare indentified by three ethnic groups of older immigrants in Melbourne, Australia.

Barrier	Ethnocultural group % (rank)		
	Greek	Italian	Chinese
Cost of dental services	2 (7)	45 (1)	52 (1)
Availability of dentists	3 (6)	17 (3)	28 (4)
Time waiting for appointments	87 (1)	38 (2)	30 (3)
Rude behavior from dentists	4 (4)	7 (8)	15 (8)
Transportation	6 (3)	10 (7)	22 (5)
Waiting time in dental office	85 (2)	19 (4)	20 (6)
Fear	4 (4)	11 (6)	17 (7)
Communication problems	3 (5)	21 (3)	38 (2)

Source: Mariño et al. (2005).

Table 14.2   Ranking of concerns of dentists in the United Kingdom treating patients from different cultural backgrounds.

Concerns	Ranking
Language barriers/communicating and interacting with patient	1
Cultural understanding	2
Casual attendance	3
Complex medical histories	4
Failed appointments	5
Extensive treatment needs	6
Obtaining consent	7

Source: Williams et al. (1995).

Culture and health interact. However, we do not know in what ways and along what domains the interactions occur (Palinkas and Pickwell, 1995). Dental professionals who work in multicultural countries are aware of the role that culture plays in the interactions they have with their patients.

Dentists and dental hygienists in the United States and in the United Kingdom (Williams et al., 1995), for instance, know that they need to understand, tolerate, and respect the cultural background of their patients (Table 14.2).

The large ethnic diversity of students in dental and dental hygiene programs in Western countries is remarkable, but it does not necessarily reflect cultural diversity because it is likely that there are uniform values and beliefs behind the ethnic facade of the students (Mariño et al., 2004). Consequently, there are likely to be major differences in values between the professionals and their immigrant patients. The health needs of a diverse society require not only a workforce that reflects the ethnic mix of society but also the cultural complexities and intermingling that exists within all industrial societies today (Mariño et al., 2004).

DIVERSITY AMONG FRAIL ELDERS

Maintaining the health of frail elders who are not part of the dominant culture is a major challenge, yet we know little about disparities in oral healthcare across different racial/ethnic groups with physical and cognitive disorders. In many cases, these elders carry a greater burden than their healthier, younger peers because their health beliefs may prevent them from obtaining the needed healthcare and indirectly threaten their survival, as in the following clinical scenario.

A clinical dilemma

Mrs. Frangelico is 85 years old and migrated to Australia from Italy about 50 years ago. She had very little access to dentists or information about mouthcare as a child. She does not have a regular dentist. However, she has vivid memories of painful tooth extractions. Recently, she had a very painful "swollen gum" and was prepared to put up with the pain. She understands English but not fluently because she lives in an Italian neighborhood of Melbourne where most people speak Italian. She has a wide circle of friends and family but she is growing frail. She postponed going to a dentist because of her fear that the dentist would extract the tooth that is surrounded by the "swollen gum." However, she agreed to go when a neighbor noticed her distress and offered to drive her to the hospital for emergency treatment when the pain became intolerable and she was having difficulty breathing.

Questions:

How does Mrs. Frangelico's cultural background affect her attitudes toward dentists and her current pain?

What might help Mrs. Frangelico get treatment more readily for her "swollen gum?"

How can her anxiety about dentists be reduced?

How does a dental practitioner help migrants who have limited English language skills to feel at ease to communicate their needs and fears about their oral healthcare?

We rely heavily on language and on our social environment, so it is very distressing when our language and interpretation of our environments are distorted. It is not unusual for immigrants with dementia to lose their ability to speak the language of the host country and to retain only their native tongue (Runci et al., 2005). Nor is it unusual for frail elders to reject healthcare unless it is provided by someone from their own cultural background. Consequently, it helps to have representatives from the minority groups, possibly through organizations advocating consumers' interest, to seek and articulate each group's healthcare needs.

Implications for oral health promotion and service provision

Lifestyles have been modified successfully even among very old and frail people, provided that their chronic diseases and disabilities are not overwhelming (Chernoff, 2001). The most common reason why older people do not attempt to improve or adopt beneficial health-related activities is that they have not been advised to do so by their physician (Resnick, 2000). Nonetheless, failure to change one's health-related behaviors could be associated also with stress, poor hearing and vision, fatigue, and other noncognitive factors (Hussain et al., 2005). Ethnic minority groups need clear, effective, and culturally appropriate information, well beyond a direct translation of brochures and manuals (Kwan et al., 1996). Typically, the literal translation of written information is linguistically inaccurate, factually incomprehensible, culturally insensitive, and occasionally offensive. For example, the concept of a medical history is not used in some cultures, so references to a "medical history" in an informational booklet for some groups will be incomprehensible to some groups. Given that advice, which is acceptable to one cultural group may not be appropriate to another, layout and presentation are important, so it is best to avoid "universal" advices or generalizations as much as possible.

Effective communication through print or digital media should be attractively designed for good visual impact, written in simple language, and presented with sensitivity to the cultural expectations and customs of the target group. This normally requires extensive consultation with several representatives of the group. Focus groups and direct face-to-face interviews are useful for gathering information before informational brochures or digital presentations are produced. Several strategies are available for making culturally appropriate materials (Table 14.3).

Clinical resolution

Dentists in a mobile clinic designed to serve ethnically, cognitively, and physically diverse elders agreed that it was important to include staff and volunteers representing most of the communities they served. They recruited students from a local dental school and from local dental hygiene and dental assisting programs—all with different ethnic and language backgrounds. They hired a clinical coordinator from a Vietnamese community and who could speak Vietnamese, English, and several dialects of Chinese.

The dentists visited frail elders in local nursing homes and were able to communicate freely in the native language of most of the residents, and had informed help to understand various cultural and health beliefs. Moreover, the residents valued the opportunity to share their background and to speak with health providers in their native language. Consequently, the experience was so pleasant for even the frailest resident that most of the elders looked forward to regular visits by the mobile clinic and never missed their recall appointments.

Table 14.3 Developing and presenting transcultural health promotional materials.

- Conduct a comprehensive background search of information already available
- Profile the normative and perceived needs of the targeted ethnic group
- Seek advice from the ethnic community during the production process
- Present content that is appropriately formatted and contextually complete
- Use visually attractive and culturally sensitive material
- Use simple and preferably bilingual language
- Select for translation information that is cross-culturally appropriate with high conceptual functional and linguistic equivalence
- Provide adequate material, positive suggestions, and additional references and support
- Avoid errors in the text and layout

Source: Kwan et al. (1996).

FUTURE CHALLENGES

Some of the barriers to oral healthcare identified here are relevant also to the indigenous populations of the host countries. However, the impact may be dramatically different among ethnic minorities and immigrant populations. Ethnic groups are not culturally homogeneous, and each group feels distinctive. This heterogeneity, both between and within groups, poses a challenge to generalizing the issues and difficulties facing elders of culturally and linguistically distinct communities.

The dental team should recognize the implications of cultural differences. Good communication skills and empathy help to foster a good dentist–patient relationship, regardless of the patient's ethnic or cultural background, but these professional characteristics are particularly important when helping older patients who remain attached to their original values and health practices.

REFERENCES

Amruthesh S. 2008. Dentistry and Ayurveda—IV: Classification and management of common oral diseases. *Indian J Dent Res* 19:52–61.

Australian Institute of Health and Welfare (AIHW). 2006. *Australia's Health 2006*. AIHW cat. no. AUS 73. Canberra: AIHW.

Berry JW, Kim U, Minde T, and Mok D. 1987. Comparative studies of acculturative stress. *Int Migr Rev* 21:491–11.

Cacioppo JT and Hawkley LC. 2003. Social isolation and health, with an emphasis on underlying mechanisms. *Perspect Biol Med* 46 (3 Suppl):S39–52.

Chen Y. 2001. Chinese values, health and nursing. *J Adv Nurs* 36:270–3.

Chernoff R. 2001. Nutrition and health promotion in older adults. *J Gerontol* 56:47–53.

Croucher R and Sohanpal R. 2006. Improving access to dental care in East London's ethnic minority groups: Community-based, qualitative study. *Community Dent Health* 23:95–100.

Dorling D and Thomas B. 2004. *People and Places. A 2001 Census Atlas of the UK*. Bristol: The Policy Press.

Dummont JC and Lemaître G. 2005. *Counting Immigrants and Expatriates in OECD Countries: A New Perspective*. OECD Social, Employment and Migration Working Paper No. 25. Available at www.oecd.org/dataoecd/34/59/35043046.pdf (accessed January 23, 2009).

Erens B, Primatesta P, and Prior G (eds.). 2001. *Health Survey for England: The Health of Minority Groups*. Department of Health. London: The Stationery Office.

Erez M and Early PC. 1993. *Culture, Self-Identity and Work*. New York: Oxford University Press.

Giddens A. 2006. *Sociology*, 5th edn. Cambridge, UK: Polity.

Guillemin F, Bombardier C, and Beaton D. 1993. Cross-cultural adaptation of health-related quality of life measures: Literature review and proposed guidelines. *J Clin Epidemiol* 46:1417–32.

Holm-Pedersen P, Vigild M, Nitschke I, and Berkey DB. 2005. Dental care for aging populations in Denmark, Sweden, Norway, United Kingdom, and Germany. *J Dent Educ* 69:987–97.

Hussain R, Mariño R, and Coulson I. 2005. The role of health promotion in healthy ageing. In: Minichiello V and Coulson I (eds.), *Contemporary Issues in Gerontology: Promoting Positive Ageing.* Sydney: Allen & Unwin, pp. 34–52.

Ip F. 2008. Immigrant Population of British Columbia. 2006 Census Fast Facts. Victoria: Service BC, Ministry of Labour and Citizens' Services. http://www.bcstats.gov.bc.ca/pubs/immig/imm073sf.pdf (accessed August 9, 2010).

Julian R. 2004. Migrant and refugee health. In: Grbich C (ed.), *Health in Australia: Sociological Concepts and Issues.* NSW: Pearson Education Australia, pp. 101–27.

Kedar N, Dwivedi KD, and Varma VP. 1996. *Meeting the Needs of Ethnic Minority Children. A Handbook for Professionals.* London: Jessica Kingsley.

Kiyak HA. 1986. Explaining patterns of dental service utilization among the elderly. *J Dent Educ* 50:679–87.

Kiyak HA. 1987. An explanatory model of older persons' use of dental services. Implications for health policy. *Med Care* 25:936–52.

Kwan SYL and Bedi R. 2000. Transcultural oral healthcare and the Chinese— An invisible community. *Dent Update* 27:296–9.

Kwan SYL and Holmes MAM. 1999. An exploration of oral health beliefs and attitudes of Chinese in West Yorkshire: A qualitative investigation. *Health Educ Res* 14:453–60.

Kwan SYL and Williams SA. 1998. Attitudes of Chinese people towards obtaining dental care in the UK. *Br Dent J* 185:188–91.

Kwan SYL, Williams SA, and Duggal M. 1996. An assessment of the appropriateness of dental health education materials for ethnic minorities. *Int Dent J* 46(Suppl. 1):277–85.

Lai DW and Hui NT. 2007. Use of dental care by elderly Chinese immigrants in Canada. *J Public Health Dent* 67:55–9.

Lai DWL and Chappell NL. 2007. Use of traditional Chinese medicine by older Chinese immigrants in Canada. *Fam Pract* 24:56–64.

Lam TP. 2001. Strengths and weaknesses of traditional Chinese medicine and Western medicine in the eyes of some Hong Kong Chinese. *J Epidemiol Community Health* 55:762–5.

Laroche M, Kim C, Hui MK, and Tomiuk MA. 1998. Test of a nonlinear relationship between linguistic acculturation and ethnic identification. *J Cross Cult Psychol* 29:418–34.

Lee KL, Schwarz E, and Mak KYK. 1993. Improving oral health through understanding the meaning of health and disease in Chinese culture. *Int Dent J* 43:2–8.

Leininger M. 1993. Towards conceptualization of transcultural healthcare systems: Concepts and a model. *J Transcult Nurs* 4:32–40.

Liou D and Contento IR. 2001. Usefulness of psychosocial theory variables in fat-related dietary behavior in Chinese Americans: Association with degree of acculturation. *J Nutr Educ* 33:322–31.

Lucas R. 1987. *Secrets of the Chinese Herbalist*. New York: Parker.

MacEntee MI, Stolar E, and Glick N. 1993. The influence of age and gender on oral health and related behaviour in an independent elderly population. *Community Dent Oral Epidemiol* 21:234–9.

Mallard AGC, Lance CE, and Michalos AC. 1997. Culture as a moderator of overall life satisfaction—Life facet satisfaction relationships. *Soc Indic Res* 40:259–84.

Mariño R, Stuart GW, Wright FAC, Minas H, and Klimidis S. 2001. Acculturation and dental health among Vietnamese living in Melbourne, Australia. *Community Dent Oral Epidemiol* 29:107–19.

Mariño R, Wright FAC, Minichiello V, and Schofield M. 2002a. Oral health beliefs and practices among Greek and Italian older Australian: A focus group approach. *Australas J Ageing* 21:193–8.

Mariño R, Wright FAC, Minichiello V, and Schofield M. 2002b. Oral health through the life experiences of older Greek and Italian adults. *Aust J Primary Health* 8:20–9.

Mariño R, Stuart G, Morgan M, Winning T, and Thompson M. 2004. Cultural consistency in Australian dental students from different ethnic backgrounds. *J Dent Educ* 11:1178–84.

Mariño R, Wright FAC, Schofield M, Minichiello V, and Calache H. 2005. Factors associated with self-reported use of dental health services among older Greek and Italian migrants. *Spec Care Dentist* 25:12–9.

Marmot MG and Syme L. 1976. Acculturation and coronary heart disease in Japanese-Americans. *Am J Epidemiol* 104:225–47.

McDonald JT and Kennedy S. 2004. Insights into the 'healthy immigrant effect': Health status and health service use of immigrants to Canada. *Soc Sci Med* 59:1613–27.

Migrant-friendly Hospitals. 2005. *Project Summary*. University of Vienna, Vienna, Austria. Vienna: Ludwig Boltzmann Institute, WHO Collaborating Centre for Health Promotion in Hospitals and Healthcare, Institute of Sociology. Available at www.mfh-eu.net/public/files/mfh-summary.pdf (accessed August 9, 2010).

Minichiello V and Coulson I. 2005. The context of promoting positive ageing. In: Minichiello V and Coulson I (eds.), *Contemporary Issues in Gerontology: Promoting Positive Ageing*. Sydney: Allen and Unwin, pp. xi–xvi.

Newbold KB and Patel A. 2006. Use of dental services by immigrant Canadians. *J Can Dent Assoc* 72:143.

Newton JT, Gibbons DE, and Gelbier S. 1999. The oral health of older people from minority ethnic communities in South East England. *Gerodontology* 16:103–9.

Newton JT, Thorogood N, Bhavnani V, Pitt J, Gibbons DE, and Gelbier S. 2001. Barriers to the use of dental services by individuals from minority ethnic communities living in the United Kingdom: Findings from focus groups. *Prim Dent Care* 8:157–61.

Newton JT, Corrigan M, Gibbons DE, and Locker D. 2003. The self-assessed oral health status of individuals from White, Indian, Chinese and Black

Caribbean communities in South-east England. *Community Dent Oral Epidemiol* 31:192–9.

ONS. 2003. *Ethnicity 2001 Census*. London: Office for National Statistics.

Palinkas LA and Pickwell SM. 1995. Acculturation as a risk factor for chronic disease among Cambodian refugees in the United States. *Soc Sci Med* 40:1643–53.

Parrillo VN. 1994. *Strangers in These Shores: Race and Ethnic Relations in the United States*, 4th edn. New York: Macmillan.

Passel JS and Cohn D. 2008. *U.S. Population Projections: 2005–2050*. Pew Research Center Report. Available pewhispanic.org/files/reports/85.pdf (accessed on June 25, 2009).

Pearson N, Croucher R, Marcenes W, and O'Farrell M. 1999. Dental service use and the implications for oral cancer screening in a sample of Bangladeshi adult medical care users living in Tower Hamlets, UK. *Br Dent J* 186:517–21.

Persson GR, Persson RE, Hollender LG, and Kiyak HA. 2004. The impact of ethnicity, gender, and marital status on periodontal and systemic health of older subjects in the Trials to Enhance Teeth and Oral Health (TEETH). *J Periodontol* 75:817–23.

Pickett KE and Wilkinson RG. 2008. People like us: Ethnic group density effects on health. *Ethn Health* 13:321–34.

Purnell L and Paulanka B. 1998. *Transcultural Health Care. A Culturally Competent Approach*. Philadelphia: F.A. Davis Company.

Redfield R, Linton R, and Herskovits MJ. 1936. Memorandum for the study of acculturation. *Am Anthropol* 38:149–52.

Resnick B. 2000. Health promotion practices of the older adult. *Public Health Nurs* 17:160–8.

Rudd R and Horowitz AM. 2005. The role of health literacy in achieving oral health for elders. *J Dent Educ* 69:1018–21.

Runci S, Redman J, and O'Connor D. 2005. Language needs and service provision for older persons from culturally and linguistically diverse backgrounds in south-east Melbourne residential care facilities. *Australas J Ageing* 23:157–61.

Schwarz E and Lo ECM. 1995. Oral health and dental care in Hong Kong. *Int Dent J* 45:169–76.

Searle W and Ward C. 1990. The prediction of psychological and sociocultural adjustment during cross-cultural transitions. *Int J Intercult Relat* 14:449–64.

Shah SM and Cook DG. 2008. Social determinants of casualty and NHS direct use. *J Public Health* 30:75–81.

Shuler CF. 2001. Inherited risks for susceptibility to dental caries. *J Dent Educ* 65:1038–45.

Simpson L, Purdam K, Taylor A, Feildhouse E, Gavalas V, Tranmer M, Pritchard J, Dorling D. 2006. *Ethnic Minority Populations and the Labour Market: An Analysis of the 1991 and 2001 Census*. Research Report 333. Department of Work and Pension. Leeds: Corporate Document Services.

Smith GD, Chaturevedi N, Harding S, Nazroo J, and Williams R. 2000. Ethnic inequalities in health: A review of UK epidemiological evidence. *Crit Public Health* 10:375–408.

Soldov M and Poon ML. 2001. Elderly Chinese in public housing: Social integration and support in Metro Toronto Housing Company. In: Chi I, Chappell NL, Lubben J (eds.), *Elderly Chinese in Pacific Rim Countries: Social Support and Integration*. Hong Kong: Hong Kong University Press, pp. 221–239.

Sproston K and Mindell J (eds.). 2006. *Health Survey for England 2004. Volume 1: The Health of Minority Ethnic Groups*. Leeds: The Information Centre.

Sproston KA, Pitson LB, and Walker E. 2001. The use of primary care services by the Chinese population living in England: Examining inequalities. *Ethn Health* 6:189–96.

Summers RM, Williams SA, and Curzon MEJ. 1994. The use of tobacco and betel quid ('pan') among Bangladeshi women in West Yorkshire. *Community Dent Health* 11:12–6.

Summers RM, Prendergast MJ, Williams SA, and Ahmed IH. 1996. Betel quid chewing amongst Bangladeshi women in West Yorkshire, UK: Characteristics of women who included tobacco in the quid compared with those who did not. *Int Dent J* 46:251–6.

Swoboda J, Kiyak HA, Persson RE, Persson GR, Yamaguchi DK, MacEntee MI, Wyatt CCL. 2006. Predictors of oral health quality of life in older adults. *Spec Care Dentist* 26:137–44.

Triandis HC and Brislin RW. 1984. Cross-cultural psychology. *Am Psychol* 39:1006–16.

United Nations. 2004. *World Economic and Social Survey 2004: International Migration*. New York: United Nations. Available at www.un.org/esa/policy/wess/wess2004files/part2web/part2web.pdf (accessed December 13, 2009).

Vega WA, Gil AG, and Wagner E. 1998. Cultural adjustment and Hispanic adolescent drug use. In: Vega WA and Gil AG (eds.), *Drug Use and Ethnicity in Early Adolescence*. New York: Plenum Press, pp. 125–37.

Victorian Ethnic Affairs Commission. 1995. *Statistical Profile of NESB Victorians*. Melbourne: VEAC.

Warnakulasuriya KAAS and Johnson NW. 1996. Epidemiology and risk factors for oral cancer: Rising trends in Europe and possible effects of immigrants. *Int Dent J* 5:93–8.

Waxler-Morrison NA, Anderson J, and Richardson E. 2005. *Cross-Cultural Caring: A Handbook for Health Professionals in Western Canada*. Vancouver: UBC Press.

Williams SA, Godson JH, and Ahmed IA. 1995. Dentists' perceptions of difficulties encountered in providing dental care for British Asians. *Community Dent Health* 12:30–4.

Palliative care and complications of cancer therapy

Martin Schimmel, Michael A. Wiseman, Stephen T. Sonis, and Frauke Müller

INTRODUCTION

The World Health Organization (WHO) defines palliative care as "an approach that improves the quality of life of patients and their families facing the problems associated with life-threatening illness ... and treatment of pain and other problems, physical, psychosocial and spiritual" (WHO, 2008).

Patients who are terminally ill should benefit from care that focuses on alleviating discomfort and pain, improving quality of life, and avoiding unnecessary and invasive treatments (Lefebvre-Chapiro and Sebag-Lanoë, 1999). Pain and opportunistic infections should be controlled when possible, while physical, functional, psychosocial, and spiritual restrictions should be addressed with care and empathy (Walsh, 1994). Palliative care is a holistic and multidisciplinary service by which the care team treats both the patient and the extended family, typically in specialized hospitals, hospices, geriatric wards, or at home with appropriate support. The team usually involves a physician as head with help from nurses, pharmacist, dietitian, spiritual counselors, and social workers, but dental professionals usually contribute beyond the inner circle of the team (Figure 15.1).

Palliative medicine was introduced for cancer patients who were terminally ill, but today, most patients in the terminal phase of any lethal disease are eligible for palliative care (Van Nees, 1996). The mouth is one of the most frequently distressed parts of the body among patients in palliative care, due in large part to analgesics, antidepressants, and antiemetic

Oral Healthcare and the Frail Elder: A Clinical Perspective.
Edited by Michael I. MacEntee © 2011 Blackwell Publishing Ltd.

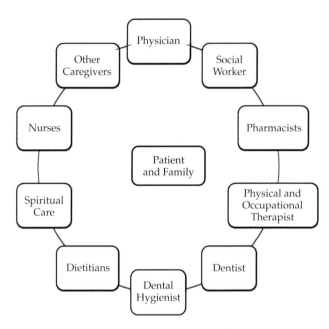

Figure 15.1 A composition of relationships within family-centered care.

Table 15.1 Distribution of oral problems in palliative care patients.

| | Prevalence percentage | | |
Symptoms	314 HIV positive patients (Larue, 1994)	197 cancer patients (Jobbins et al., 1992a)	20 hospice patients (Aldred et al., 1991)
Xerostomia	77	58	97
Oral soreness	33	42	31
Candidiasis	85	70	nr
Dysphagia	35	37	51
Difficulty talking	nr	nr	66
Denture problems among those wearing dentures	45	71	40

nr, not reported.

medications that precipitate salivary gland hypofunction, candidiasis, and uncomfortable dentures (Table 15.1).

However, dental consultations in palliative care are often requested mostly for toothaches rather than for a dry mouth or uncomfortable dentures (Figure 15.2).

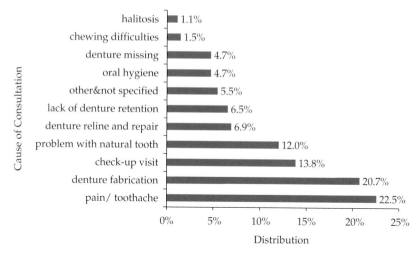

Figure 15.2 Distribution of motives for 275 dental consultations in a palliative care unit. (Adapted from Schimmel et al., 2008.)

PALLIATIVE DENTAL TREATMENT

Dental treatment as part of palliative care aims to maintain function and comfort in and around the mouth by oral hygiene and controlling pain and infections as the terminal illness progresses. Dental restorations, prosthodontics, periodontal curettage, and other surgery should be rendered only after considering carefully the patient's general condition, motivation, life expectancy, and overall propensity for treatment (Mojon and MacEntee, 1994).

Requests to replace or repair dentures are motivated frequently by requests to maintain the dignity of normal appearance and to improve a patient's chewing ability. The functional, psychological, and psychosocial implications of head and neck disfigurement have significant emotional effects on the patient and the patient's carers (Dropkin et al., 1983). Consequently, palliative care, when needed, can be very demanding and emotionally stressful for everyone involved. Surgical scars, trismus, xerostomia, opportunistic infections, rampant "radiation" caries, and neglected oral hygiene can cause pain and major loss of function, while loss of appetite, malnourishment, and other manifestations of a general weakness or cachexia can seriously disturb quality of life (Jobbins et al., 1992a). It is worth noting also that patients who are cognitively impaired or unconscious, when compared with patients who are cognitively intact, tend to receive less pain control medications, probably because communication between patient and carers is so difficult (Pautex et al., 2006).

MOUTH PROBLEMS WITH TERMINAL ILLNESS

Oral mucositis

Oral mucositis is among the most common and clinically significant toxicities of drug and radiation therapy for cancer. Depending on the type, dose, and frequency of radiation treatment, the mucositis appears in various ways ranging from localized erythema to diffuse, contiguous, and deep ulcers. However, the mucosa will be injured to some extent in nearly everyone who receives radiation and chemotherapy. About one-third of recipients of conditioning regimens for hematopoietic stem cell transplants, for example, usually develop mucositis, whereas one-fifth of the patients receiving their first course of conventional cycled chemotherapy for solid tumors, such as breast cancer, develop mucosal ulcers. Moreover, if the dose of chemotherapy remains high in subsequent cycles, the prevalence of ulcerative mucositis rises to more than half the patients who had mucositis during the first cycle. While the frequency of ulcerative mucositis is relatively low in patients with solid tumors, the mucosa is nearly always painful.

The pain associated with oral mucositis is often unbearably painful and debilitating (Figure 15.3).

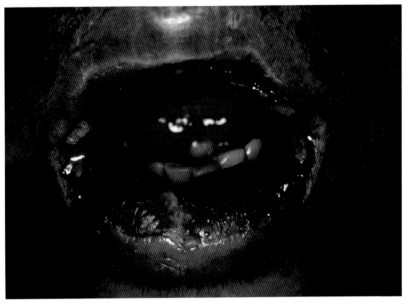

Figure 15.3 Generalized mucositis of the lips in a patient receiving chemotherapy.

Patients with severe mucositis require opioid analgesics, but even morphine might not adequately control the pain. At times, patients have to interrupt their treatment for the cancer because the mouth pain makes additional treatment intolerable. The clinical ramifications of mucositis are significant when patients cannot swallow solid foods and liquid diets are required, and, worse still, parenteral nutrition or gastrostomy (G-tube) feedings are needed when it is impossible to take food by mouth. Indeed, the pain of mucositis is probably the most severe complication of myeloablative or bone marrow chemotherapy or head and neck radiation therapy. The loss of an intact mucosal barrier in myelosuppressed cancer patients increases the risk of bacteremia and sepsis in large part because the mouth is a potent source of pathogenic bacteria.

Mucositis has an increased impact on resource use and healthcare costs associated with cancer treatment when compared with patients unaffected by mucositis, mostly because they use more narcotics and antibiotics. In addition, if patients need parenteral or enteral feedings, they have higher numbers of unplanned physician and emergency room visits and more hospital admissions, and they spend longer periods in the hospital. The influence on health economics is dramatic with the incremental cost of mucositis among head and neck cancer patients in excess of US$20,000 (Elting et al., 2007).

Radiation therapy

The most common regimen for radiation therapy used in the treatment of head and neck cancer is a cumulative radiation dose of about 65–70 Gy. Gray (Gy) measures the radiation energy deposited in biological tissues. It is given incrementally in daily doses of around 2 Gy 5 days per week until the planned course is finished. Usually, the radiation is accompanied weekly or every 3 weeks by cisplatin, a platinum-containing chemical compound, to heighten the sensitivity of the tumor cells to the radiation. However, the chemotherapy is avoided in patients who are very frail to avoid additional toxicity.

Oral erythema and, occasionally, superficial necrosis appear usually by the end of the first week of treatment following a cumulative dose of 10 Gy. Patients complain initially that the mouth feels as if it has been burned, and by the end of the third week and a cumulative dose of 30 Gy, erosion and ulceration appear with increasing pain. Ulcers may be covered by a pseudomembrane comprised of dead cells, fibrin, and bacteria (Figure 15.4).

Lesions are limited to the movable mucosa with the buccal mucosa, lateral and ventral tongue, floor of mouth, and soft palate most frequently affected. At this point, patients will begin to select food that is bland and soft. In general, mucositis does not occur on the gingiva, dorsal surface of the tongue, or hard palate. The extent of the mucositis, pain, and difficulty eating increases typically as the radiation continues to the point where it

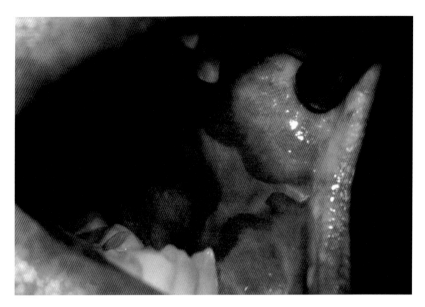

Figure 15.4 Erosive mucositis of the buccal mucosa following a cumulative dose of 30-Gy radiation therapy.

is necessary to stop until the mucosa recovers a little. Mucosal injury persists for 2–3 weeks after radiation is finished, and then healing occurs spontaneously.

Chemotherapy

Mucositis from chemotherapy is similar in appearance and distribution to radiation-induced mucositis, but it differs in two important ways. First, the course of chemotherapy-induced mucositis is more acute. Symptomatic mucosal changes typically begin 3 or 4 days following drug infusion, peak in another couple of days, persist for 2–3 days, and then gradually resolve. Second, there is usually accompanying evidence of myelosuppression, which is especially significant because neutropenic changes coincide largely with the development of the oral ulcers and increase the risk of secondary infections, bacteremia, and sepsis.

Scoring mucositis

Measuring the severity of mucositis helps in the communication among caregivers, patient management, and clinical research. The WHO criteria and the National Cancer Institute's Common Terminology Criteria for Adverse Events (NCI-CTCAE v3.0) in the United States are the most widely recognized grading scales for assessing mucositis. The NCI scale

Table 15.2 Comparison of the scoring scales for mucositis offered by the World health Organization (WHO) and the National Cancer Institute (NCI).

Grade	WHO	NCI clinical
0	Normal	Normal
1	Erythema and pain	Erythema
2	Ulceration[a] and diet with solid food	Patchy ulceration
3	Ulceration[a] and diet with only liquids	Confluent ulceration
4	Ulceration[a] and no food by mouth	Tissue necrosis and bleeding

[a]Ulceration and/or formation of a pseudomembrane.

uses criteria based on clinician assessment and on patient function, whereas the WHO scale produces a single score by combining the clinical and functional assessments together (Table 15.2).

In general, scores greater than 3 are severe, although the suffering of patients often exceeds the scores derived by clinicians.

Preventing and treating mucositis

Treatment guidelines have been published by the Multinational Association for Supportive Cancer Care (O'Keefe et al., 2007). In general, mucositis is exacerbated by local irritation; therefore, promotion of good oral hygiene is helpful along with removal of sharp edges from teeth and dentures. Consistent use of saline or bicarbonate rinses should be encouraged also. A chlorhexidine mouthrinse might benefit patients receiving chemotherapy, but it is not recommended for radiated patients. Removable dentures should be avoided if possible, and recommendations given for a soft diet of blended foods and commercially available diet supplements.

Cryotherapy, in the form of ice chips, administered before and during chemotherapy might help patients with mucositis, especially those receiving 5-fluorouracil or melphalan. Although there is very little information supporting the use of medications to ease the symptoms of mucositis, topical agents can help to improve or control burning symptoms during early phases of mucositis. Rinsing with a 50/50 mixture of benadryl and kaopectate, or Maalox (not to be swallowed), or viscous xylocaine can be helpful, or Caphosol (EUSA Pharma, Oxford, UK), a lubricant and remineralizing solution might help to diminish symptoms, especially for patients with xerostomia. Hospitalized patients are often offered a "magic mouthwash" that typically contains viscous xylocaine, benadryl, a topical steroid, an antifungal, and an antibiotic, although the mixture is no more efficacious than saline (Dodd et al., 2000). Kepivance (Biovitrum, Stockholm, Sweden)—a keratinocyte growth factor—is approved by the Food and Drug Administration (FDA) in the United States for the prevention and treatment of mucositis, but it is very aggressive physiologically and inappropriate for frail elders.

The WHO pain ladder (Macleod, 2008) is useful for controlling painful mucositis. Topical therapy will not control the symptoms of ulcerative mucositis for most patients. Acetaminophen and other nonsteroidal anti-inflammatory drugs are comforting as soon as patients experience pain that exceeds the benefits of topical analgesics, and more aggressive opioid analgesics by mouth, patch, or injection help when mucosal ulcers appear.

ORAL HYGIENE

Managing daily mouthcare is a necessary task in palliative care because of the high risk for aspiration pneumonia, especially for patients with compromised immune systems (Imsand et al., 2002). An effective oral hygiene regimen will lower this risk by reducing bacterial counts in the mouth (Yoneyama et al., 1999; Sjogren et al., 2008), although there is much uncertainty about how best to manage oral hygiene for this population (Table 15.3).

There are encouraging possibilities with a daily spray (~1 mL) of 0.2% chlorhexidine into the mouth that certainly warrants further exploration (Clavero et al., 2003), but we still rely largely on toothbrushes and the ability of frail elders or their carers to remove the bacterial plaque from the teeth, mucosa, and dentures (Thorne et al., 2001; Sumi et al., 2002;

Table 15.3 Procedures for promoting daily mouthcare for patients in palliative care (adapted from GABA, 2003; Nitschke, 2000).

Oral hygiene	Procedures
1. Patient can perform oral hygiene	• Motivate patient for self-care • Monitor hygiene and assist if needed • Select toothbrushes and floss holders to compensate for disabilities
2. Patient is bedridden and cannot perform oral hygiene	• Prevent aspiration by supporting patient to sit upright in bed; use kidney dish under patient's chin • Sit behind patient to stabilize the head with one arm and reach forward to the mouth with toothbrush or floss holder in the other hand
3. Denture hygiene	• Remove denture and clean with soap and water every day • Rinse dentures with water after each meal; soak dentures in a 1:6 NaOCl:H2O solution for 30 min each week • Store denture in a dry container when not in the mouth

Bellomo et al., 2005). Patients who cannot rinse the mouth will be comforted by frequent applications of gauze soaked in a mouthwash or other refreshment to the lips and mouth and by artificial saliva introduced to the mouth every hour or so on a cotton swab (Persson et al., 1991, 2007; Nitschke, 2000; GABA, 2003).

CARIES

Palliative care is frequently associated with caries because of salivary gland dysfunction as a side effect of medications or radiation therapy. Management of caries in this context requires (1) substitution of sugar with sucrose substitutes, such as xylitol and sorbitol, to reduce the acidogenic potential of dental plaque (Amaechi et al., 1999); (2) daily use of a 0.2% sodium fluoride mouthrinse to enhance the resistance of teeth to the demineralizing impact of acid (Wyatt and MacEntee, 2004); (3) effective oral hygiene; and (4) restorative dentistry to repair teeth and eliminate dental cavities and other loci of bacteria (Lo et al., 2006). There is some doubt about the effectiveness of sugar substitutes as a strategy to prevent demineralization of teeth when a fluoride mouthrinse is used (Giertsen et al., 1999). However, the threat and consequences of caries to frail elders demands any action that might be helpful, especially for patients who are xerostomic and who might be unable to use a mouthrinse reliably.

INTOLERANCE TO DENTURES

The benefits of removable dentures are reduced in most palliative care patients due to lack of motivation, cognitive deficiency, loss of muscular control, or hypersensitive and painful mucosa (Taji et al., 2005). Xerostomia and salivary gland hypofunction is probably the most common cause of intolerance to dentures in this population. Fortunately, patients can eat nutritiously without teeth, although it demands a special effort to select and prepare food correctly (Bradbury et al., 2006). A practical but important issue in palliative care is to prevent loss of dentures, whether they are worn regularly or not. There are several simple ways to identify removable dentures, and in some jurisdictions, this is a legal requirement, so that they can be located if misplaced (see Chapter 12 by Frenkel et al.).

XEROSTOMIA

Xerostomia—subjective sense of oral dryness—is very common among patients in palliative care mostly because of the side effects from medications or as a consequence of cancer treatments (Thomson, 2005). It can be a very distressing disorder and difficult to manage. First, the patient's environment, including oxygen intake, should be maintained at a relatively high humidity. The lips and mouth can be swabbed with water-soluble products such as Biotene Oral Balance Moisturizing Gel (GlaxoSmithKline [GSK], Brentford, UK), K-Y Jelly (Johnson & Johnson, New Brunswick, NJ), or Muko Gelly (*Ingram* and *Bell* Medical, Don Mills, ON). Petroleum-based ointments should be avoided because they dry the mucosa further, and they prevent saliva from washing pathogens from the mucosa.

Patients with salivary gland hypofunction causing inadequate salivary flow can keep the mouth moist by sipping water or spraying the mouth with water from a vaporizer. Some patients who complain of constant thirst are suffering from a dry mouth rather than dehydration, and if they drink large quantities of water, they can upset the distribution of salts in the blood and sodium in the plasma, which can lead to the neurological disturbances of hyponatremia (Brunner, 1993). Salivary flow can be stimulated by sugarless chewing gum or flavored sugar-free lozenges. However, sugar and other refined carbohydrate products that increase the risk of caries must be avoided when attempting to stimulate salivary flow. Edentulous patients can use lemon drops on the tongue, but this is not recommended in patients with natural teeth because the low pH produced will also increase the risk of caries. Of course, foods must be moist with sauces, gravies, and accompanying sugarless drinks to help chewing and swallowing.

Clinical scenario 1

A woman was transferred to palliative care in a semicomatose state and unable to swallow with advanced lung cancer. She was on 4 L of oxygen by nasal prongs and had a very dry mouth with spontaneous bleeding from her lips, tongue, and gingiva (Figure 15.5). A water-soluble lubricant was applied to hydrate the tissues. She died 24 h later.

CANDIDIASIS

Fungal infections are very prevalent in patients with defective or depleted immune systems (Jobbins et al., 1992b; Larue, 1994; Akpan and Morgan, 2002; MacEntee et al., 2004; Davies et al., 2008) and, particularly, in the palate under upper complete dentures (Figure 15.6).

Dental prostheses, corticosteroids, and xerostomia greatly increase the risk factors for fungal infections (Budtz-Jørgensen et al., 2000; Schimmel et al., 2008). The fungi proliferate quickly, and they reinfect rapidly following a course of antifungal therapy; consequently, they are difficult to manage (Sweeney and Bagg, 1995). Candidiasis can be treated topically or systemically (Table 15.4).

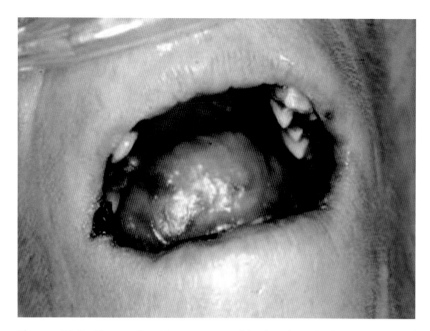

Figure 15.5 Xerostomia with spontaneous bleeding from the lips, tongue, and gingiva of a patient with advanced small cell carcinoma of the lung.

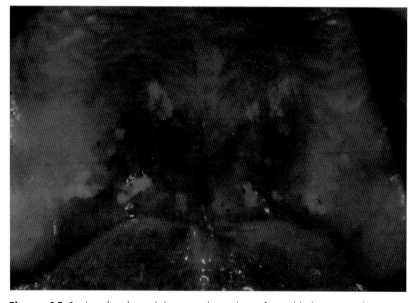

Figure 15.6 Localized candidiasis in the palate of an elderly man with a compromised immune system following radiation therapy.

Table 15.4 Treatments for candidiasis.

	Dose
Topical treatments	
Nystatin	
• Liquid or frozen suspension	200,000–500,000 IU, swished and swallowed three to five times per day for 14 days
• Suppository	100,000 IU, sucked four times per day for 14 days
Clotrimazole	
• Suppository	100 mg, once per day for 7 days
• Troche	10 mg, five times per day for 14 days
• 1% cream applied to denture	Three to four times per day for 7 days
Systemic treatments	
Ketoconazole	
• Orally	200–400 mg/day for 7–14 days
Fluconazole	
• Orally	100–200 mg on first day and 50–100 mg/day orally for 7–14 days
Itraconazole	
• Orally	100–200 mg/day for 7–14 days
Amphotericin B	
• Intravenously	0.25–1.5 mg/kg/day

The treatment choices are determined by the site and extent of infection. Topical agents can be mixed and frozen with water and juice on a stick. The ice provides cryotherapy, to relieve the pain associated with the sensation of a burning mouth. As the ice cools, the mouth is hydrated, and the nystatin is released slowly to the mucosa (Wiseman, 2006). Many of the topical suspensions of nystatin contain sugar for taste, which nourishes the fungi and increases the risk of caries, but it is possible to produce a sugar-free suspension of nystatin to eliminate this problem (Table 15.5).

Systemic antifungal agents are used only in severe generalized infestations. They are used with caution because toxic reactions can occur when taken with sedatives, such as midazolam or triazolam (Olkkola et al., 1994). If topical treatment is ineffective, a microbiological sample from the infected site should be cultivated to identify the pathogen and the most effective antifungal agent. Patients who are unconscious can aspirate topical agents if the agents are not incorporated within a viscous jelly or paste when applied to the mouth (Wiseman, 2006). Acrylic dentures with fungal infections should be disinfected daily in a 1:6 sodium hypochlorite:water solution for about 15 min, and rinsed thoroughly in clean water before replacing in the mouth. Removable partial prostheses with metal components might corrode if soaked in sodium hypochlorite (bleach), so they should be cleaned with soap and water. Acrylic removable prostheses

Table 15.5 Formulation for a sugar-free 100,000 IU nystatin suspension.

Ingredients	Procedure
• 6,000,000 IU nystatin • 120 mg stevioside 90% powder • 100 mg potassium acesulfame • 45 mg sodium saccharin • 120 mg xanthan gum • 120 mg sodium benzoate	Triturate in glass mortar and pestle
• Glycerine paste • 2 mL flavoring • Purified water • 0.1–0.2 ml peppermint oil if needed for flavor	Add glycerine to make a smooth paste to eliminate all of the brown bumps from the xanthan gum, and add purified water

should be stored in a dry environment to help control the growth of *Candida* when not in the mouth (Stafford et al., 1986).

Yeast infection of the facial skin or facial wounds may result in frequent itching or burning. Thus, antifungal treatment might help in avoiding secondary bacterial infection through picking and itching of the infected skin (Faergemann and Dahlen, 2009).

Clinical scenario 2

Mr. Weber presented with severe angular cheilitis and oropharyngeal candida-associated stomatitis.

He was treated initially with a topical antifungal (nystatin) mixed in frozen "popsicles" and with an antibacterial soap plus a topical ointment with nystatin applied to the corners of the mouth.

This treatment did not control the fungus, so after 10 days, a systemic triazole antifungal agent fluconazole was prescribed along with an artificial salivary solution (Glandosane®, Fresenius Kabi Ltd, Cheshire, UK) to ease the discomfort of his dry mouth.

TASTE DISORDERS AND DYSPHAGIA

A large proportion of patients in palliative care have a disturbed sense of taste (Twycross, 1986). Saliva helps to stimulate taste; consequently, salivary gland hypofunction increases the disturbance, whereas rinsing the mouth with water or artificial saliva (e.g., Glandosane) will improve the perception of taste. Chemotherapy and radiotherapy to the head and neck can damage taste receptors in the nose and mouth, and monosodium glutamate may help stimulate the damaged receptors (Schiffman, 2000; Ravasco, 2005). There are other physical impairments to food passing through the mouth ranging from tumors of the tongue to damage to the hypoglossal nerve that can alter taste, but they are relatively rare when compared with salivary gland hypofunction.

COMMUNICATIONS

Patients and their families generally appreciate honesty in the final stage of life; therefore, discussions about dying and death should not be avoided. Honest and empathetic communications are central to effective palliative care. Nonetheless, it is very difficult, if not impossible, to communicate directly with a patient who is in an advanced stage of dementia; consequently, an astute clinician will draw upon close observation and various indirect methods of exchange (Chalmers, 2000). Short words and sentences presented in a clear, slow, and low-toned voice are most effective, and each question should be answered before proceeding to the next. Steady eye contact, smiles, and a gentle touch are also helpful to maintain attention. Erratic and aggressive behavior, such as restlessness, refusing food, moaning, or shouting are all indications of personal discomfort and pain, and frequently serve as the only overt indication of pain in a severely demented patient (Ettinger, 2000). When pain is suspected, icons and other communication aids can help to move further toward the source of the pain (Pautex et al., 2005). In any event, communication to detect the source of pain can be very challenging in a patient who is obviously distressed but withdrawn.

REFERENCES

Akpan A and Morgan R. 2002. Oral candidiasis. *Postgrad Med J* 78:455–9.

Aldred MJ, Addy M, Bagg J, and Finlay IG. 1991. Oral health in the terminally ill: A cross-sectional pilot survey. *Spec Care Dentist* 11:59–62.

Amaechi BT, Higham SM, and Edgar WM. 1999. Caries inhibiting and remineralizing effect of xylitol in vitro. *J Oral Sci* 41:71–7.

Bellomo F, de Preux F, Chung JP, Julien N, Budtz-Jørgensen E, and Müller F. 2005. The advantages of occupational therapy in oral hygiene measures for institutionalised elderly adults. *Gerodontology* 22:24–31.

Bradbury J, Thomason JM, Jepson NJA, Walls AWG, Allen PF, and Moynihan PJ. 2006. Nutrition counselling increases fruit and vegetable intake in the edentulous. *J Dent Res* 85:463–8.

Brunner FP. 1993. Pathophysiology of dehydration. *Schweiz Rundsch Med Prax* 82:784–7.

Budtz-Jørgensen E, Mojon P, Rentsch A, and Deslauriers N. 2000. Effects of an oral health program on the occurrence of oral candidosis in a long-term care facility. *Community Dent Oral Epidemiol* 28:141–9.

Chalmers JM. 2000. Behavior management and communication strategies for dental professionals when caring for patients with dementia. *Spec Care Dentist* 20:147–54.

Clavero J, Baca P, Junco P, and Gonzalez M. 2003. Effects of 0.2% chlorhexidine spray applied once or twice daily on plaque accumulation and gingival inflammation in a geriatric population. *J Clin Periodontol* 30:773–7.

Davies AN, Brailsford SR, Beighton D, Shorthose K, and Stevens VC. 2008. Oral candidosis in community-based patients with advanced cancer. *J Pain Symptom Manage* 35:508–14.

Dodd MJ, Dibble SL, Miaskowski C, MacPhail L, Greenspan D, Paul SM, Shiba G, and Larson P. 2000. Randomized clinical trial of the effectiveness of 3 commonly used mouthwashes to treat chemotherapy-induced mucositis. *Oral Surg Oral Med Oral Pathol Oral Radiol Endod* 90:39–47.

Dropkin MJ, Malgady RG, Scott DW, Oberst MT, and Strong EW. 1983. Scaling of disfigurement and dysfunction in postoperative head and neck patients. *Head Neck* 6:559–70.

Elting LS, Cooksley CD, Chambers MS, and Garden AS. 2007. Risk, outcomes, and costs of radiation-induced oral mucositis among patients with head-and-neck malignancies. *Int J Radiat Oncol Biol Phys* 15:1110–20.

Ettinger RL. 2000. Dental management of patients with Alzheimer's disease and other dementias. *Gerodontology* 17:8–16.

Faergemann J and Dahlen G. 2009. Facial skin infections. *Periodontol 2000* 49:194–209.

GABA. 2003. *Gesund im Alter auch im Mund Audiovisual Material. Fortbildungs- und Lern-CD-ROM für Pflegekräfte, Ärzte und pflegende Angehörige.* Grabetsmattweg, CH-4106 Therwil, Switzerland: GABA International AG.

Giertsen E, Emberland H, and Scheie AA. 1999. Effects of mouth rinses with xylitol and fluoride on dental plaque and saliva. *Caries Res* 33:23–31.

Imsand M, Janssens JP, Auckenthaler R, Mojon P, and Budtz-Jørgensen E. 2002. Bronchopneumonia and oral health in hospitalized older patients. A pilot study. *Gerodontology* 19:66–72.

Jobbins J, Bagg J, Finlay IG, Addy M, and Newcombe RG. 1992a. Oral and dental disease on terminally ill cancer patients. *Br Med J* 304:1612.

Jobbins J, Bagg J, Parsons K, Finlay I, Addy M, and Newcombe RG. 1992b. Oral carriage of yeasts, coliforms and staphylococci in patients with advanced malignant disease. *J Oral Pathol Med* 21:305–8.

Larue F. 1994. Pain and symptoms during HIV disease—A French nation study. *J Palliat Care* 10:95.

Lefebvre-Chapiro S and Sebag-Lanoë R. 1999. Soins palliatifs chez les personnes âgées. *Rev Prat* 49:1077–80.

Lo EC, Luo Y, Tan HP, Dyson JE, and Corbet EF. 2006. ART and conventional root restorations in elders after 12 months. *J Dent Res* 85:929–32.

MacEntee MI, Nolan A, and Thomason JM. 2004. Oral mucosal and osseous disorders in frail elders. *Gerodontology* 21:78–84.

Macleod R. 2008. Management of breakthrough pain in patients with cancer. *Drugs* 68:913–24.

Mojon P and MacEntee MI. 1994. Estimates of time and propensity for dental treatment among institutionalized elders. *Gerodontology* 11:99–107.

Nitschke I. 2000. Zahnmedizinische Grundlagen zur geriatrischen Rehabilitation—eine Einführung in die Alternszahnmedizin. *Z Gerontol Geriatr* 33:45–9.

O'Keefe DM, Schubert MM, Elting LS, Sonis ST, Epstein JB, Raber-Durlacher JE, Migliorati CA, McGuire DB, Hutchins RD, and Peterson DE. 2007. Mucositis Study Section of the Multinational Association of Supportive Care in Cancer and the International Society for Oral Oncology. *Cancer* 109:820–31. Available at www.mascc.org/mc/page.do?sitePageId=87007 (accessed January 12, 2010).

Olkkola K, Backman J, and Neuvonen P. 1994. Midazolam should be avoided in patients receiving systemic antimycotics ketoconazole or itraconazole. *Clin Pharmacol Ther* 55:481–5.

Pautex S, Herrmann F, Le Lous P, Fabjan M, Michel JP, and Gold G. 2005. Feasibility and reliability of four pain self-assessment scales and correlation with an observational rating scale in hospitalized elderly demented patients. *J Gerontol A Biol Sci Med Sci* 60:524–9.

Pautex S, Michon A, Guedira M, Emond H, Le Lous P, Samaras D, Michel JP, Herrmann F, Giannakopoulos P, and Gold G. 2006. Pain in severe dementia: Self-assessment or observational scales? *J Am Geriatr Soc* 54:1040–5.

Persson GR, Yeates J, Persson RE, Hirschi-Imfeld R, Weibel M, and Kiyak HA. 2007. The impact of a low-frequency chlorhexidine rinsing schedule on the subgingival microbiota (the TEETH clinical trial). *J Periodontol* 78:1751–8.

Persson RE, Truelove EL, LeResche L, and Robinovitch MR. 1991. Therapeutic effects of daily or weekly chlorhexidine rinsing on oral health of a geriatric population. *Oral Surg Oral Med Oral Pathol* 72:184–91.

Ravasco P. 2005. Aspects of taste and compliance in patients with cancer. *Eur J Oncol Nurs* 9(Suppl. 2):S84–91.

Schiffman SS. 2000. Intensification of sensory properties of foods for the elderly. *J Nutr* 130(Suppl. 4S):927S–30S.

Schimmel M, Schoeni P, Zulian G, and Müller F. 2008. Utilisation of dental services in a university hospital palliative and long term care unit in Geneva. *Gerodontology* 25:107–12.

Sjogren P, Nilsson E, Forsell M, Johansson O, and Hoogstraate J. 2008. A systematic review of the preventive effect of oral hygiene on pneumonia and respiratory tract infection in elderly people in hospitals and nursing homes: Effect estimates and methodological quality of randomized controlled trials. *J Am Geriatr Soc* 56:2124–30.

Stafford GD, Arendorf T, and Huggett R. 1986. The effect of overnight drying and water immersion on candidal colonization and properties of complete dentures. *J Dent* 14:52–6.

Sumi Y, Yasunori N, and Yukihiro M. 2002. Development of a systematic oral care program for frail elderly persons. *Spec Care Dentist* 22:151–5.

Sweeney MP and Bagg J. 1995. Oral care for hospice patients with advanced cancer. *Dent Update* 22:424–7.

Taji T, Yoshida M, Hiasa K, Abe Y, Tsuga K, and Akagawa Y. 2005. Influence of mental status on removable prosthesis compliance in institutionalized elderly persons. *Int J Prosthodont* 18:146–9.

Thomson WM. 2005. Issues in the epidemiological investigation of dry mouth. *Gerodontology* 22:65–76.

Thorne S, Kazanjian A, and MacEntee MI. 2001. Oral health in long-term care: The implications of organizational culture. *J Aging Stud* 15:271–83.

Twycross RG. 1986. Care of the dying. Symptom control. *Br J Hosp Med* 36:244–6, 248–9.

Van Nees MC. 1996. Les soins palliatifs dans un service aigu de gériatrie. *Infokara* 41:33–9.

Walsh D. 1994. Palliative care: Management of the patient with advanced cancer. *Semin Oncol* 21:100–6.

WHO. 2008. *WHO Definition of Palliative Care*. Available at www.who.int/cancer/palliative/definition/en/ (accessed January 5, 2010).

Wiseman M. 2006. The treatment of oral problems in the palliative patient. *J Can Dent Assoc* 72:453–8.

Wyatt CCL and MacEntee MI. 2004. Caries management for institutionalized elders using fluoride and chlorhexidine mouthrinses. *Community Dent Oral Epidemiol* 32:322–8.

Yoneyama T, Yoshida M, Matsui T, and Sasaki H. 1999. Oral care and pneumonia. Oral Care Working Group. *Lancet* 354:515.

A framework for assessing the outcome of oral healthcare in long-term care facilities

Matana Kettratad-Pruksapong, Arminée Kazanjian, B. Lynn Beattie, and Michael I. MacEntee

THE DILEMMA

The assessment of any health program can usually be conducted because assessors know what the program is like and how it should work. We use the term "assessment" rather than "evaluation" because the latter implies measurement, whereas assessment can accommodate both health status measurements and other qualitative outcomes that cannot be measured but nonetheless are essential components and outcomes of healthcare. In addition, the term "evaluation" is sometimes misunderstood to be restricted to summative measurements. Similarly, implementers of a program would be more confident about how to provide care when there is evidence of effectiveness gathered from an outcome assessment. However, in the case of oral healthcare for frail elders, care providers and assessors are neither sure how to provide care nor how to assess it. Without gold standard for care, the following questions arise:

- What should be the objectives of care?
- How does the healthcare program function?
- Is it working and meeting expected needs?
- How do we know if what we do is making a difference?

In this chapter, we will explain the concepts and challenges in developing outcome assessments for mouthcare programs in long-term care (LTC)

Oral Healthcare and the Frail Elder: A Clinical Perspective.
Edited by Michael I. MacEntee © 2011 Blackwell Publishing Ltd.

facilities, and offer a comprehensive framework for assessing outcomes of mouthcare in the facilities.

ASSESSING ORAL HEALTHCARE PROGRAMS

There are methods for assessing the oral status of elderly people (Kayser-Jones et al., 1995; MacEntee and Wyatt, 1999; Bauer, 2001) and methods for assessing the psychosocial impact of oral impairment, disease, and disability (Atchison and Dolan 1990; Slade, 1997; Slade et al., 1998). However, the methods have been used mostly to identify the needs for care, but there has been remarkably little effort to assess the benefits of oral healthcare services in LTC, and there are no guidelines or best practices for assessing the effectiveness of the services (Dolan, 1993; MacEntee et al., 1999).

Caring for frail elders involves complicated biophysical, psychosocial, and organizational elements. Consequently, assessment of outcomes is far from straightforward. Mouthcare products and techniques can be efficacious—they can operate effectively—in the controlled context of clinical trials, but whether or not their benefits are sustainable within the much less controlled operations of LTC is doubtful (Chalmers et al., 2004). Similarly, the dental knowledge and skills acquired by nursing staff during in-service educational programs also appear to be unsustainable within the conflicting demands of most nursing facilities (MacEntee et al., 1999, 2007; Watt et al., 2006; Pruksapong and MacEntee, 2007).

The lack of demonstrable benefits from oral healthcare programs for frail elders is worrisome, particularly in an era where the very sustainability of healthcare in any context is under close scrutiny, and depends on accountability demonstrating practical effectiveness and value for money (Romanow, 2002).

KEY CONCEPTS

Basic concepts of outcome assessment

There are two main concepts of how healthcare programs should be assessed: one is "quality of care" and the other "program evaluation." They both emerged separately from demands for improved quality and accountability. Initially, quality of care focused mostly on the performance of people, while evaluation attempted to measure the results or outcome of the program. However, they have many similarities, and, more recently, both have been expanded to consider a wide range of the components that are integral to the operations and success of a program.

According to the Institute of Medicine (2001) in the United States, quality of care typically identifies "the degree to which health services increase the likelihood of outcomes that are consistent with current professional knowledge." Donabedian (2003) created a very useful framework with three levels for assessing the quality of care. On Level 1, he proposed an assessment of the *structure* of the human, financial, and other material resources within which care is delivered; on Level 2, he judged the *process* of care, including the technical and interpersonal activities; and on Level 3, he considered the *outcomes* from the perspectives of both the recipients and the providers of care. He recommended also that the results of the assessment at each level should lead to corrective actions when the quality is deemed to be inadequate.

Considerations of quality assurance go beyond the limits of a unique performance and outcome judgement to include a range of organizational variables. It provides a continuous rather than a unique assessment of care and improvement of quality. Some administrators of programs refer to this as a "continuous quality improvement" or "total quality management" (McLaughlin and Kaluzny, 2006).

Evaluation of a healthcare program, on the other hand, aims to judge merit, enhances effectiveness, and provides information for further improvements (Weiss, 1998; Patton, 2002). Formative evaluation is linked usually to the process of development, whereas summative evaluation is associated more with outcome measures or final tallies when the program functions successfully. It too, like quality of care, has expanded to include a range of information about the characteristics of a program, in addition to developments and outcomes.

Essentially, both quality assessment and program evaluation are systematic inspections of the structure, activity, and outcome of a service or organization. When information about the program comes from a comprehensive investigation based on a combination of quality assurance and program evaluation, there is the hope that both accountability and improvement of quality are addressed.

Oral healthcare

The success of oral healthcare as a part of LTC depends at least as much on the organizational culture, philosophy, and connectivity of everyone involved as it does on the dental treatment available for the residents (MacEntee et al., 1999). Indeed, oral healthcare as an integral part of the general care provided to residents is an important quality indicator of the overall care offered by a nursing facility. Unfortunately, the nursing and dental personnel all too frequently operate independently of one another with an "us and them" perspective. When asked what makes oral healthcare challenging, typically the nurses complain about the difficulty of getting dentists or dental hygienists to attend residents in the facility, about the high cost of dental treatment, and about the disinterest and different healthcare values among the residents and their families. On the other hand, families are apt to complain about nurses who do not provide the help and care needed. Overall, the conflicting values and expectations of all the participants make it exceedingly difficult to introduce new programs of any kind, and especially programs for which nurses and care-aides have very little training.

A MODEL FOR ASSESSING AN ORAL HEALTHCARE FOR FRAIL ELDERS

Assessing multiple components

Several key components of an oral healthcare program in LTC influence how it operates. The existing healthcare system and social structure are major influences, but they are shaped in various important ways by the expectations of the residents and by the competence and resources of the staff (Figure 16.1).

Each component can be assessed by various indicators, such as the philosophy and management of the administration, the financial support for different personnel, the comprehensiveness of operational and health records, and, of course, the ease of access to dental personnel (Figure 16.2).

More specific information can be gleaned from how the residents' oral hygiene is monitored. Contracts with dental consultants provide insights to how interdisciplinary teams are structured and the role of dental personnel. The type, location, and focus of continuing education courses for staff indicate how well administrators recognize the limitations of professional training. Biological indicators of mouthcare, such as plaque and gingival indices offer more detailed information on mouthcare, but they are difficult

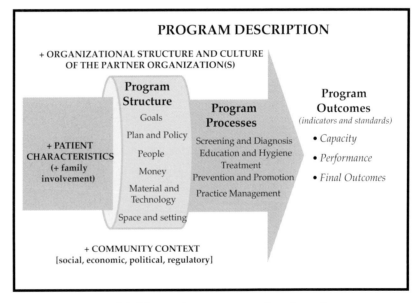

Figure 16.1 A model of the mouthcare assessment based on a "structure–process–outcome" framework. (Adapted from Pruksapong and MacEntee, 2007.)

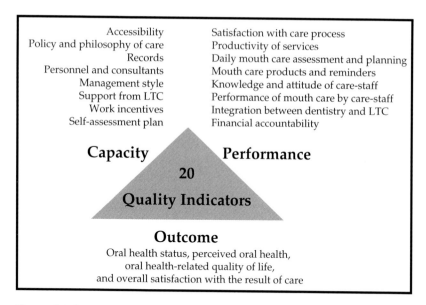

Accessibility
Policy and philosophy of care
Records
Personnel and consultants
Management style
Support from LTC
Work incentives
Self-assessment plan

Satisfaction with care process
Productivity of services
Daily mouth care assessment and planning
Mouth care products and reminders
Knowledge and attitude of care-staff
Performance of mouth care by care-staff
Integration between dentistry and LTC
Financial accountability

Capacity   **Performance**

20

Quality Indicators

Outcome
Oral health status, perceived oral health,
oral health-related quality of life,
and overall satisfaction with the result of care

Figure 16.2 Categories and subcategories of quality indicators in long-term care. (Adapted from Pruksapong and MacEntee, 2007.)

to interpret in elderly populations. Finally, and possibly most significantly, the satisfaction expressed by everyone involved gives a good overall indication of professional camaraderie and the extent to which concerns and needs are addressed.

The range of this assessment requires a balanced consideration of all the components, recognizing that some issues will be more important than others as circumstances and expectations dictate. In any event, it is worth noting that traditional biological measures of treatment outcomes are insufficient to reflect the complexity of an oral healthcare program in an LTC facility, which probably explains, in a large part, why we do not have good guidelines or best practices for assessing the effectiveness of oral healthcare for older people (Dolan, 1993; MacEntee et al., 1999).

Outcome assessment for a complex program

The assessment method we propose is rooted in a broad range of ideas (Palmer et al., 1991; Weiss, 1998; MacEntee et al., 1999; Institute of Medicine, 2001; Patton, 2002; Donabedian, 2003) and in personal experiences with an oral healthcare program for LTC facilities in Vancouver (Pruksapong, 2008). By means of a "continual assessment worksheet," the steps required to amass all of the information needed for a comprehensive assessment are considered (Appendix). The comprehensive oral health program delivered to elders in LTC was designed originally as an assessment model for managers and personnel. The evaluation process and quality indicators can be modified and applied to any area of the program. For example, the facility administrator and nurse leaders can use the model to audit daily mouth-care provided by the nursing staff.

Continual assessment

The assessment begins with the administration, nursing staff, residents, and other interested parties discussing the purpose of the assessment, and constructing probing questions specific to each aspect of the program (Figure 16.3).

Sometimes, the goals of care are acceptable to all during this initial assessment, but more typically, they require compromise and negotiation. Engaging a wide range of participants at this early stage helps to ensure that results will be accepted and valued by most of the interested parties. A systematic review of each step should identify all of the contributions to the complicated process and encourage both introspection and change as situations evolve.

The aim of this assessment method is to offer everyone an opportunity to identify the scope of information needed, the interpretative and reporting process, and the potential for implementing improvements (assessment overview).

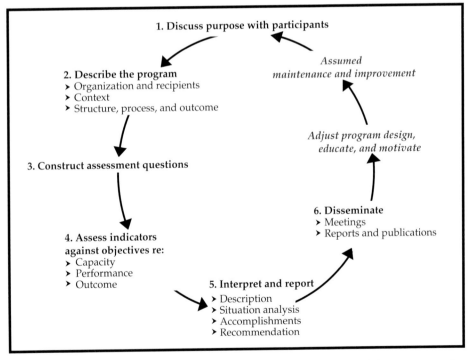

Figure 16.3 Incremental steps for continual assessment of the outcomes of a complex program. (Adapted from Pruksapong and MacEntee, 2007.)

Continual assessment overview.

Step 1   Discuss the purpose of the assessment with the participants.
Step 2   Describe the program.
Step 3   Construct assessment questions.
Step 4   Assess indicators against objectives.
Step 5   Interpret and report results.
Step 6   Disseminate findings, adjust the program, and continue the iterative
          loop back to Step 1.

Objectives of Care	Minimal Standards
Oral hygiene	• Residents should be given an opportunity for oral hygiene at least once a day. • Residents should be encouraged and assisted if needed to clean the mouth and teeth before going to bed at night.
Overall oral health status	• Everyone should be free of infection and pain, and be able to chew and swallow without discomfort. • All natural teeth and dentures should be comfortable, secure, and complement the resident's natural appearance.

Figure 16.4 Examples of minimal oral healthcare standards specific to local conditions. (Adapted from Pruksapong, 2008.)

When the assessment begins, information comes from clinical and administrative records, interviews, questionnaires, and direct observation of the day-to-day activities in the facility. The participants are asked to clarify the goals of the program and describe how they would achieve the goals (Steps 1). Also, they would select appropriate assessment questions in keeping with the program's circumstances and stage of development (Step 3). Later, the assessors can select indicators among the three components: program's capacity, performance, and outcome reflecting the program quality (Step 4). Our framework provides guidelines for seeking information about the objectives of care, examining against minimal standards of care specific to the local conditions in which care is rendered (Figure 16.4).

Next, the interpretation and report of the initial findings should again involve as many participants as possible in an effort to achieve a consensus on progress, accomplishments, and deficiencies (Step 5), which leads in turn to discussions on the dissemination of the findings (Step 6).

At the end of the first six steps, the findings should encourage the participants to maintain the quality achieved and initiate change to

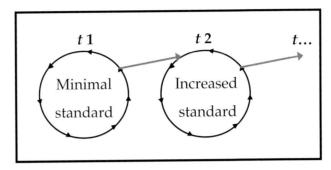

Figure 16.5 Incrementally increasing standard of care for each assessment time (*t*). (Adapted from Pruksapong and MacEntee, 2007.)

overcoming deficiencies. The initial standards of care are based usually on the goals that were set when the program starts. However, goals change with time and experience. Therefore, following this initial assessment of progress, improvements are needed at each assessment cycle to meet everyone's expectations for change (Figure 16.5).

A realistic expectation at the outset of a daily mouthcare program, for example, might be to obtain a toothbrush, toothpaste, and a fluoridated mouthrinse for each resident without too much concern for how they are used. Subsequently, as this limited goal is reached, the next cycle might change realistically to implement and sustain an effective regimen of oral hygiene for all. Subsequently, after further assessment and progress, arrangements can be made with dental professionals to provide specific treatments.

Clinical scenario: resolving worries at Active Hollow Lodge

Ms. Worry Jaw, the Director of Care at Active Hollow Lodge has been able, through the Regional Health Authority, to get financial support to pay Dr. Wisdomdent and his dental assistant for examining the elderly residents once a year. She also persuaded Ira Pain, the Chief Administrator of the facility, to use the residents' comfort fund to pay for Mr. John Whitechord, a dental hygienist, who also attends the residents regularly, and to buy mouthcare supplies such as toothbrushes and fluoridated mouthwashes.

This dental and dental hygiene program has been working for about 4 years with reasonable appreciation from the residents and their relatives, but Dr. Wisdomdent and Mr. Whitechord knew that it had glitches. In particular, they were concerned about the apparent neglect of daily oral hygiene among the residents and the high incidence of caries and gingivitis.

One day, Ms. Jaw told Dr. Wisdomdent that "the new Board at the Regional Health Authority is revising the budget for everything over the next 4 years, and they asked for a report to justify the cost of the dental program." She looked worried and a little confused as she asked, "Doc, do you know of the best way to do this? We know that most people here like the program but is there a dental standard against which we can assess the service?"

At first, Dr. Wisdomdent himself appeared worried as he discovered that only one-third of the residents received the dental treatment he recommended the previous year—"not a convincing figure to report to some penny-pinching government bureaucrat" he thought. He consulted with Mr. Whitechord who suggested that the care-aides with additional training could help the residents with daily mouthcare when necessary. This was a good idea; however, he also realized that he had to be more persuasive to the residents and their families about his own recommendations for treatment, and that this would require improved support from physicians, nurses, and care-aides.

A few days later, Dr. Wisdomdent phoned Ms. Jaw joyfully, requesting a combined meeting with the nurse leaders and the head of the family council. He explained to Ms. Jaw that he had worked out what to report to the Health Authority to secure the budget and to assess the dental services more effectively than before.

At the hastily assembled meeting, Dr. Wisdomdent presented a model for assessing an oral healthcare program in LTC facilities. He explained with diagrams and photographs that there is no gold standard of care for the mouth, probably because the dental status of frail elders varies greatly for good and for bad. He stressed further that "standard implies context, and we should agree as a group on the goal of care and the standard appropriate to our residents' needs." He showed them how the model indicates all the possible points of assessment and offers suggestions for data collection as the program evolves. He emphasized further how the standards of care they determined at the outset of the program are likely to change "as we increase the bar following each cycle of assessment."

The meeting ended with lots of questions and enthusiastic debate before agreeing that the immediate goal at Active Hollow Lodge was to keep the oral health status of the residents stable and free of infection. They would achieve this through ongoing training of the care-aides and sensitizing of the nondental staff to the significance of oral healthcare as a primary preventive strategy against aspiration pneumonia, and as a key component of overall well-being. The nurse leaders assumed responsibility for continuously assessing the program of oral healthcare in the Lodge, and for setting up a subcommittee to design an audit of the daily mouthcare given to the residents. Finally, Ms. Worry Jaw announced that she was more than happy with this plan to recommend to the Regional Health Authority that funding of the dental program be continued and, if possible, increased.

Dr. Wisdomdent and Mr. Whitechord left the meeting feeling very collegial and cheerful in the renewed hope that perhaps—just perhaps—they were recognized now as significant players on the multidisciplinary team that influences everything at Active Hollow Lodge. But mostly, they left feeling good that the residents would benefit from the implementation of this model of oral healthcare and assessment. Dr. Wisdomdent did remark to his wife later that evening that he wondered why Ms. Jaw did not offer the support to the program without all this fuss and innovation. She replied that he was a wonderful dentist and recommended him "not to worry about the politics of institutional life!"

SUMMARY

Many healthcare decisions are made on a daily basis in LTC facilities by different decision makers who have different concerns. The facility administrator is concerned about affordability, return on investment, and the risks of inaction. The health professional is concerned about evidence for medical benefit and whether the intervention is truly an advance on standard practice. These separate decisions ultimately translate into programs and interventions in the facility and have impact on the oral health of the frail elderly.

Using an explicit assessment model assists in developing a common understanding of the properties, effects, and outcomes of programs or interventions in a local context. In addition, it facilitates the inclusion of all stakeholders, therefore providing the opportunity to incorporate a multiplicity of perspectives, and the negotiation of what will work best for the frail residents, given current resources and professional capacity. The assessment model is designed to determine whether the achievements and deficiencies—usually both are present—are due to the planning or the implementation processes, or more likely to a combination of both processes. It will remind assessors, for example, to investigate the effectiveness, rather than simply the efficacy, of the interventions. It can help to diagnose problems associated with the program and offer reasonable recommendations for improvements. At the present time, there is no gold standard for oral healthcare in long-term facilities, but by implementing a methodical framework, standards for care can be built and improved.

REFERENCES

Atchison KA and Dolan TA. 1990. Development of the geriatric oral health assessment index. *J Dent Educ* 54:680–7.

Bauer JG. 2001. The index of ADOH: Concept of measuring oral self-care functioning in the elderly. *Spec Care Dentist* 21:63–7.

Chalmers J, Johnson V, Tang JH, and Titler MG. 2004. Evidence-based protocol: Oral hygiene care for functionally dependent and cognitively impaired older adults. *J Gerontol Nurs* 30:5–12.

Dolan TA. 1993. Identification of appropriate outcomes for an aging population. *Spec Care Dentist* 13:35–9.

Donabedian A. 2003. *An Introduction to Quality Assurance in Health Care*. Oxford: Oxford University Press.

Institute of Medicine. 2001. *Committee on Quality of Health Care in America. Crossing the Quality Chasm: A New Health System for the 21st Century.* Washington, DC: National Academy Press.

Kayser-Jones J, Bird WF, Paul SM, Long L, and Schell ES. 1995. An instrument to assess the oral health status of nursing home residents. *Gerontologist* 35:814–24.

MacEntee MI and Wyatt CCL. 1999. A clinical index of oral dysfunction in elderly populations (CODE). *Gerodontology* 16:85–96.

MacEntee MI, Thorne S, and Kazanjian A. 1999. Conflicting priorities: Oral health in long-term care. *Spec Care Dentist* 19:164–72.

MacEntee MI, Wyatt CCL, Beattie BL, Paterson B, Levy-Milne R, McCandless L, and Kazanjian A. 2007. Provision of mouth-care in long-term care facilities: An educational trial. *Community Dent Oral Epidemiol* 35:25–34.

McLaughlin CP and Kaluzny AD. 2006. *Continuous Quality Improvement in Health Care: Theory, Implementations, and Applications*, 3rd edn. Sudbury, MA: Jones and Bartlett.

Palmer RH, Donabedian A, and Povar GJ. 1991. *Striving for Quality in Health Care: An Inquiry into Policy and Practice*. Ann Arbor, MI: Health Administration Press.

Patton MQ. 2002. *Qualitative Research and Evaluation Methods*, 3rd edn. Thousand Oaks, CA: Sage Publications.

Pruksapong M. 2008. *Development of a Model for Assessing the Quality of an Oral Health Program in Long-Term Care Facilities*. PhD dissertation. Vancouver: University of British Columbia.

Pruksapong M and MacEntee MI. 2007. Quality of oral health services in long-term care: Towards an evaluation framework. *Gerodontology* 24:224–30.

Romanow RJ. 2002. *Building on Values: The Future of Health Care in Canada—Final Report*. Ottawa: Government of Canada Publications. Available at www.cbc.ca/healthcare/final_report.pdf (accessed January 1, 2010).

Slade G (ed.). 1997. *Measuring Oral Health and Quality of Life*. Chapel Hill, NC: University of North Carolina, Dental Ecology.

Slade GD, Strauss RP, Atchison KA, Kressin NR, Locker D, and Reisine ST. 1998. Conference summary: Assessing oral health outcomes—Measuring health status and quality of life. *Community Dent Health* 15:3–7.

Watt RG, Harnett R, Daly B, Fuller SS, Kay E, Morgan A, Munday P, Nowjack-Raymer R, and Treasure ET. 2006. Evaluating oral health promotion: Need for quality outcome measures. *Community Dent Oral Epidemiol* 34:11–7.

Weiss CH. 1998. *Evaluation: Methods for Studying Programmes and Policies*, 2nd edn. Upper Saddle River, NJ: Prentice Hall.

Appendix: Quality assessment worksheets

Matana Kettratad-Pruksapong,
Arminée Kazanjian, B. Lynn Beattie,
and Michael I. MacEntee

Quality Assessment Worksheet
Step 1
Discuss Purpose of Assessment

Programme name: _____

Assessment period: Beginning: _____ Ending: _____ Assessment Cycle #

Stage of Development
☐ Planning
☐ Initial implementation
☐ Adaptive implementation
☐ Matured implementation
☐ Expansion

Partnership Programme: ☐ YES   ☐ NO

Identify partners in the assessment:
☐ administrators: government, organizations, educational institutions, long-term care facilities, hospitals
☐ sponsors: funding agencies, donors
☐ programme manager, co-ordinator, other administrative staff
☐ providers: nursing personnel, dental personnel
☐ recipients and families: friends, power of attorney, public trustee, insurance company
☐ allied health professionals: PT, OT, dietician, social worker, etc
☐ others: unit clerk, pastoral care, recreational staff
☐ advocacy groups:
☐ others (please specify):
_____

Purpose of Assessment
☐ What is happening? [Gain insight for planning]
☐ Analyse capacity? [Gap/Asset or SWOT*]
☐ Is it working? What works? What doesn't? [Assess effect, summative evaluation, accountability]
☐ How can we make it better? [Quality improvement]
☐ To raise awareness among staff [Quality improvement through accountability]
☐ Others [Please specify] _____

_____

* SWOT = Strength, Weakness, Opportunity, Threat

Quality Assessment Worksheet
Step 2
Describe the Programme

Sources of information:
☐ meetings with participants;
☐ focus groups of participants;
☐ individual interviews;
☐ questionnaire and open-ended reflective survey;
☐ observation during site visits;
☐ analysis of administrative documents (e.g. annual reports; newspapers; memoranda, Minimum Data Set, Resident Assessment Instrument; financial records; insurance claims; complaint records).

Present findings in the form of logic models using text, tables and diagrams as appropriate. A description of the programme will help to select suitable objectives for each stage of development, and to interpret the findings relative to the objectives.

Step 3
Assessment Questions

Develop a set of specific assessment questions.

Quality Assessment Worksheet
Step 4
Assess Indicators Against Objectives

[**NOTE:** Indicators when used alone are descriptive and neutral. However, standards need judgment. You will probably begin the assessment based on minimal standards, but increase the standards incrementally as the objectives of the programme change.]

Sources of Information:
☐ meetings with participants;
☐ focus groups of participants;
☐ individual interviews;
☐ questionnaire and open-ended reflective survey;
☐ observation during site visits;
☐ analysis of administrative documents (e.g. annual reports; newspapers; memoranda, Minimum Data Set, Resident Assessment Instrument; financial records; insurance claims; complaint records).

Samples of Reflective Open-ended Questions:
■ What are the strengths of the programme?
■ What was missing when the programme started?
■ What needs to improve?
■ What strategies would improve the programme?
■ What advice can you offer others who are planning a similar programme?

Quality Assessment Worksheet
Step 5
Interpret and Report Results

[**NOTE:** Please refer to national or local agencies to integrate with existing long-term care framework.]

Interpret:
☐ the programme's capacities and SWOT;
☐ successes;
☐ failures;
☐ factors contributing to successes;
☐ problems and barriers contributing to failures;
☐ future intervention targets;
☐ action plans.

Step 6
Disseminate Findings, Adjust the Programme, and Continue Iterative Loop Back to Step 1

Meetings, focus groups, presentation to local community representatives, and publications are well-suited in specific ways to discuss strategies for:
■ infra-structural changes;
■ service protocol changes;
■ motivational activities;
■ educational activities.

Index

Page numbers in *italics* refer to Figures; those in **bold** to Tables.

Oral Healthcare and the Frail Elder: A Clinical Perspective.
Edited by Michael I. MacEntee © 2011 Blackwell Publishing Ltd.